Integrative Health

A Holistic Approach for Health Professionals

Cyndie Koopsen, MBA, RN, HN-BC
ALLEGRA Learning Solutions, LLC
San Diego, California

Caroline Young, MPH
ALLEGRA Learning Solutions, LLC
San Diego, California

JONES AND BARTLETT PUBLISHERS
Sudbury, Massachusetts
BOSTON TORONTO LONDON SINGAPORE

World Headquarters
Jones and Bartlett Publishers
40 Tall Pine Drive
Sudbury, MA 01776
978-443-5000
info@jbpub.com
www.jbpub.com

Jones and Bartlett Publishers
Canada
6339 Ormindale Way
Mississauga, Ontario L5V 1J2
Canada

Jones and Bartlett Publishers
International
Barb House, Barb Mews
London W6 7PA
United Kingdom

Jones and Bartlett's books and products are available through most bookstores and online booksellers. To contact Jones and Bartlett Publishers directly, call 800-832-0034, fax 978-443-8000, or visit our website, www.jbpub.com.

Substantial discounts on bulk quantities of Jones and Bartlett's publications are available to corporations, professional associations, and other qualified organizations. For details and specific discount information, contact the special sales department at Jones and Bartlett via the above contact information or send an email to specialsales@jbpub.com.

Production Credits
Publisher: Kevin Sullivan
Acquisitions Editor: Emily Ekle
Acquisitions Editor: Amy Sibley
Associate Editor: Patricia Donnelly
Editorial Assistant: Rachel Shuster
Associate Production Editor: Amanda Clerkin
Associate Marketing Manager: Rebecca Wasley
Manufacturing and Inventory Control Supervisor: Amy Bacus
Composition: Paw Print Media
Cover Design: Kristin E. Ohlin
Cover Image Credit: © Alex James Bramwell/ShutterStock, Inc.
Printing and Binding: Malloy, Inc.
Cover Printing: Malloy, Inc.

Library of Congress Cataloging-in-Publication Data
Koopsen, Cyndie.
Integrative health : a holistic approach for health professionals / Cyndie Koopsen, Caroline Young.
p. ; cm.
Includes bibliographical references and index.
ISBN 978-0-7637-5761-8 (pbk.)
1. Integrative medicine. 2. Holistic medicine. I. Young, Caroline, MPH. II. Title.
[DNLM: 1. Complementary Therapies. WB 890 K82i 2009]
R733.K587 2009
613—dc22

2008029804

6048

Printed in the United States of America
14 13 12 10 9 8 7 6 5 4

Life is either a daring adventure or nothing at all.
—Helen Keller

To all our families and friends, and to the many great people we have met who have provided us with inspiration, guidance, and support during our exciting life journeys. Thank you for making our world so full of love and joy!

Acknowledgments

As we reflect on our lives and our journeys, we are aware of individuals who, from our earliest memories, have nurtured our spirits. They have provided a healing presence, offered us inspiration, and provided unwavering love and support. We recognize that our relationships with families, friends, colleagues, patients/clients, and even ourselves have all contributed to our work and this book. We have gleaned immeasurable inspiration from individuals who are no longer in an earthly form but who continue to guide and inspire us from their own special place. We are aware that many other individuals helped us with this book, but they are too numerous to mention. Their support, love, and unique gifts allowed this book to come into being, and we gratefully acknowledge their contribution.

We are grateful to all of those at Jones and Bartlett Publishers who believed in our project and provided unwavering support. Thank you, Kevin Sullivan, Emily Ekle, and Rachel Shuster. You are a pleasure to work with.

We remain incredibly blessed to know Gail Fink, a wonderful colleague and calming presence during all of our creations—and certainly this book. Gail provides invaluable editorial expertise and words of wisdom. She is an amazing woman and we are grateful to know her and call her friend. Thank you, Gail. We could not have done it without you.

We are incredibly lucky to be business partners and best friends. To be able to write, create, and experience all this with each other has been a fabulous experience. We continue to look forward to more exciting adventures!

Contents

Preface

Integrative Health: A Holistic Approach for Health Professionals was developed to provide students, teachers, healthcare providers, and interested laypeople with a comprehensive, unique resource for understanding integrative health care and delivering effective, compassionate informed care to their current and future clients. It was also designed so interested readers with no healthcare background can find well-researched, pertinent information that can help them improve the quality of their lives through a holistic approach to health and well-being. This book is the result of our extensive training, research, and experience in the fields of nursing, nutrition, stress management, psychology, public health, physical activity, energy medicine, spirituality, and education, as well as our direct clinical, research, writing, and consulting experience in these areas.

Individuals, groups of students, and seasoned professionals in disciplines such as nursing, medicine, holistic healing arts, social work, physical therapy, psychology, and theology can use this book. In addition, interested laypeople will find the content invaluable in their search for reliable integrative healthcare information. It is an excellent resource for clinical and classroom instructors alike and a valuable addition to any instructor's library.

Each of the 12 chapters in this book can be used independently of the others. The beginning of each chapter contains learning objectives, and the end contains key concepts, questions for reflection, and references.

Introduction

The doctor of the future will give no medicine, but will interest his patients in the care of the human frame, in diet, and in the cause and prevention of disease.

—Thomas Edison

The philosophy of complementary and alternative medicine (CAM) and integrative medicine is not new. It has been discussed for hundreds of years across many disciplines. Long before the advent of high technology, magnetic resonance imaging and robotic surgery, Aristotle (384–322 BC) reflected on the human condition through observation, assessment, and reflection. During the last century, accepted medical care overlooked CAM, but that stance is changing as healthcare providers realize the benefits of combining the external, technical aspects of curing with the internal, nonphysical aspects of healing (Rakel & Weil, 2007).

The use of complementary and alternative therapies has escalated, along with growing concerns about health care in the United States. It is no secret that the contemporary conventional American healthcare system is in need of a revision. While it excels at treating medical emergencies, identifying microscopic elements like genomes, and addressing complex surgical cases, conventional medicine has failed in addressing disease prevention and management. Over $1 trillion a year is spent on health care in the United States, making it the most expensive healthcare system in the industrialized world (Bright, 2002). Americans pay more for medical care than people in most other nations of comparable living standards, and we accomplish less while our costs continue to spiral out of control. The client–provider relationship is deteriorating and technology is overutilized.

As more and more Americans become discouraged by an increasingly inadequate healthcare system, a growing number are turning to CAM and integrative therapies to address their needs. These individuals recognize the effectiveness of an integrated approach to health, and they appreciate the blend of body and mind, science and experience, and traditional and cultural perspectives for diagnosis and treatment. They prefer the emphasis on the individual as a whole, rather than conventional medicine's emphasis on diagnostic testing and treatment with medications.

Traditional medicine is getting the message. In 1993, a study published in the *New England Journal of Medicine* found that more than 33% of those surveyed chose alternative medicine over conventional treatments (Eisenberg et al., 1993). In that same year, an office of alternative medicine was started within the National Institutes of Health (NIH) with an initial budget of $2 million. The office was later upgraded to the National Center for Complementary and Alternative Medicine (NCCAM), and by 2006 its budget was $122 million to allow for much-needed research (Rakel & Weil, 2007).

In 1997 alone, U.S. citizens spent more than $27 billion on alternative treatments. They paid most of this out of pocket, since health insurance does not cover these treatments (Bright, 2002; Trivieri & Anderson, 2002). During that same year, Andrew Weil, MD, started the first fellowship program in integrative medicine at the University of Arizona. In 2004, data from the NCCAM and the National Center for Health Statistics (NCHS) showed that 36% of adults used some form of complementary and alternative treatment to manage their health (that number rises to 62% if megavitamin therapy, meditation, chiropractic care, yoga, diet-based therapies, massage, and prayer for health reasons are included) (Rakel & Weil, 2007; Second Opinion, 2007). However, nearly 70% of clients reported not talking to their doctors about complementary or alternative treatments, either because of skepticism about how much they think their physicians know or because their physicians don't ask (Crute, 2008).

By 2005, approximately 27% of U.S. hospitals offered complementary and alternative medicine therapies, up from 8% in 1998. Federal and foundational research funds are now close to $225 million per year (Comarow, 2008). By 2007, more than 30 medical schools across the United States and Canada were part of the Consortium of Academic Health Centers for Integrative Medicine. The consortium brings academic leaders together "to transform health care through rigorous scientific studies, new models of clinical care, and innovative educational programs that integrate biomedicine, the complexity of humans, the intrinsic nature of healing, and the rich diversity of therapeutic systems" (Rakel & Weil, 2007, p. 5).

THE ROOTS OF CONVENTIONAL MEDICINE

The roots of conventional medicine, including drug and surgery procedures common in Western (allopathic) medicine, came into being in the early 20th century and can be traced to the famous scientist, spiritual mathematician, and philosopher René Descartes (1596–1650). His work led to the development of Cartesianism, or the Cartesian split, a philosophy characterized by a rationalistic, dualistic view of the world. Concerned that prevailing scientific materialistic thought would reduce the conscious mind to something that could be manipulated and controlled, Descartes did his best to separate the mind and the body to protect the spirit from science. He believed that the mind and spirit should be the focus of the church, leaving science to address the body (Rakel & Weil, 2007; Trivieri & Anderson, 2002). His philosophy resulted in a separation of mind and body that ultimately led to the fields of specialization common in Western medicine today. Each specialization focuses exclusively on its particular organ or system, usually without regard to how the human organism and life itself are intertwined.

During the 1600s and 1700s, philosophers John Locke and David Hume influenced the reductionistic movement, which suggested that we could better understand a larger whole if we reduced natural phenomena to smaller parts (Rakel & Weil, 2007). The mid-19th century saw the discovery of microbes, followed by the development of the microscope, X-rays, and antibiotics, as well as the organization of medical schools into specialized departments such as cardiology and nephrology (Trivieri & Anderson, 2002). Samuel Hahnemann (1755–1843), a German physician and chemist, coined the term *allopathy* (meaning "other suffering") to describe what he thought was a misguided approach to the care of disease and health prevention. Today the term *allopathic medicine* is used to describe modern conventional medical methods.

Only recently has modern science taken the steps to reunite the mind and body that Descartes separated 360 years ago. Albert Einstein's revolutionary unified field theory, which was widely regarded at the time as ludicrous, led Western science back to the ancient idea that all points (energy and matter) connect and that each significantly affects the others. Human beings (with their emotional, mental, spiritual, and physical components) are very much a part of this connection (Seaward, 2006). The American Holistic Medical Association was founded in 1978 to promote a common community to treat the whole person (Trivieri & Anderson, 2002). This reunification is important, especially in the study of stress and its relationship with the mind, body, and spirit.

Micozzi (2006) asserts that, in our efforts to make medicine scientific, Western medicine in particular has emphasized that knowledge about the world, including nature and human nature, must meet the following criteria:

- *Objectivism:* The observer is separate from the observed.
- *Reductionism:* Complex phenomena are explainable in terms of simpler, component phenomena.
- *Positivism:* All information can be derived from physically measurable data.
- *Determinism:* Phenomena can be predicted from a knowledge of scientific law and initial conditions.

Micozzi further states that we all know this is not the only way of knowing.

CONCEPTS OF COMPLEMENTARY AND ALTERNATIVE MEDICINE

The concepts of alternative, holistic, and integrative medicine have their roots in various healing traditions that have been around since as early as 5000 BC. Nursing pioneer Florence Nightingale embraced this philosophy when she included herbs as an essential tool in her nurse's bag and stressed the need for clean water, fresh air, light, compassionate care, and spiritual support (Hendricks, 2007).

Although many diverse healthcare systems fall within the category of integrative and complementary and alternative medicine, they share some similarities in their views of health and healing. According to Micozzi (2006), this "overall philosophy can be called a *new ecology of health*, sustainable medicine, or 'medicine for a small planet'" (p. 3). The key elements of this philosophy include the following (Micozzi, 2006; Trivieri & Anderson, 2002):

- *There is a strong emphasis on wellness versus medicalization.* Medicalization is the process by which health behaviors are defined and treated as medical issues and, as such, they are within the purview of healthcare professionals. The goal of preventing disease is crucial, but there is also a strong focus on engaging the individual's inner resources as an active and conscious participant in his or her own health. No outside person or entity gives the state of health to an individual; rather, health results from a balance of internal resources and external natural and social environments. An emphasis on lifestyle changes, self-care, and education adds to the options of care.
- *There is an emphasis on self-healing.* The belief is that the body heals itself. While this principle may seem obvious to some, it is one of the foundational beliefs of CAM systems. The body's ability to heal is tied to its inner resources and the external environment. The evidence for self-healing can be seen in clinical observations of the placebo effect or spontaneous remissions. Evoking the healing powers of love, hope, humor, and enthusiasm and releasing the toxic consequences of shame, guilt, greed, depression, fear, anger, and grief are encouraged. The relationship between the physician and the client considers the needs, desires, awareness, and insight of *both*.
- *The body is an energetic system and a living entity.* Disruptions in the balance and flow of energy cause illness, and the body's response to energy imbalance leads to disease. Because the body can make itself sick, it can also heal itself. Holism focuses as much on the kind of client who has a disease as it does on the kind of disease a client has. Illness is viewed as a manifestation of a dysfunction of the whole person, not an isolated event.

- *Nutrition and natural products are essential to health.* The reliance on nutrition and natural products is not merely an adjunct to therapy but an essential aspect of wellness. Nutrients are taken into the body in the most literal sense and provide calories as well as energy and resources to help the individual stay healthy or get well. Micozzi (2006) notes that "because the basic plan of the body, as a physical entity and as an energy system, evolves and exists in an ecological context, what the body needs it obtains from the environment in which it grew" (p. 6).
- *Plants are an essential element of health and a dominant aspect of the environment in which human beings evolved.* Plants produce the oxygen we breathe and essential oils. They are a source of vibrational energy as well as medicines.
- *CAM systems emphasize individuality, along with an emphasis on the whole person and his or her unique resources.* Concepts of normalization, standardization, and generalization are difficult to apply to CAM research and clinical practice. If the body has its own energy and is uniquely individual, then the emphasis is on the healed, not on the healer. This is quite a different paradigm from traditional allopathic health systems. In CAM, optimal health is viewed as the "conscious pursuit of the highest qualities of the physical, environmental, mental, emotional, spiritual, and social aspects of human experience" (Trivieri & Anderson, 2002, p. 7).

Sociopolitical forces have also shaped the CAM philosophy. Examples of these profound shifts in culture, science, technology, and communication that caused an altered consciousness and required a new understanding and approach to living include the following (Bright, 2002):

- The civil rights movement, addressing forces of cruelty, injustice, and fragmentation in culture
- The women's rights movement and issues of unequal personhood
- The consumer rights movement, examining fairness and legal protection in health care
- The ecology movement, citing a growing awareness of the damage being done worldwide to the health of humans, animals, and vegetation by the unrestrained growth and exploitation of natural resources
- The wellness movement, with its focus on educating people to change their beliefs, attitudes, and lifestyles
- The holistic movement, which views living things as greater than the sum of their parts

THE MOVE TOWARD INTEGRATIVE HEALTH CARE

The terms *complementary* and *alternative* are often used interchangeably but their meanings are not similar. *Complementary* implies a therapy that is used *in conjunction with* a conventional therapy. An *alternative* therapy is one that is used *instead of* a conventional therapy. Bright (2002) notes that "complementary/alterative therapies cover a broad range of healing philosophies, approaches, and therapies that conventional Western medicine does not commonly use, accept, study, understand, or make available" (p. 7). Some CAM therapies are also called *holistic* because they address the whole person, including physical, mental, emotional, and spiritual facets (Bright, 2002).

What has been labeled *alternative medicine* in the United States is a social phenomenon and consumer movement of significant proportions (Micozzi, 2006). Rakel and Weil (2007) note that, with the growth of good scientific research regarding many CAM therapies, "the labels once used to classify these therapies are no longer needed" (p. 6). They add that the terms *complementary* and *alternative* "only serve to detract from a therapy by making it sound second class" (p. 6). Therapies labeled under the CAM heading include nutrition, spirituality, and stress management. Rakel and Weil argue that sound science underlies these therapies, and none of them can be considered less significant than conventional therapies. They further state that labeling these as CAM contributes to healthcare fragmentation and the problems associated with multiple providers treating the client in multiple ways. They believe we need a medical model built on relationship-centered care that fosters healing by allowing practitioners to gain insight into the client's situation and to build the client's trust and confidence in the practitioner (Rakel & Weil, 2007).

The move now is toward using the term *integrative medicine*, which stresses the importance of using evidence to understand how best to integrate both complementary and alternative therapies into our current healthcare model so we can facilitate health and healing and effect positive change in our healthcare system. Popularized by Andrew Weil, the term *integrative medicine* includes the concept of "communication among all health providers who share the responsibility in coordinating the best possible treatment plan for a client, including the client's choices for care and the providers' expertise in understanding and managing the complexities of conventional-complementary treatment interactions" (Bright, 2002, pp. 9, 11). Integrative medicine focuses on healing rather than on disease; Rakel and Weil (2007) describe it as a "healing oriented medicine that takes account of the whole person (body, mind, and spirit), including all aspects of lifestyle. It emphasizes the therapeutic relationship and makes use of all appropriate therapies, both conventional and alternative" (p. 7).

The philosophy of integrative medicine is not new; it has been explored and discussed for ages across many disciplines. In fact, Aristotle is considered one of the first holistic physicians because he believed that every person was a combination of both physical and spiritual properties with no separation between body and mind. However, we are now experiencing a shift toward recognizing the benefits of combining the external, physical, and technologic successes of medicine with the internal, nonphysical exploration of healing (Rakel & Weil, 2007).

REFERENCES

Bright, M. A. (2002). Paradigm shifts. In M. A. Bright, *Holistic health and healing* (pp. 3–30). Philadelphia: F. A. Davis.

Comarow, A. (2008, January 21). Embracing alternative care: Hospitals put unorthodox therapies into practice. *U.S. News and World Report, 144*(2), 31–40.

Crute, S. (2008, March/April). The best medicine. *AARP The Magazine*, 58–64.

Eisenberg, D. M., Kessler, R. C., Foster, C., Norlock, F. E., Calkins, D. R., & Delbanco, T. L. (1993). Unconventional medicine in the United States: Prevalence, costs, and patterns of use. *New England Journal of Medicine, 328*(4), 246–252.

Hendricks, M. (2007, Spring). Nursing the whole patient. *Johns Hopkins Nursing, 5*(1), 25–32.

Micozzi, M. S. (2006). Characteristics of complementary and integrative medicine. In M. S. Micozzi, *Fundamentals of complementary and integrative medicine* (3rd ed., pp. 3–8). St. Louis, MO: Saunders Elsevier.

Rakel, D., & Weil, A. (2007). Philosophy of integrative medicine. In D. Rakel, *Integrative medicine* (2nd ed., pp. 3–13). Philadelphia: Saunders Elsevier.

Seaward, B. L. (2006). *Managing stress: Principles and strategies for health and well-being* (5th ed.). Sudbury, MA: Jones and Bartlett.

Second opinion: Why recommend complementary and alternative medicine (CAM)? (2007, Spring). *Johns Hopkins Nursing, 5*(1), 3.

Trivieri, L., Jr., & Anderson, J. W. (Eds.). (2002). *Alternative medicine: The definitive guide.* Berkeley, CA: Celestial Arts.

About the Authors

Caroline and Cyndie's journey continues to be a source of inspiration and joy for both of them. They first met almost 20 years ago when they worked together in the community health and wellness department of a large metropolitan hospital. Discovering that they shared a mutual interest in other cultures and in the integrative aspects of care that were not well addressed in the healthcare environment in which they practiced, they instantly connected and began a marvelous and deeply satisfying business partnership and friendship.

In 1994, Caroline and Cyndie founded ALLEGRA Learning Solutions, LLC, to provide print and online professional education courses for nurses and other healthcare professionals. Their journey continues to lead them down many interesting paths. They have integrated knowledge gained through unique cultural and diverse healthcare experiences with other people. They have traveled extensively throughout the world and found their lives enriched by the many cultures, health traditions, and wonderful people they met along the way. Their journey has included attention to personal healthcare practices, academic courses, workshops, continued study and sharing of diverse healthcare traditions and practices, reading, and experiencing and practicing modalities of care as they continue to learn that integrating the various aspects of who they are and how they may be healed is an integral part of health and healing.

• • •

Cyndie Koopsen, MBA, RN, HN-BC, is a registered nurse with a certification in public health and holistic nursing and a master of business administration degree. Her professional nursing career has involved caring for clients in many settings and from many walks of life. Cyndie has been involved in nursing leadership and administration, staff development and education, community education, and holistic care. In addition, she has managed large-scale clinical preventive programs and has designed, developed, and presented clinical programs for multicultural audiences spanning the spectrum of health promotion and disease prevention.

Caroline Young, MPH, holds a bachelor's degree in psychology and a master of public health degree with an emphasis in health promotion. Her extensive public health background includes expertise in research, design, development, marketing, implementation, and evaluation of community health programs. She also has expertise in developing education and health promotion programs for culturally diverse populations, senior populations, and faith communities.

The authors of *Spirituality, Health, and Healing*, Caroline and Cyndie have served as adjunct faculty members with several colleges and have coauthored distance education texts on cultural diversity, alternative medicine, and gerontology. They have conducted workshops, led seminars, and given presentations on numerous healthcare topics. They have developed more than several hundred online professional continuing education courses for vocational, baccalaureate, and master's level degree programs. They have also designed and developed certificate programs in the areas of spirituality, complementary and alternative medicine, gerontology, and end-of-life issues.

CHAPTER 1

Holistic Stress Management

The act of caring is the first true step in the power to heal.
—Phillip Moffitt

LEARNING OBJECTIVES

1. Describe the concept of stress.
2. Identify the stages of the general adaptation syndrome (GAS).
3. Explain the effects of stress on the individual.
4. Describe the physiology of stress.
5. Explain the concept of psychoneuroimmunology.
6. Identify the ways self-awareness can help an individual manage stress.
7. Describe the roles of cognitive restructuring and effective communication in stress management.
8. Explain the role of guided imagery in stress management.
9. Describe the impact of social support on health.
10. Describe art therapy and its role in stress management.
11. Explain how journaling affects health and can address stress.

INTRODUCTION

Each and every day, we face stressors. Events, people, circumstances, concerns, and a certain amount of stress are part of our normal daily lives. Some of us rise to the occasion and thrive in these situations. Others experience a combination of negative physical and psychological effects. Why do we react differently to stressors? Despite much research on the topic, the answer is not clearly understood, but a key element is how we manage the stressors we face.

Stress is a reaction to any stimulus or challenge that upsets our normal function and disturbs our mental or physical health. Stress is brought on by internal circumstances (such as illness, pain, or emotional upset) or by external circumstances (such as death, family or financial problems, or job challenges) (Trivieri & Anderson, 2002). Attitudes, beliefs, and emotional states ranging from love to anger can trigger chain reactions that affect blood chemistry, heart rate, and the activity of every cell and organ in the body (Pelletier, 1993).

ORIGINS AND DEFINITIONS OF STRESS

The concept of the mind's influence on health has been recognized since the time of Hippocrates. As the founder of Western medicine and the originator of the Hippocratic oath, Hippocrates equated health to the harmonious balance between mind, body, and environment. During the Renaissance, English physician Thomas Sydenham furthered this concept. Recognized as a founder of clinical medicine and epidemiology, Sydenham observed the "healing power of nature" and asserted that a person's internal responses to external forces were a major factor in disease and health (Pelletier, 1993).

For many years after Hippocrates and Sydenham, very little was published or discussed about stress. Prior to the 1960s, it was difficult to find any articles on the topic; now the term *stress* is as common as the term *computer*.

Originally, the word *stress* was used in the context of physics and described the amount of tension or force placed on an object to bend or break it. Hans Selye was the first to apply the notion of stress to human beings (Seaward, 2006). Known as the father of stress research, Selye developed much of the foundation for what we know today about stress. During the 1950s, he developed what he called the general adaptation syndrome (GAS), which states that all organisms have a similar response when confronted with a challenge to their well-being, regardless of whether they see the challenge as positive or negative. GAS is comprised of three stages of response (Eliopoulos, 2004; Payne, 2005; Seaward, 2006; Trivieri & Anderson, 2002):

1. The first stage is the *alarm reaction*, also known as the fight-or-flight response. First described during the 19th century by Harvard physiologist Walter B. Canon, the fight-or-flight response is the body's internal adaptive response to a threat (Seaward, 2006). In this stage, the body "gears up" physically and psychologically for a real or perceived threat. This response was essential to survival in a time when human beings faced all types of physical threats, such as wild animals (Eliopoulos, 2004; Leddy, 2006).
2. In the *stage of resistance*, the body maintains its state of readiness, but not to the extent of the initial alarm phase.
3. If the body has to maintain the heightened state of readiness, it reaches a *stage of exhaustion*. At this point, the body has no further energy reserves, is unable to sustain the workload required by constant vigilance, and fails. Illness and possibly death can ensue (Eliopoulos, 2004).

Today the word *stress* has many different definitions and connotations. According to Seaward (2006), in Eastern philosophies stress is considered to be the absence of inner peace; in Western culture it is considered the loss of control. Serge Kahili King, a noted healer, describes stress as any change experienced by the individual. Researcher Richard Lazarus calls it a state of anxiety produced when events and responsibilities exceed one's ability to cope with them. Selye added to this definition that "stress is the nonspecific response of the body to any demand placed upon it to adapt, whether that demand produces pleasure or pain" (Seaward, 2006, p. 4). Seaward also states that the most recent definition of stress is "the inability to cope with a perceived (real or imagined) threat to one's mental, physical, emotional, and spiritual well-being, which results in a series of physiological responses and adaptations" (p. 4).

While the definitions of stress vary, most agree that stress is not what happens to someone—those outside forces are the stressors. What matters is how the person reacts to what happens.

THE BODY'S REACTION TO STRESS

In the 1950s and early 1960s, psychiatrists Thomas Holmes and Richard Rahe at the University of Washington School of Medicine found ways to quantify the effects of stressful events. They found that events like divorce, a death in the family, a job change, pregnancy, obtaining a large mortgage, marriage, and retirement can take their toll. The more stress people experience, the more likely they are to become sick in the months following the stressful events. When life brings many stressors at once, a prolonged, intense, and potentially dangerous reaction is even more likely (Pelletier, 1993).

Scientists now believe that the body responds differently to different types of stress:

- *Good stress*, which Selye called *eustress*, motivates us, has pleasant or enjoyable effects, keeps us excited about life, and can be fulfilling. Examples include falling in love, getting a job promotion, watching a scary movie, taking a roller coaster ride, or having a surprise birthday party (Seaward, 2006). While such events may cause a short alarm response, its strength and duration are limited.
- *Bad stress*, called *distress* by Selye, fully initiates the fight-or-flight response and may have a prolonged impact on a person's life. A divorce, having a loved one involved in an accident, and a job loss are possible examples. Usually when individuals talk about stress, they are referring to distress (Eliopoulos, 2004). Signs of distress include headaches, heart palpitations, pain, a constricted throat, weariness, nausea, and diarrhea (Trivieri & Anderson, 2002).

- *Neustress* describes sensory stimuli that have no consequential effects and are considered neither good nor bad (Seaward, 2006).

What one person considers distress can be considered eustress by another. For example, one person may consider a long commute to be a great way to unwind from a hectic day at work while another person may consider the long drive to be tiring and a barrier to time spent with the family.

Types of Stress

While the body's reactions can vary, there are four types of stress (Trivieri & Anderson, 2002):

- *Physical stress* can include trauma, illness, intense physical labor, environmental pollution, inadequate light, childbirth, noise, toxins, inadequate oxygen supply, hypoglycemia, hormonal or chemical imbalances, dietary stress, substance abuse, and dental problems.
- *Psychological stress* can include fear, resentment, information overload, worry, shame, guilt, jealousy, self-criticism, and anxiety. It can also include the loss of a sense of control, beliefs and attitudes, and a worldview.
- *Psychosocial stress* can include relationship difficulties, a lack of social support, and isolation.
- *Psychospiritual stress* can include a joyless life; meaningless work; and a crisis of values, meaning, and purpose.

Seaward (2006) also discusses *technostress*, a term used to describe the ability or inability to cope with the rapid pace of technology. Prior to 1955 the most common causes of death were infectious diseases such as polio, rubella, tuberculosis, typhoid, and encephalitis, most of which have been eradicated due to vaccines or medications. After World War II, the age of high technology introduced modern conveniences like the microwave, television, DVD player, laptop computer, and cell phones. Cited as luxuries that would allow more free time, they seem to have increased our drive to remain productive, decreased leisure time, and led to all types of unhealthy lifestyles—and increasing technostress. In addition to its 24/7 nature, technostress has other characteristics that may lead to more stress, illness, disease, and dysfunction and a greater imbalance in life:

- *Information overload* due to floods of e-mails, faxes, Web site advertisements, instant messaging, text messaging, voice mail, and other waves of incoming data

- *The lack of clear boundaries between personal and professional lives* because of the accessibility offered by cell phones, pagers, palm computers, and other devices
- *The increasing lack of privacy* due to the use of Internet cookies, ever-increasing information storage and data mining, and other means of obtaining personal information
- *Ethical issues* regarding our personal information falling into the wrong hands, such as insurance companies who then revoke polices based on genetic profiling

Stress and Individual Personality Types

The typical people associated with stress are also associated with heart disease. These *type A personalities* drive themselves hard to achieve one goal after another, have free-floating hostility, have a fiercely competitive spirit, create action plans with deadlines, and perform activities as quickly as possible. They have a preoccupation or obsession with the passage of time and are impatient. They usually engage in more than one thought or activity at a time (polyphasia or multitasking) and have rapid speech patterns. Type A personalities are also excessively alert, feel a need to control (often manipulatively), and have a constant need to be recognized (Payne, 2005; Seaward, 2006; Williams, 1993. They often obtain great material wealth, expect immediate gratification, are competitive (e.g., for sales goals or salaries), are highly analytical, see people as numbers, are less socially connected, and watch a lot of television. While the type A personality often has a negative connotation, our society typically values the achievements of a type A (Seaward, 2006).

Two of the key traits that predict higher-than-normal death rates among type A individuals are hostility and hostile aggression. Anger leads to a deterioration of the heart's pumping efficiency, reducing the body's and the heart's blood supply and increasing the risk of sudden death (Seaward, 2006; Williams, 1993).

Type B individuals are more relaxed than type A personalities and do not exhibit the same traits. Type Bs have been found to be almost immune to coronary heart disease.

There is also a type D (depression) personality that some call psychocardiology, linking anxiety and depression to cardiac function (Seaward, 2006).

If negative psychological traits can intensify the effects of stress, positive ways of coping may buffer the body from its effects. What seems to be important is the ability to manage the traits. Psychologist Suzanne Kobasa at City University of New York identified a type of person she described as a "hardy" individual, who typically possesses three traits:

- A sense of control over his or her life and of having the right information to make decisions that can make a crucial difference
- A feeling of being committed to his or her work, hobby, or family
- A sense of challenge in which change is viewed as an opportunity to develop the self rather than as a threat to his or her equilibrium

These traits make such an individual less likely to suffer from stress-related diseases (Payne, 2005; Pelletier, 1993; Seaward, 2006).

The sense of control seems to be especially important in avoiding illness, even in animal experiments, a point that was highlighted in a study conducted by University of Pennsylvania psychologist Martin E. P. Seligman. In Seligman's study, laboratory mice were subjected to electrical shocks they could not escape, to no electrical shocks, and to escapable shocks. Seventy-three percent of the mice who received shocks they could not escape developed at least some tumors while only 37% of the mice who could escape suffered tumor growth. In humans, a similarly high rate of heart disease has been linked to "job strain" of certain jobs (such as air traffic controllers, secretaries, or bus drivers), where people felt high pressure but little or no control over how they met the job's demands (Pelletier, 1993).

PHYSIOLOGY OF STRESS

When the body perceives a threat, a series of chemical and physical responses occur. The first response is the activation of the autonomic nervous system (ANS) (Pelletier, 1993), a part of the nervous system that is not normally under our control. The sympathetic branch of the autonomic nervous system regulates the stress response while the parasympathetic nervous system controls the relaxation response. When the stress response occurs, the body secretes catecholamines (stress hormones) that help prepare the person to either fight or turn from the threat and run. The most well known of these stress hormones are epinephrine, secreted by the adrenal glands (medulla) located on top of the kidney, and norepinephrine, also secreted by the adrenal glands and nerve endings throughout the body (Seaward, 2006). The release of these hormones triggers the fight-or-flight response.

The anterior pituitary gland secretes adrenocorticotropic hormone (ACTH), which stimulates the adrenal glands to release aldosterone and cortisol. The pituitary gland also secretes vasopressin, or antidiuretic hormone.

- *Aldosterone* and *vasopressin* preserve blood volume by reducing the amount of sodium and water that the kidneys excrete (Eliopoulos, 2004; Leddy, 2006). Heart rate increases, blood pressure rises, breathing rate and depth increase, the liver releases glucose, and blood vessels in vital organs dilate while the vessels of nonessential organs (like the skin and digestive tract) constrict. The entire body is focused on keeping the brain, heart, lungs, and major muscles ready to fight or flee.

- *Cortisol* increases glucose production and helps break down fats and proteins to provide the body with the needed energy for dealing with the event (Eliopoulos, 2004; Leddy, 2006).

Responses to Short- and Long-Term Stress

There are two forms of stress:

- *Short-term (acute) stress* is intense, disappears quickly, and is caused by events such as a near miss on the highway or a loud noise. The body responds with the typical fight-or-flight response (Leddy, 2006; Seaward, 2006).
- *Long-term (chronic) stress* occurs over a longer period of time (e.g., hours, days, weeks, or months). The responses experienced are prolonged, often leading to the development of chronic disease. Examples include living with a horrible college roommate; looming credit card bills; dealing with a difficult boss; or having relationship problems with a close friend, spouse, or family member.

With long-term stress, the immune system is often suppressed or less vigilant than normal, blood cholesterol levels rise, and calcium is lost from the bones. The individual can become hypertensive; experience chronic pain, headaches, constipation or diarrhea, weight loss or gain, tiredness, sleep problems, crying, changes in eating, drinking, or smoking behaviors; feel irritable, depressed, or restless; and have difficulty thinking, concentrating, or remembering things. Social withdrawal and changes in the quality of relationships can also occur (Leddy, 2006; Seaward, 2006).

In addition to these conditions, stress can cause individuals to experience physiological effects like nausea, reduced libido, amenorrhea, and teeth grinding. Emotionally, they may experience irritability, anger, withdrawal from activities they enjoy, anxiety, a tendency to be easily startled, and drug or alcohol use. Intellectually, individuals can be forgetful, have difficulty being productive, experience reduced creativity, be less attentive to detail, and be preoccupied (Eliopoulos, 2004; Payne, 2005; Seaward, 2006).

Stress and Disease

The link between body and mind is a powerful one, but research has yet to effectively explain the link between stress and disease. However, it is widely recognized that chronic stress can affect the human body and increase the risk for developing heart disease, asthma, arthritis, cancer, hypertension, migraine headaches, and ulcers. Some statistics state that 50–90% of health-related problems are aggravated by stress (Eliopoulos, 2004). Other conditions aggravated by stress include colitis, speech problems, emphysema, neuromuscular syndromes, gastritis, and hypoglycemia (Trivieri & Anderson, 2002). Stress can increase one's susceptibility to illness, suppress the immune system, and create hormonal imbalances that can further interfere with immune function (Trivieri & Anderson, 2002).

Psychoneuroimmunology

The field of *psychoneuroimmunology* explores the relationship between psychological factors and health. There is a tremendous amount of information on this relationship, and entire books have been written about it. This section provides an overview of the topic; those interested in further study are encouraged to explore the references at the end of this chapter.

In the 1970s, psychologist Robert Ader and immunologist Nicholas Cohen were the first to show that the immune system "learned" associations and therefore affected health (Kiecolt-Glaser & Glaser, 1993). As previously discussed, individuals react to their environments, and the brain signals the rest of the body through the nervous, endocrine, and immune systems.

The Nervous System

The nervous system is comprised of the central nervous system (CNS) and peripheral nervous system (PNS). The CNS consists of the brain and spinal cord; the PNS consists of 31 pairs of spinal nerves and 12 pairs of cranial nerves that branch off from the brain and spinal cord. The PNS also includes the autonomic nervous system (ANS) or neurons that innervate the muscles and glands that automatically maintain bodily homeostasis (Freeman, 2004).

The human brain is further divided into three levels: the vegetative level, the limbic system, and the neocortical level (Seaward, 2006).

- The *vegetative level* consists of both the brain stem and the reticular formation, which connects the brain to the spinal cord.
- The *limbic system* is the emotional center of the brain and contains the thalamus, hypothalamus, pituitary gland, and a structure called the amygdala (Seaward, 2006). The amygdala links our emotional responses to our memories and has strong connections to the hypothalamus. The hypothalamus modulates heart activity, body temperature, blood pressure, and endocrine activity, and it also contains the centers that

modulate a person's emotional condition and basic biologic drives (sex, thirst, and hunger). When the amygdala responds to danger or stress, it signals the hypothalamus to initiate the fight-or-flight response by the sympathetic nervous system (Freeman, 2004).

- The *neocortical level*, the highest and most sophisticated level of the brain, is where our sensory information is processed (decoded) as a threat or nonthreat and where cognition (thought process) takes place. The neocortex houses the neural mechanisms that allow us to analyze; imagine; and create and employ intuition, memory, and organization (Seaward, 2006).

The Endocrine System

The endocrine system is comprised of glands (pituitary, thyroid, parathyroid, adrenal, pineal, and thymus), organs (pancreas, ovaries, testes, hypothalamus), and tissues (pockets of cells in the small intestines, stomach, kidneys, and heart) that produce hormones that act as needed to monitor or alter bodily processes (Freeman, 2004). These glands and tissues help regulate metabolic functions that require endurance rather than speed, and they release the chemical messengers (hormones) that attach to specific cell receptor sites to alter cell metabolism. The hypothalamus has direct influence over the pituitary (or "master") gland (Seaward, 2006).

The Immune System

The immune system shares anatomic connections and signal molecules with the nervous and endocrine systems (Bartol & Courts, 2005). It is made up of the thymus and spleen, as well as lymphocytes and other white blood cells. The immune system has two major components (Levy, 2002):

- The *innate (nonspecific) immune system* is the body's first line of defense against threatening organisms. Included in this system are granulocytes and macrophages; these phagocytic white blood cells recognize and destroy threatening organisms. The innate system also includes natural killer (NK) cells, which attack and destroy virally infected cells and cancer cells.
- The *acquired (specific) immune system* is made up of certain white blood cells (lymphocytes) and the antibodies they produce. Lymphocytes circulate throughout the blood or lymphatic tissue, patrolling the body for signs of danger. All these cells are produced in the bone marrow throughout life (Freeman, 2004). Kiecolt-Glaser and Glaser (1993) explain that "all of these immunological organs have now been

shown to contain networks of nerve cells, which provide a pathway for the brain and central nervous system to influence immunity" (p. 41).

The immune systems interact by means of two distinct mind- or brain-mediated pathways that are activated by stress.

- The first and most direct brain pathway is the *sympathetic-adrenal-medullary (SAM) axis*, which activates the ANS. The motor neurons of the ANS use neurotransmitters and neuropeptides for information and thus communicate directly with immune cells and tissue to alter immune system responses (Freeman, 2004). Neurotransmitters are substances that transmit nerve impulses across a synapse. Neuropeptides are unique messenger hormones, produced in the brain (and other body organs), that fit into the receptor sites of lymphocytes. Immune cells have built-in receptor sites for the several hundred or so neuropeptides, which can either increase or decrease the cells' metabolic function (Seaward, 2006). Disease or health can result.
- The second and indirect brain pathway is the *hypothalamic-pituitary-adrenal (HPA) axis*, which alters both the physiology and immune functions by signaling the endocrine system to release hormones. Once the hormones are released, the physiologic and immune responses occur.

When an individual's CNS responds to internal or external stressors or stimuli, informational substances (such as neurochemicals) are produced. The body interprets these substances and determines which informational substances to produce and release (Freeman, 2004). Other parts of the body react and affect everything from heart rate to sexual function to immunity.

EFFECTIVE STRESS MANAGEMENT TECHNIQUES

Like every chapter in this book, this section includes techniques to help the reader effectively manage stress.

Self-Awareness

Rew (2005) defines self-reflection as "the process of turning one's attention or awareness inward to examine thoughts, feelings, beliefs, and behaviors" (p. 429). It is a deliberate process with a goal of discovery and learning. *Self-awareness*, or being aware of the self, is the tendency to focus attention on the private aspects of the self. It includes self-exploration, recognizing one's strengths and weaknesses, and knowing one's self. Payne (2005) notes that increasing self-knowledge comes from listening to ourselves: what we are, who we are, and how we are.

By increasing our self-awareness, we understand our outward behavior and how others respond to it, thereby improving our personal relationships. Self-awareness is closely linked to the concept of living in the present, since that is where we make our impact. Lessons learned from the past are important in helping us perform our best in the present. Living this way produces greater peace of mind; self-awareness can thus be seen as a stress management tool (Payne, 2005).

Payne (2005) lists several ways to improve self-awareness:

- *Become aware of your personal thinking style:* Sometimes people think in a focused way, and at other times they think more broadly. Mode of thinking is connected to self-esteem. Those with an internal locus of control (that is, a tendency to believe they have control over their lives and environment) tend to have higher self-esteem than those who have an external locus of control (little or no control over the environment). Thinking is more positive with an internal locus of control.
- *Be aware of your intuitive powers:* Intuition can provide much information about the inner self and involves "an intense feeling of certainty that may be accompanied by a sense of mystery or confusion" (Rew, 2005, p. 432).
- *Be aware of your emotions and feelings:* This principle is not about self-indulgence but instead about self-examination and an exploration of ways in which you might need to change. This method examines emotional patterns: how people express themselves spontaneously or in controlled ways, how they share their feelings, and how they use catharsis to move forward.
- *Be aware of your body:* This awareness includes how you are breathing and how your digestion, skin, or muscles feel.
- *Be aware of the environment:* How are you obtaining information through sight, sound, smell, touch, and taste?
- *Be aware of how you relate to others:* People can tell a lot about you by what you show of yourself, your appearance, your general demeanor, and what you say. Verbal and nonverbal behavior also tells a story about who you are. Your level of assertiveness is an aspect of relating and a means of insisting on having your interests respected while others advance their goals.

Cognitive Restructuring

Holocaust survivor and noted author and psychoanalyst Victor Frankl once said, "Everything can be taken away from man but one thing—the last human freedom, to choose one's attitude in any given set of circumstances." We know that stressors abound in life and that an individual's *perception* of the stressor, not the stressor itself, makes for either a mountain or a molehill. *Cognitive restructuring* is a coping technique that substitutes negative, self-defeating thoughts with positive, affirming thoughts to change the perception of the stressor from threatening to nonthreatening (Seaward, 2006).

Negative thoughts often result from low self-esteem and perpetuate the problem by suppressing or obliterating feelings of self-worth and self-acceptance. Some studies have shown that, on average, a child hears 400 negative comments for every positive one. Negative comments become conditioned (learned) responses that are carried into adulthood in the form of negative thoughts. Catastrophic headlines and negative media messages are also part of our everyday lives, and this negative perspective leads to negative thinking that can have an addictive and destructive quality (Seaward, 2006).

Two personality traits are closely related to locus of control, which has been shown to affect health:

- *Pessimism*, a personality trait heavily grounded in negativism, promotes toxic thoughts, a term coined in the 1980s.
- *Victimization* is an attitude where one feels specifically targeted by events or circumstances and believes that he or she has no choice but to suffer the consequences. "Victims" seek pity and sympathy from friends and validate their own perceptions of personal violation.

Thoughts and attitudes such as these have been shown to depress the immune system, decrease the longevity of cancer clients, and affect mental health. Psychologists use the term *self-fulfilling prophecy* to describe the link between perceptions, beliefs, and related behaviors (Seaward, 2006).

Cognitive restructuring can be achieved through four simple steps:

1. *Be aware* of stressors and acknowledge them. Identify why these situations and events are stressors and identify the emotions associated with them.
2. *Reappraise the situation.* See whether a different (more objective) viewpoint restructures the situation. Understand which situations you can control and which must be accepted as out of your control.
3. *Adopt the new frame of mind*, substituting a negative perspective for a positive one.
4. *Evaluate* whether this process worked and, if so, how beneficial it was so you can use it again (Seaward, 2006).

Effective Communication

The ability to effectively communicate is an essential tool in managing stress. If most people were to list their top 10 stressors, they would probably find that at least half of them dealt with relationships with family, friends, and coworkers. Strong relationships require good communication skills. The average person spends 75% of the day communicating with others. The degree of perception and interpretation required, as well as the many layers of meaning in every interaction, leave much room for misinterpretation and therefore stress (Seaward, 2006).

Effective communication includes the ability to express thoughts and feelings in understandable words and the ability to listen, clarify, and process information as it is intended. *Verbal communication* is actually a series of thoughts and perceptions described through words, and it has two components:

- *Encoding* is the process by which the speaker attempts to frame thoughts and perceptions into words.
- *Decoding* is the process by which the listener translates, dissects, analyzes, and interprets the message (Seaward, 2006).

Nonverbal communication is any communication that does not include words. Examples include clothing and appearance, the use of paralanguage (the meaning conveyed by voice tone and pitch, such as "uh-hum" or "hmmm"), bodily contact and proximity, respect for personal space, eye contact, and facial expressions (Evans, 1996).

Effective communication involves accurate listening, the use of silence, appropriate body language, reflecting (e.g., repeating the person's words to demonstrate listening), summarizing what was said, and self-awareness (Evans, 1996).

Effective listening, attending, and responding involve several key elements (Seaward, 2006):

- *Pay total attention to what the speaker is saying*, not to one's own thoughts. Do not prepare rebuttals or comments while someone is speaking.
- *Maintain eye contact* but do not stare continually.
- *Avoid the use of words that are emotional or prejudiced* to keep the listener from becoming disinterested.
- *Use minimal encouragers* (such as "oh" or "uh-huh") to tell the speaker you are both on the same wavelength.
- *Paraphrase* what is said to help ensure understanding.
- *Ask questions* to clarify statements.
- *Use empathy* to reflect and share feelings and galvanize the listening experience.
- *Provide feedback* to the speaker as appropriate.
- *Use language appropriate to the audience* and attack issues, not people.

- *Avoid information overload* so the information presented can be effectively received.
- *Enhance your vocabulary* to effectively articulate your issues, and resolve problems as they arise so they do not fester.

Benson's Method

During the 1970s, Herbert Benson was studying high blood pressure at Harvard's Thorndike Laboratory. He was approached by a group who practiced Transcendental Meditation (TM) and who believed their meditations could lower blood pressure. Benson discovered that TM could lower heart rate, breathing rate, oxygen consumption, blood lactate levels, and blood pressure. Upon further study, he realized that these results were common to all meditation practices and found several key elements to achieving what he called the relaxation response (Pelletier, 1993). These elements include a quiet environment, a comfortable position, a mental device (such as a word to focus on), and a passive attitude (Payne, 2005; Smith, 2006). Many of these are the same elements used in guided imagery. Based on his findings, Benson developed a simple method of meditation known as the Benson method.

Imagery

The imagination is probably an individual's least initialized health resource. It can be used to remember and re-create the past, develop insight into the present, influence physical health, enhance creativity, inspire, and anticipate the future (Trivieri & Anderson, 2002).

Trivieri and Anderson (2002) define *imagery* as a "flow of thoughts that one can see, hear, feel, smell, or taste in one's imagination" (p. 245). Imagery is the natural way for the nervous system to store, access, and process information. It is a rich, symbolic, highly personal language that involves fantasy as well as experience and is the interface between the mind and the body (Trivieri & Anderson, 2002). Imagery and intuition are part of our nonlogical thinking and they connect us with our inner subjective reality (Zahourek, 2002).

Historically, people have believed that imagery could magically influence present and future health and prosperity. Indigenous cultures and shamans use it with ancient healing rituals since they view the mind, body, and spirit as a whole. They believe that rituals, visions, and images are the bridge between the physical world and the healing power of the spiritual realm (Zahourek, 2002).

Imagery can be used on its own or in conjunction with therapeutic touch, meditation, biofeedback, Reiki (pronounced *ray kee*), reflexology, and other holistic practices (Schaub & Dossey, 2005).

Therapeutic Characteristics of Imagery

Imagery has three main characteristics that provide value to healthcare providers and assist in the healing process:

- It directly affects physiology.
- It provides insight and perspective into health through the mental processes of association and synthesis.
- It is intimately connected to the emotions, which are at the root of many health conditions.

Imagery can affect heart rate, blood pressure, respiratory patterns, oxygen consumption, carbon dioxide elimination, brainwave rhythms, the electrical characteristics of the skin, local blood flow and temperature in tissues, gastrointestinal motility and secretions, sexual arousal, levels of hormones and neurotransmitters in the blood, and immune system function (Schaub & Dossey, 2005; Trivieri & Anderson, 2002).

In addition, imagery helps people find meaning in events and situations and helps them understand and control their patterns of thinking. It makes the mind more receptive to new information; helps reduce fear, anxiety, and pain; and directly affects physiology, especially the sympathetic nervous system stress responses.

Imagery is a versatile therapeutic intervention that is often used in conjunction with hypnosis, biofeedback, desensitization, and cognitive behavioral techniques. It can be used at any stage of a therapeutic process but healing patterns are more easily established when individuals are relatively healthy than when they are faced with a serious disease. No research has yet been able to determine the specific kind of imagery that works best for a given type of client, symptom, illness, or disease (Trivieri & Anderson, 2002; Zahourek, 2002).

Types of Imagery

Of the different forms of imagery (Leddy, 2006; Zahourek, 2002), the experiential types include active, receptive, process, and end-state imagery.

- *Active imagery* uses conscious and deliberate effort to develop concrete and symbolic images. These images can be either a wise entity or inner guide or general healing images that include events, people, places or things, light, warmth, or heat. This approach is best used to address symptoms.
- *Receptive imagery* addresses the emotional significance of symptoms. This form occurs spontaneously and allows images to "bubble up" into

the conscious mind without a specific effort. It often occurs in the early stages of sleep or just prior to awakening.
- *Process imagery* uses a step-by-step approach to achieve the individual's goal. It is the rehearsal of a procedure or event.
- *End-state imagery* asks individuals to imagine their final, healed state.

Guided Imagery

Guided imagery involves the purposeful use of mental images by working with another person to achieve a desired therapeutic goal. It does not require elaborate equipment and it is safe and noninvasive (Payne, 2005). In this method, a person deliberately forms mental images while in a deeply relaxed state.

Guided imagery has been used to reduce phobias, complement other therapies, and facilitate a peaceful death. It has also been used to reduce chronic pain, allergies, high blood pressure, stress-related gastrointestinal symptoms, and functional urinary and reproductive irregularities (including premenstrual syndrome and dysmenorrhea); accelerate healing from acute injuries (including sprains, strains, broken bones, and symptoms of the flu, cold, and infections); and help with addictions, bulimia, and psoriasis (Leddy, 2006; Trivieri & Anderson, 2002; Zahourek, 2002).

In guided imagery, specific words, symbols, and ideas are used to elicit images. For example, imagine holding a juicy, bright yellow lemon. Feel its coolness, its weight, and the texture of its skin. Now imagine cutting it open, bringing it to your nose, and smelling it. Imagine biting into it and sucking the sour juice into your mouth. What did you experience as you imagined this? Did you salivate? Did you have any other physical reactions? Guided imagery draws on all the senses: sound, taste, movement, vision, touch, and inner sensation. They work best when integrated thoroughly with the person's entire being. You probably salivated more with the description of the lemon image than you would if you were told simply to imagine salivating.

Guided imagery sessions often use a preexisting scripted process that usually lasts 20–25 minutes and begins with a general relaxation technique that helps to center the mind. A typical format includes identifying the problem, goal, or disease and then incorporating the following (Leddy, 2006):

- The individual finds a comfortable place to recline or sit.
- Extremities are uncrossed and the eyes are closed or focused on one spot or object in the room.
- The person focuses on his or her breath, uses abdominal breathing, and with each breath says "in" and "out."
- The individual may feel the body becoming heavy and warm.

- The images of the problem, goal, or disease are developed, as well as the inner and external (treatment or healing) resources.
- If the thoughts wander, the individual brings the mind back to thinking of his or her breathing and relaxed body.
- The session ends with images of the desired state of well-being.

Effective suggestions for the sessions include the following (Leddy, 2006):

- In your mind, go to a place that feels good and that you enjoy.
- What do you see, feel, taste, hear?
- Take a few deep breaths.
- Imagine yourself the way you want to be (describe the desired goal specifically).
- Imagine the steps you need to take to be how you want to be.
- Practice these steps now in the place where you feel good.
- What is the first thing you will do to help yourself be how you want to be?
- Remember that you can return to this place, this feeling, this way of being whenever you need to.
- When you are ready, you may return to the room we are in.
- You will feel relaxed and refreshed and ready to resume your activities.
- You may open your eyes slowly and tell me about the experience when you are ready.

To facilitate relaxation, individuals can use commercial audiotapes of verbal suggestions, music, sounds of nature, pictures of objects or places, aromas, scented candles or oils, or another person giving suggestions in a soft, pleasant voice to assist in the image formation (Leddy, 2006). Examples of imagery include beaches with waves, a salty sea breeze, warm sand, and the colors of the sunset or lush green meadows with blue skies and puffy clouds. Mountain images, including lakes and flowers, singing birds, and the smell of pine trees or the sound of a stream, are also helpful. For healing, images can include visualizing good monsters eating bad monsters or personifying the immune system's cells as soldiers destroying cancer cells. For self-esteem building, some use the image of a tightly closed flower bud that opens to become a beautiful flower (Leddy, 2006).

Several types of words can help the practitioner during the guided imagery session (Leddy, 2006):

- *Metaphors* imply comparisons. For example, "You feel relaxed, like a warm waterfall."
- *Truisms* are statements that the intellect accepts as accurate. For example, "As you take in your next breath, oxygen is flowing into your lungs and into every cell in your body."

- *Synesthesia* is the combination of several senses simultaneously. For example, "Can you feel the color of the sky?"
- *Linkages* connect certain statements, behaviors, and actions with thoughts. For example, "Once more . . . relax deeply . . . and feel yourself really sinking into the surface of the floor and feel supported by this surface."
- *Mirroring* involves repeating the client's words or descriptions instead of using your own.

Social Support

While we know that stress can affect health, studies in the 1960s and 1970s also showed that social isolation was repeatedly associated with increased risk of mortality and morbidity. Just as an individual's hardiness is an important factor in his or her ability to cope with stress, the strength of the individual's social networks is also crucial (Freeman, 2004; Pelletier, 1993; Spiegel, 1993).

In 2000, Shelly Taylor and her colleagues wanted to explore whether women and men responded differently to stress. They proposed a new theory for the female stress response called *tend and befriend.* The theory asserts that, although both men and women have a built-in dynamic for the survival of physical danger, women also have an inherent nurturing response for offspring as well as a means to befriend others. As a result, they create strong social support systems and are thereby able to cope better with stressful situations. Taylor suggests this characteristic is due to DNA, a combination of brain chemistry and hormones, and generational social factors (Seaward, 2006).

As human beings, we benefit from our social relationships and they challenge our adaptability and health. We strive to connect with others, and the number of contacts we make with others (including friends, acquaintances, and family members) best predicts both our physical and our emotional health. Our social support acts as a buffer or protective layer against the wide variations of transitions we experience during our lives (Pelletier, 1993). Studies show that higher levels of social support correlate with lower levels of cholesterol and improve immune function (Freeman, 2004; Spiegel, 1993). Even having a pet is a form of connection that is important to a person's health (Pelletier, 1993).

Studies have also demonstrated that poor relationships and social support can adversely affect the immune system (Kiecolt-Glaser & Glaser, 1993). People with supportive social networks have better overall health, lower rates of cancer and heart disease, less coronary blockage (as measured by angiograms), shorter hospital stays when they do get sick, and better resistance to infection than those whose social bonds are not as supportive. People who are isolated have higher-than-average rates of many types of illnesses, including arthritis, hypertension, heart disease, viral infections, cancer, and tuberculosis (Pelletier, 1993; Scheiber, 2008). In the first study of its kind, University of California, Los Angeles researchers found that feelings of isolation are linked to alterations in the activity of genes that drive inflammation (one of the body's first immune responses). What mattered was not the size of the person's network but how many people the individual felt close to over time (Scheiber, 2008).

In other studies, women with cancer who had minimal social contact were 2.2 times more likely to die of cancer over a 17-year period than the most socially connected individuals. Having a spouse tripled the chances that a person with coronary artery disease would be alive 5 years later. Married people live longer on average than those who are single, widowed, divorced, or never married (Spiegel, 1993).

Why is this so? One theory holds that social support leads to physical consequences by influencing behavior since people who believe that others care about them are more likely to take the basic steps needed to stay healthy. Social support also helps people avoid bad habits (Williams, 1993). Friends and a wide social network may also shield the body from the consequences of stress. Women with breast cancer who attended support groups survived for an average of 18 months longer than those who did not attend. Support groups provide social support, a place for emotional ventilation, and education. They also help people change their perspectives on their situation and their responses to it (cognitive restructuring) (Spiegel, 1993).

Art Therapy

Nearly everyone has found themselves doodling while talking on the phone, keeping a personal journal, or painting or sculpting as a hobby. As people do these things, they find that their feelings and ideas change and they may even feel themselves transported away from their everyday problems. Involvement with art can alter feelings, clear the mind, and raise consciousness. Involvement with art is, indeed, a therapeutic process (Lippin & Micozzi, 2006).

The ability of the arts to enhance health has been known since the beginning of time. Early, preliterate human beings naturally embodied feelings, attitudes, and thoughts in symbols. Many anthropologists believe that singing and dancing preceded verbal exchanges in humans. The ancient Greeks recognized the connection between healing and the arts through their use of aesthetics in buildings, healing gardens, and temples, where the arts played a predominant role in healing (Lippin & Micozzi, 2006). Florence Nightingale, an advocate for aesthetics, healing, and recovery, talked about the importance of beautiful objects of all colors and their effect on recovery.

At the turn of the 20th century, art therapy as one aspect of the creative arts movement came into being as a therapy in its own right. Sigmund Freud and Carl Jung engaged several of their clients in drawing to better understand their psychological disorders. Margaret Naumburg, in association with Dr. Nolan Lewis, conducted research on children with troublesome behaviors at the New York State Psychiatric Unit. Art therapy emerged as its own discipline in the 1960s when specialists became trained and certified in the theoretical basis and application of art.

The 21st century has already seen a dramatic increase in attempts to inject variety into healing environments in the form of color, design, and art and in the use of music, movement, and healing gardens. Healthcare providers now realize that interventions need to take place at the level of the spirit as well as the level of the body and the cell (Donnelly, 2007).

All across the United States, the therapeutic aspect of art is gaining recognition. In cooperation with The Joint Commission and the Americans for the Arts, the Society for Arts in Healthcare (SAH) completed a survey that found 2,500 hospitals using the arts to create healing environments, support client mental health and emotional recovery, and develop positive working environments (Knutson, 2006). The hospital arts movement continues to grow through architectural design, interior design, and the placement of fine art in strategic healthcare setting locations such as lobbies, waiting rooms, client rooms, and high-tech intervention areas (Lippin & Micozzi, 2006).

What Is Art Therapy?

Established in 1969, the American Art Therapy Association describes *art therapy* as the use of art in a creative process, providing the opportunity for nonverbal expression and communication and fostering self-awareness and personal growth. Art therapy initiates a strengthened partnership between the nonverbal, artistic, spatial right-brain function and the more analytical, logical, and verbal left-brain function, and it serves to balance and integrate these two cognitive functions (Seaward, 2006).

During the 1900s, psychologists explored the unconscious and found that the creative process can play an important role in revealing and healing health issues. Shealy (1996) notes that "emotions are experienced—without the filter of words—in the body itself, and emotional memories are encoded and stored there. The psychotherapeutic use of the creative arts enables us to connect with the material directly, and give nonverbal expression to what is driving or crippling us" (p. 110).

The field of *expressive arts* is based on the belief that each person has worth, dignity, and the capacity for creative self-direction (Cantwell, 2006). Art therapy is based on the premise that many thoughts, feelings, and insights cannot be expressed verbally because several abstract constructs of the mind lack the necessary vocabulary to describe the focus, intensity, and understanding of encounters that the mind tries to process and grasp (Seaward, 2006). Creative arts allow that to happen. As Donnelly (2007) explains, "The arts distinguish us among species and make us uniquely human" (p. 165). When we use art as a technique that allows inner knowing to explore freely, we create a balance between our inner and outer paradigms (Wetzel, 2006). Engaging in the arts is life affirming and life enhancing (Lippin & Micozzi, 2006).

In *active, creative art therapy,* the client engages in the creative process. Lippin and Micozzi (2006) explain that this creative process enhances an individual's life force "through classic biophysiological responses such as movement, relaxation, and emotional catharsis, as well as through self-discovery and awareness; increased self-esteem, pleasure, hope, and optimism; and the achievement of transcendence . . . Perhaps most important, the creation of beauty itself is a profound and powerful source of health and well-being" (p. 332).

Passive exposure to the arts, including music, dance, painting, sculpture, poetry, and drama, has also been shown to have healing properties. Passive exposure provides a means of imaginative expression that circumvents the blocks between the conscious and unconscious mind (Shealy, 1996).

Benefits of Art Therapy

Art therapy has been shown to improve relaxation and help participants be more aware of physical and emotional issues (Repar & Patton, 2007). One of the greatest impacts of art could be the potential to synthesize and integrate issues such as pain, loss, and death (Lippin & Micozzi, 2006). Ultimately, clients find their way to a deeper understanding of their own issues. Many people find that the spontaneous, uncensored nature of art therapy provides a powerful, healing, and revealing therapeutic release (Kim, 2006; Nieves, 2006; Shealy, 1996). Because it works on a nonverbal level, art therapy is an excellent form of therapy and relaxation for individuals whose traumas are buried too deep for words or for children who do not have the words to describe their distress.

Art therapy has been shown to have a number of other effects:

- It decreases perceived pain, reduces the amount of pain medication needed, decreases anxiety levels, and lowers blood pressure, heart rate, and respiratory rates (Kim, 2006; Nieves, 2006; Shealy, 1996).

- Use of the arts leads to self-knowledge, self-discovery, mood change, and emotional catharsis (e.g., weeping, laughing, sexual activity) that can induce pleasure and relaxation.
- Drawing can serve as a bridge between the healthcare provider and the client, family, and surrounding world. It can increase pleasure, motivation, and learning, and ultimately influence behaviors. It can provide a sense of hope and optimism that has been linked to positive effects on the immune system (Lippin & Micozzi, 2006).
- Art therapy can also provide a means of reducing guilt, facilitating impulse control, and strengthening the ego through discovery of personal and growth interests (Seaward, 2006).

Types of Art Therapy

Drawing, painting, craftwork, and model making are all forms of art therapy that have been utilized. There is no formula to determine which techniques are best to use. The decision can be based on the healthcare provider's experience or the individual's preference (Cantwell, 2006). Clients may draw parts of their bodies that unconsciously concern them or they may draw something they have been unable to verbalize. The goal is not to produce a skillful finished work of art but to follow spontaneous impulses as they utilize form, lines, colors, and textures. Realizing that there is no right or wrong form of expression, because it comes directly from the person, supports the goal of having clients engage in art without fearing shame, ridicule, derision, or embarrassment so they can cast off their "inner critic" (Lippin & Micozzi, 2006).

Some have suggested that the colors an individual selects in art therapy have associated meanings: red (passionate emotional peaks), orange (life change), yellow (energy), blue and green (happiness and joy), purple (highly spiritual nature), brown (stability), black (grief or personal empowerment), and gray (ambiguity) (Seaward, 2006).

Art Therapy Settings

Art therapy, primarily drawing and illustrations, has been used in many types of settings, including drug rehabilitation centers, eating disorder clinics, veterans' hospitals, prisons, oncology units, and clinics for the emotionally disturbed (Seaward, 2006). While art therapy can be applied to most client populations, several specific populations may receive special value from its application.

- Pediatric clients are often more freely expressive and engage in play more easily than adult clients.

- Geriatric clients who are especially vulnerable to pharmaceutical and surgical interventions can use art therapy as a supplement or complementary therapy.
- Sufferers of certain central nervous system disorders, such as Alzheimer's disease, may benefit from the creative process of art therapy.
- AIDS clients and their families have found art therapy (e.g., the quilt project) to be extremely helpful in dealing with the losses associated with this disease.
- Health professionals can use art therapy to cope with the physical and psychological stressors of their profession.
- Individuals with chronic diseases and chronic pain find that art therapy provides hope, pleasure, and beauty and improves their quality of life.
- Dying clients often use art therapy to resolve lifelong psychological and spiritual issues, express conflict and desires, address their pain, and leave their loved ones with something of value (Lippin & Micozzi, 2006).

The Future of Art Therapy

Advances in neuroscience, psychoneuroimmunology, and psychoneurocardiology have provided some important tools to support solid research on creative arts therapy. Research issues for the future could (Lippin & Micozzi, 2006):

- Evaluate the impact of aesthetic stimuli (such as color, form, sound, rhythm, words, and beauty itself) on human physiology
- Examine how the human brain perceives, processes, integrates, and reacts to aesthetic stimuli
- Explore the neurophysiological nature of creativity and its relationship to human health
- Evaluate how arts contribute to the development of self and cultural self-esteem as well as individual mental health and brain development
- Determine which steps must be taken to ensure that arts medicine topics are included in formal medical and nursing curricula.

Journaling

For centuries, people have kept personal records or logs of important information about everything from lunar eclipses, famines, and changes in world leaders to personal information about the trials and tribulations of life in many different settings. Originating from the French word *journée*, meaning "from sunrise to sunset," journals began as a means of guidance on long trips or as a way to orient the traveler home. Journalists have long described events, and explorers such as Christopher Columbus, Meriwether Lewis and William Clark, and Admiral Robert Peary all kept diaries (Seaward, 2006).

Today, U.S. presidents and space shuttle astronauts keep daily journals (Seaward, 2006). Many of us wrote in diaries as adolescents, when we may have written about mundane thoughts or deeply moving events. As we transitioned to adulthood, we may have left the diary behind but still kept to-do lists, appointment books, notes on calendars, or perhaps boxes of poems, short notes, ideas for another day, and lists of goals or dreams. Even these abbreviated entries provide sketches of our lives (Rew, 2005).

Journaling is a creative, fulfilling, insightful, and therapeutic exercise (Freeman, 2004). Rew (2005) writes that "diaries, journals, logs, reviews, stories, and letters help us keep track of and enhance the pattern of our lives" (p. 427). Weil (2005) adds that "journaling, or expressive writing, is a simple, gentle, and inexpensive healing technique" (p. 6). Rakel (2007) notes that journaling is "the process of writing about times in our lives that are stressful or traumatic" (p. 1043). Seaward (2006) defines therapeutic journaling as "a series of written passages that document the personal events, thoughts, feelings, memories, and perceptions in one's journey throughout life leading to wholeness" (p. 231).

By writing about an experience, we help make it our own, we explore its meaning, and we ultimately experience the way we can release it (Rew, 2005). Journaling can be termed a *transpsychological experience;* that is, an experience that describes the therapeutic effects of self-discovery through active awareness, allowing the individual to access personal resources and promoting wholeness (Seaward, 2006).

Benefits of Journaling

Journaling has been found to improve physical health, enhance the immune system, improve lung function in asthmatics, improve wound healing and memory function, and result in fewer visits to medical practitioners. It can relieve stress and improve relaxation, lessen fatigue and pain, reduce high blood pressure, and improve sleep (Rakel, 2007; Weil, 2005). In studies of students who kept journals in which they wrote about traumatic or disturbing events, the students had better immune system function and fewer visits to the university's health clinic than those who did not keep journals (Kiecolt-Glaser & Glaser, 1993).

Although Seaward (2006) states that "confessions of the mind lighten the burden of the soul" (p. 231), in some instances disclosure may not improve mental health. When the mind suppresses something traumatic, it often does so for a reason, and uncovering the events can be difficult for the conscious mind to handle. In these situations, working with a licensed therapist is important because the timing of disclosure can be crucial (Rakel, 2007).

Interestingly, in an attempt to understand the pathophysiology behind "the clinical effects of disclosure," James Pennebaker interviewed polygraphers (lie detector operators) who worked for the Federal Bureau of Investigation and the Central Intelligence Agency (Rakel, 2007). Pennebaker learned that polygraphers look for changes (particularly reductions) in heart rate, blood pressure, respiratory rate, and skin conductance when people confess. These drops in responses also occur when people relax. Polygraphers believe that people have to work to inhibit their thoughts, behaviors, and feelings and that this work, over time, causes stress that can lead to immune suppression and disease. That assumption may help explain why journaling (a form of disclosure) can reduce stress and support immune function.

Journaling provides an opportunity to take repressed thoughts from the unconscious to the conscious level, allowing the individual to control and organize his or her thoughts and, by transferring the thoughts to paper, to avoid low-grade stress. Since most people naturally have an inability to fully express the entire range of human emotions, journaling provides an opportunity to experience an emotional catharsis by releasing toxic thoughts (Seaward, 2006). A striking example of this can be seen from a review of the online journal entries made before and after the World Trade Center destruction in New York City on September 11, 2001. There were fewer visits to healthcare professionals after the event; one reason is believed to be that the event opened people up and stimulated communication and a sense of "we" versus "I," bringing the community together and reducing social isolation (Rakel, 2007).

Journaling should not replace medical treatment but it is effective in working through issues that might otherwise stay hidden or suppressed. Deep-seated emotional issues may surface and cause sadness but, over time, the process of writing down thoughts and insights makes people feel calmer, happier, and more accepting of themselves. Journaling helps individuals look inward, in private, and hopefully gain new insights to solve problems (Weil, 2005).

Tips for Successful Journaling

Journaling does not require much time, equipment, or training and it can be done anytime and anywhere. According to Seaward (2006), the only requirements are:

- A notebook dedicated solely to the journal writing
- A writing implement (pen or pencil)
- A quiet, private, undisturbed environment where you can collect your thoughts

Before you begin to write, center yourself by taking a moment to relax and connect to the here and now. Sometimes soft music can help you center and create a conducive environment in which to write. Then:

- Label your journal entries with the month, day, and year to track any patterns or tendencies. Writing each entry should take about 20 minutes.
- Begin by writing about something difficult or troubling in your life, either past or present; describe how you feel about the event; and reflect on how it affects you physically and mentally. Choose something that you have not shared at length with anyone else.
- Honesty and openness about feelings are essential. Describe the event in detail including the situation, surroundings, and sensations you remember. You may use a prescribed format or simply let the thoughts stream.
- Describe your deepest feelings about the event and let you emotions run freely in your writing. Be spontaneous, write continuously, and don't censor your writing.
- Don't be concerned about grammar, punctuation, sentence structure, spelling, or neatness. Just let the thoughts flow, since these pages are for your eyes only.
- Keep your journal private. Sharing it might compromise your vow of honesty.
- Include descriptions of both stressful events and positive experiences.
- Include artwork, drawings, poems, or prayers if you wish.

At the end of the session, try to reflect on what you have learned or how you have grown from the event. Try journaling for at least 3–4 days in a row, writing about either the same experience or a different one. You can journal regularly or as needed (Freeman, 2004; Rakel, 2007; Seaward, 2006; Weil, 2005).

Adleman (2006, p. 15) suggests using the following affirmations when journaling:

- It is safe for me to write about my feelings.
- I easily express my feelings through my writings.
- I am writing my way to increased health.
- I gain valuable insights through my writing.
- I am healing from within through writing.
- Writing is an empowering process.

Healthcare providers do not need to read what their clients write; the therapeutic benefit comes from the expression of the emotions themselves. Healthcare practitioners need to avoid creating guilt when helping individuals explore past experiences. If they do evaluate writings, they should be aware of certain journaling characteristics that reflect a shift toward a healthier outlook (Rakel, 2007):

- An evolving story that has a beginning, middle, and end
- The development of insight in the client's writings and the use of words such as *understand* and *realize*
- The demonstration of optimism through the use of positive words
- A change in pronouns, as the writing progresses, from first person to second person (reflecting the writer's connection to others)

KEY CONCEPTS

1. Stress is the inability to cope with a perceived (real or imagined) threat to one's mental, physical, emotional, and spiritual well-being, resulting in a series of physiological responses and adaptations.
2. People react to their environments, and the brain signals the rest of the body through the nervous, endocrine, and immune systems.
3. There are many holistic stress management techniques including self-awareness, cognitive restructuring, effective communication, guided imagery, social support, art therapy, and journaling.

QUESTIONS FOR REFLECTION

1. How does stress affect the body physiologically?
2. How does stress affect the individual?
3. How do self-awareness, cognitive restructuring, guided imagery, art therapy, and journaling impact an individual's ability to manage stress?

REFERENCES

Adleman, C. S. (2006, Spring). A write choice for stroke recovery. *AHNA Beginnings, 26*(3), 14–15.

Bartol, G. M., & Courts, N. F. (2005). The psychophysiology of bodymind healing. In B. M. Dossey, L. Keegan, & C. E. Guzzetta, *Holistic nursing: A handbook for practice* (4th ed., pp. 111–133). Sudbury, MA: Jones and Bartlett.

Cantwell, J. (2006, Spring). Expressive arts in a hospice setting. *AHNA Beginnings, 26*(3), 18–20.

Donnelly, G. F. (2007). From the editor. The arts in healthcare: Healing through creativity. *Holistic Nursing Practice, 21*(4), 165.

Eliopoulos, C. (2004). *Invitation to holistic health: A guide to living a balanced life.* Sudbury, MA: Jones and Bartlett.

Evans, E. (1996). Communication skills and counseling. In D. F. Rankin-Box (Ed.), *The nurses' handbook of complementary therapies* (pp. 75–81). Edinburgh: Churchill Livingstone.

Freeman, L. (2004). *Mosby's complementary and alternative medicine: A research-based approach* (2nd ed.). St. Louis, MO: Mosby.

Kiecolt-Glaser, J. K., & Glaser, R. (1993). Mind and immunity. In D. Goleman & J. Gurin (Eds.), *Mind-body medicine: How to use your mind for better health* (pp. 39–61). Yonkers, NY: Consumer Reports Books.

Kim, K. J. (2006, Spring). Diversity in art expression. *AHNA Beginnings, 26*(3), 10–11.

Knutson, L. (2006). Bringing art into a healthcare facility. *AHNA Beginnings, 26*(3), 24.

Leddy, S. K. (2006). *Integrative health promotion: Conceptual bases for nursing practice* (2nd ed.). Sudbury, MA: Jones and Bartlett.

Levy, E. M. (2002). Psychophysiology of mind-body healing. In M. A. Bright, *Holistic health and healing* (pp. 55–69). Philadelphia: F. A. Davis.

Lippin, R. A., & Micozzi, M. S. (2006). Arts therapy. In M. S. Micozzi, *Fundamentals of complementary and integrative medicine* (pp. 332–350). St. Louis, MO: Saunders Elsevier.

Nieves, C. (2006, Spring). Using art to help hospital patients. *AHNA Beginnings, 26*(3), 12.

Payne, R. A. (2005). *Relaxation techniques: A practical handbook for the health care professional* (3rd ed.). Edinburgh: Churchill Livingstone.

Pelletier, K. R. (1993). Between mind and body: Stress, emotions, and health. In D. Goleman & J. Gurin (Eds.), *Mind-body medicine: How to use your mind for better health* (pp. 19–38). Yonkers, NY: Consumer Reports Books.

Rakel, D. (2007). Journaling. In D. Rakel, *Integrative medicine* (2nd ed., pp. 1039–1043). Philadelphia: Saunders Elsevier.

Repar, P. A., & Patton, D. (2007). Stress reduction for nurses through arts-in-medicine at the University of New Mexico Hospitals. *Holistic Nursing Practice, 21*(4), 182–186.

Rew, L. (2005). Self-reflection: Consulting the truth within. In B. M. Dossey, L. Keegan, & C. E. Guzzetta, *Holistic nursing: A handbook for practice* (4th ed., pp. 429–447). Sudbury, MA: Jones and Bartlett.

Schaub, B. G., & Dossey, B. M. (2005). Imagery: Awakening the inner healer. In B. M. Dossey, L. Keegan, & C. E. Guzzetta, *Holistic nursing: A handbook for practice* (4th ed., pp. 567–613). Sudbury, MA: Jones and Bartlett.

Scheiber, C. S. (2008, March/April). Loneliness connects to genes for immune support. *Spirituality and Health, 11*(2), 27.

Seaward, B. L. (2006). *Managing stress: Principles and strategies for health and well-being* (5th ed.). Sudbury, MA: Jones and Bartlett.

Shealy, C. N. (Ed.). (1996). *The complete family guide to alternative medicine: An illustrated encyclopedia of natural healing.* Shaftesbury, Dorset, UK: Element Books.

Smith, N. (2006, November). Stress less. *Real Simple*, 285–289.

Spiegel, D. (1993). Social support: How friends, family, and groups can help. In D. Goleman & J. Gurin (Eds.), *Mind-body medicine: How to use your mind for better health* (pp. 331–349). Yonkers, NY: Consumer Reports Books.

Trivieri, L., Jr., & Anderson, J. W. (Eds.). (2002). *Alternative medicine: The definitive guide.* Berkeley, CA: Celestial Arts.

Weil, A. (2005, September). Journaling: Self-healing through writing. *Dr. Andrew Weil's Self-Healing*, 6.

Wetzel, W. (2006, Spring). You gotta have art! *AHNA Beginnings, 26*(3), 4.

Williams, R. B. (1993). Hostility and the heart. In D. Goleman & J. Gurin (Eds.), *Mind-body medicine: How to use your mind for better health* (pp. 65–83). Yonkers, NY: Consumer Reports Books.

Zahourek, R. P. (2002). Imagery. In M. A. Bright, *Holistic health and healing* (p. 113–120). Philadelphia: F. A. Davis.

CHAPTER 2

Health and the Human Spirit

Just as a person casts off worn-out clothes and puts on new ones, so also the embodied Self casts off worn-out bodies and enters others which are new.

—Bhagavad Gita

LEARNING OBJECTIVES

1. Discuss theories of spirituality.
2. Examine the connection between spirituality and health.
3. Describe the spiritually healing processes of mystery, love, suffering, hope, forgiveness, peacemaking, and grace.
4. Identify areas of research on spirituality, religion, and health.
5. Describe various spiritual rituals.
6. Discuss spirituality and the aging population.
7. List and describe six spiritual areas of interest within the healthcare system.
8. Describe the role of spiritual care providers in administering spiritual care.
9. Explain the elements of a spiritual assessment and healing interventions.

INTRODUCTION

All people are spiritual and, by virtue of being human, all people, regardless of age, are bio-psycho-social-spiritual beings. Widespread evidence shows that the interest in spirituality is not confined to individuals who attend church or who are identified as being religious (Shea, 2000). Spirituality is an integral part of the health and well-being of every individual.

According to DeLaune and Ladner (2006), people throughout history have dealt with pain, illness, and healing in spiritual ways. In many primitive cultures, a single person simultaneously held the positions of priest, psychiatrist, and physician. Freeman (2004) notes that "the first practices of spiritual healing were performed during the stone age by shamanic priest-doctors.

Healing practices were also recorded in ancient Egypt and in the early Jewish and Christian traditions" (p. 519).

Today many Americans believe their spirituality helps promote healing, especially when medications and other treatments cannot provide a cure for their conditions. Micozzi (2006) notes that "the blending of spirituality with the tenets of alternative, complementary, and integrative therapies provides individuals with a means of understanding how they contribute to the creation of their illness and to their healing" (p. 305). As the information age gives way to the intuition age, healthcare professionals will need to focus less on logical, linear, mechanical thinking and more on creative, lateral, and emotional thinking (Reynolds, 2001). Larry Dossey predicts that "we're going to see an integration of physical and spiritual interventions in healing, not a replacement of one by the other" (Freeman, 2004, p. 546). Kligler and Lee (2004) note that "integrative medicine is renewing the soul of medicine by combining advances of science and technology in Western medical training with the whole person approach of traditional healing systems" (p. xix).

The field of integrative health care calls for healthcare professionals to promote an environment in which the spiritual beliefs of the individual, family, and community are respected. This shift in focus means that the provision of care will encompass a more holistic perspective—one that attends to all aspects of mind, body, and spirit. A holistic foundation means that healthcare providers will assess and respond to each client's physical, emotional, mental, and spiritual dimensions.

Healthcare professionals are entrusted with the holistic care of their clients. This means nurses and other healthcare providers care for the soul and spirit as well as for the body. By caring for individuals in a way that acknowledges the mind-body-spirit connection, healthcare providers acknowledge the whole person. Spiritual care is a part of holistic care (DeLaune & Ladner, 2006).

No discussion of spirituality would be complete without referring to the concept of a supreme being or intelligent force. This being is known throughout the world by many different names, including God, Goddess, Allah, Higher Power, Universal Intelligence, Spirit, the Absolute, and Source. In using some of these names throughout this chapter, we mean no disrespect to anyone and sincerely hope none is taken.

SPIRITUALITY DEFINED

The term *spirituality* is derived from the Latin *spiritus*, meaning "breath" and related to the Greek *pneuma* ("breath"), which refers to the vital spirit or soul. Benor (2006) defines the word *spiritual* as "transpersonal awarenesses arising spontaneously or through meditative and other practices, beyond ordinary explanations, and to which are attributed an inspiring and guiding meaningfulness, often attributed to a Deity" (p. 467).

Clearly, although there is no one definition of spirituality, descriptions of its characteristics abound in the literature. Burkhardt (2007) states that "trying to define spirituality is akin to trying to lasso the wind. The wind is sensed and felt, and its effect on us and things around us is seen, but it cannot be contained within imposed boundaries, or even the best definitions" (p. 263). The following list demonstrates the range of definitions (Burkhardt & Nagai-Jacobson, 2005; Daniels, Nosek, & Nicoll, 2007; DeLaune & Ladner, 2006; Seaward, 2006; Sorajjakool & Lamberton, 2004; Stanley & Beare, 1995; Weil, 1997):

- Spirituality means believing in a power operating in the universe greater than oneself; it involves a sense of interconnectedness with all living creatures and an awareness of the purpose and meaning of life.
- Spirituality is a personal, individualized set of beliefs and practices that are not church related.
- Spirituality includes aspects of higher consciousness, transcendence, self-reliance, self-efficacy, love, faith, enlightenment, mysticism, self-assertiveness, community, and bonding as well as a supreme being or supreme intelligence that may be referred to as God, Allah, Jesus, Buddha, or otherwise.
- Spirituality is a two-dimensional concept with both vertical and horizontal dimensions. The vertical represents a relationship with a supreme being and the horizontal represents relationships with others.
- The term *spiritual* refers to the transcendental relationship between the person and a higher being, a quality that goes beyond a specific religious affiliation.
- Spirituality is a unifying force, providing meaning in life and consisting of individual values, perceptions, and faith as well as being a common bond among individuals.
- Spirituality involves the nonphysical, immaterial aspects of an individual's being—with energies, essences, and the parts that will exist after the body disintegrates. The whole picture of health involves physical, mental, and spiritual components. Whether religious or not, a person can lead a spiritual life and explore the influence of spirituality on health.
- Spirituality is the animation force, life principle, or essence of being that permeates life and is expressed and experienced in multifaceted connections with self, others, nature, and a supreme being. Shaped by cultural experiences, spirituality is a universal human experience.
- Spirituality is the essence of who people are and how they are in the world and, like breathing, is essential to human existence.

While no one has been able to provide a universally accepted definition of spirituality, theorists and researchers agree that it is a multidimensional phenomenon. It is *not* the same as religion, which is a set of beliefs and practices associated with a particular church, synagogue, mosque, or other formal organized group (DeLaune & Ladner, 2006). Spirituality is simply *being* and it impacts everything people say, think, and do (Eliopoulos, 2004).

Humans are mind-body-spirit beings by nature, and all people are spiritual beings. Spiritual healer Rosemary Altea (2006) explains that, as spiritual beings having a human experience, each of us comes into this world with breathtaking gifts such as the power of intuition, the power to sense the invisible world around us, or the power to create healing energy.

THEORIES OF SPIRITUALITY

Spirituality is reflected in everyday life as well as in disciplines ranging from philosophy and popular literature to psychotherapy, health psychology, medicine, nursing, sociology, and science (Chandler, 1999; Hatch, Burg, Naberhaus, & Hellmich, 1998; Mahoney & Graci, 1999; Tuck, Wallace, & Pullen, 2001). The theories presented in this section are a sample of some of the theories in use today, and they include concepts from theology, psychology, sociology, medicine, and nursing.

Theories from Theology, Psychology, and Sociology

Theology describes spirituality as one's belief in God, which is expressed through religious beliefs and practices.

In *psychology*, spirituality is explained as an expression of one's internal motives and desires, concentrating on the self instead of on a supreme intelligence. Psychology examines one's spiritual search for meaning, purpose, and guidance.

Sociology examines the concept of spirituality by studying groups of people. According to sociology, people strongly influence other people, who are in turn influenced by the groups in which they live. Sociology describes spirituality as the spiritual practices and rituals of groups of people as well as the social morality within personal relationships (Meraviglia, 1999).

Medical Theories

Contemporary medicine has historically given little attention to the spiritual dimension, despite its importance in the fundamental goal of healing.

Now, however, medicine focuses increased attention on exploring the relationship between clients' spiritual needs and the more traditional aspects of their medical care. Medical schools have begun offering courses in spirituality, religion, and health, with many schools receiving grants from the National Institute for Healthcare Research to develop curricula in spirituality and medicine (Freeman, 2004; Hiatt, 1986; Kligler & Lee, 2004; Koenig et al., 1999).

Trends that appear to be driving this new interest in spirituality include the many studies that have demonstrated a strong connection between spirituality and improved health, client demand for greater personal attention from their physicians, the growing importance of end-of-life care, and the increasing dissatisfaction among physicians with what they view as an increasingly depersonalized practice (Eliopoulos, 2004; Freeman, 2004; Kligler & Lee, 2004; Micozzi, 2006).

Nursing Theories

Nursing incorporates all the perspectives of theology, psychology, sociology, and medicine while also examining spirituality quantitatively from other perspectives, including spiritual health, spiritual well-being, spiritual perspective, self-transcendence, faith, quality of life, hope, religiousness, purpose in life, and spiritual coping (Meraviglia, 1999). Traditionally, nursing has always been concerned with the health care of the whole person, including the physical, psychological, social, cultural, environmental, and spiritual dimensions (Bergquist & King, 1994; Martsolf & Mickley, 1998). Nursing theoretical models in which spirituality is a major concept include Betty Neuman's Neuman systems model, Margaret Newman's theory of health, Rosemary Parse's theory of human becoming, and Jean Watson's theory of human caring.

Betty Neuman's Neuman Systems Model

This model focuses on the wellness of clients in relationship to environmental stressors and their reactions to stressors. Neuman describes the client/client system as a total system in interaction with the internal and external environments. The entire client system contains five variables: physiological, psychological, sociocultural, developmental, and spiritual. Each of these variables is a subset of all parts, which forms the whole of the client. Neuman and Fawcett (2002) write:

> The philosophic base of the Neuman Systems Model encompasses wholism, a wellness orientation, client perception and motivation, and a dynamic systems perspective of energy and variable interaction with the environment to mitigate possible harm from internal and external stressors, while caregivers and clients

> form a partnership relationship to negotiate desired outcome goals for optimal health retention, restoration, and maintenance. This philosophic base pervades all aspects of the model. (p. 12)

To address the wholeness concept of care, practitioners must consider all five variables. Several authors have expanded Neuman's model to include issues related to spiritual well-being, spiritual needs, spiritual care, and spiritual distress.

Margaret Newman's Theory of Health

Newman's theory built upon Martha Rogers' idea of humans as energy fields, expanding it to view humans as unique patterns of consciousness. Newman (1994) states that "the person does not possess consciousness—the person is consciousness" (p. 33). Her theory defines *consciousness* as the capacity of the system to interact with the environment, and she posits that the process of life involves movement toward higher levels of consciousness. The dimensions of person-environment interaction include exchanging, communicating, relating, valuing, choosing, moving, perceiving, feeling, and knowing. Newman describes expanded consciousness as a general spiritual term (Martsolf & Mickley, 1998; Newman, 1994).

Rosemary Parse's Human Becoming Theory

Rosemary Parse developed the human becoming theory to move nursing's view of the person from the medical model to a human science perspective (Martsolf & Mickley, 1998; Parse, 1999). According to Parse (1999), "This theory posits that humans live at multidimensional realms of the universe all-at-once as they prereflectively and reflectively choose from options incarnating imaged value priorities" (p. 8). Frisch (2005) describes the various aspects of Parse's theory in the following way: "*Person* is a unified, whole being. *Health* is a process of becoming; it is a personal commitment, an unfolding, a process related to lived experiences. *Environment* is the universe. The human-universe is inseparable and evolving as one" (p. 85).

Jean Watson's Theory of Human Caring

Jean Watson's theory is based on a spiritual-existential and phenomenological orientation that draws on Eastern philosophies. Focusing on nurse–client interactions and asserting that humans are energy fields with patterns of consciousness, this theory acknowledges the spiritual dimension of people. In Watson's theory, caring is considered the essence of nursing practice and requires the nurse to be personally, morally, and spiritually engaged. The one caring and the one being cared for are considered co-participants in self-healing; they each have the power to heal themselves (Falk-Rafael, 2000; Martsolf & Mickley, 1998; Saewyc, 2000; Watson, 2005).

According to Watson (2005), the original 10 "carative" factors identified in her 1985 book, *Nursing: The Philosophy and Science of Caring,* are still a guiding philosophical-ethical practice model. They are:

1. The formation of a humanistic-altruistic system of values
2. The instillation of faith-hope
3. The cultivation of sensitivity to one's self and to others
4. The development of a helping-trusting relationship
5. The promotion and acceptance of the expression of positive and negative feelings
6. The systematic use of scientific problem-solving methods for decision making
7. The promotion of interpersonal teaching-learning (later refined to read as transpersonal teaching-learning)
8. The provision of a supportive, protective, and/or corrective mental, physical, sociocultural, and spiritual environment
9. Assistance with the gratification of human need
10. Allowance for existential-phenomenological dimensions

Achieving Theoretical Unity

Achieving theoretical unity requires consistency and universality in both the terminology and the language used to describe the spiritual dimension (McSherry & Draper, 1998). The challenge for health care and spiritual care providers is to agree on such a universal theory. A universal, inclusive definition of the spiritual dimension that reflects the unique nature of all individuals will provide a basis for research and enable a more careful study of spirituality (Young & Koopsen, 2005).

SPIRITUALITY AND THE HEALING PROCESS

Spirituality plays an important role in health and healing. *Healing* occurs when we help others and ourselves, when we seek harmony and balance, and when we assess what we have forgotten about connectedness, unity, and interdependence (Dossey, Keegan, & Guzzetta, 2005). In fact, the words *healing, whole,* and *holy* are derived from the same root: the Old Saxon *hal,* meaning "whole."

Healing is a spiritual process that attends to the wholeness of a person: mind, body, and spirit (Burkhardt & Nagai-Jacobson, 2005). L. Dossey (2002) describes "spiritual" as having a sense of connectedness with a source in the universe that is infinite in space and time and both wiser and more powerful than the individual sense of self; Dossey further indicates that healing is the restoration of a sense of wholeness.

The spiritual dimension of each person is a component in the healing process. However, as Lemmer (2005) notes, "One of the greatest challenges in dealing with the spiritual dimension of the human person is that the spirit is not a concrete, objective reality" (p. 311).

Aspects of the Spiritual Dimension

According to Burkhardt and Nagai-Jacobson (2005), inherent in the spiritual domain are the following eight aspects: mystery, love, suffering, hope, forgiveness, grace, peacemaking, and prayer. The first seven are discussed in the following paragraphs (prayer is discussed later in the chapter).

1. *Mystery:* Mystery is a part of life and a part of spirituality. Mystery goes beyond understanding and explanation. Part of an individual's spiritual journey involves accepting mystery and finding a tolerable comfort level with it (Burkhardt & Nagai-Jacobson, 2005). Spirituality reassures people as they encounter troubling and unexplainable experiences, and it helps them survive the unknown.
2. *Love:* Love fuels spirituality and prompts people to live from the heart. Love includes dimensions of self-love, divine love, love for others, and love for all of life. Love includes such qualities as kindness, warmth, understanding, generosity, and tenderness. Maintaining a loving presence is an important component of spiritual care. Love is how individuals can reach out to, heal, and connect with one another. Love often underlies acts of courage and compassion that cannot be otherwise explained (Burkhardt & Nagai-Jacobson, 2005).
3. *Suffering:* Suffering occurs on physical, mental, emotional, and spiritual levels and is one of life's unexplainable elements. Attempts to understand the concept of suffering have shaped virtually all cultural and religious traditions. For some people, suffering enhances their spiritual awareness, while for others suffering appears meaningless and causes feelings of anger and frustration. Sociocultural, religious, familial, and environmental factors influence an individual's response to suffering. A knowledge of personality, culture, religious traditions, and family background may assist the healthcare professional in understanding the nature and meaning of suffering for a particular person (Burkhardt & Nagai-Jacobson, 2005).

4. *Hope:* Hope is future oriented and goes beyond believing and wishing. There are two levels of hope: specific hope and general hope. Specific hope implies a goal or desire for a particular event or outcome. General hope includes a sense that the future is somehow safe. A significant factor in overcoming illness and in living through difficult situations, hope helps people deal with fear and uncertainty and helps them envision a positive outcome (Burkhardt & Nagai-Jacobson, 2005).
5. *Forgiveness:* Religious beliefs, cultural traditions, family upbringing, and personal experiences all contribute to shaping a person's attitudes about forgiveness. A belief in God, Spirit, or a supreme intelligence may also influence one's ability to offer and receive forgiveness. Being able to release the need to berate or punish oneself for past actions is an important part of forgiveness (Burkhardt & Nagai-Jacobson, 2005).
6. *Grace:* Grace is a blessing that comes into one's life unearned. It is often thought of as a gift from God, or from life itself, and it enables, assists, and empowers a person in the midst of a difficult or overwhelming circumstance (Burkhardt & Nagai-Jacobson, 2005).
7. *Peacemaking:* Having inner peace is a way of being. It is independent of external forces. Being a peacemaker in today's world is a spiritual challenge. As persons appreciate and live in the reality of their connection with others and with all creation across distance, time, and space, the possibility of peace grows (Burkhardt & Nagai-Jacobson, 2005).

People are taken to the deepest places in their beings when spiritual or core life issues occur. Not quantifiable and usually expressed as questions or as great mysteries, these issues challenge individuals to experience life at the highest heights and deepest depths (Burkhardt & Nagai-Jacobson, 2005). Healthcare professionals are often in a position to help clients deal with their life issues. Understanding the various aspects of the spiritual dimension helps to ensure that they provide care in a holistic manner.

Spirituality's Effects on Healing

The recognition of spirituality's impact on healing has grown significantly over the past several decades. Researchers are beginning to define the complex connections between religious and spiritual beliefs and practices and an individual's physical and psychological health. They have discovered a positive relationship between religion and physical health, and they have demonstrated that spiritual beliefs and practices are beneficial to health and can help reduce the risk of developing a number of serious illnesses (Ebersole & Hess, 1997; Larson, Swyers, & McCullough, 1998). Recent studies have shown a statistically significant relationship between religious involvement, better mental health, and greater social support. They have also found that almost 80% of those who are religious have significantly greater well-being, hope, and optimism than those who are less religious (Micozzi, 2006).

As a result of these discoveries, medical schools now include courses on religion, spirituality, and health in their curricula (Micozzi, 2006). Medical students are beginning to examine their own spirituality as well as that of their clients, to study the world's major religious teachings, to learn how to take a spiritual history, and to communicate better with clients about their spiritual concerns.

Most healthcare professionals interact with all three dimensions of a person: physical, mental, and spiritual. While most professionals are competent at assessing the physical and mental aspects, it is equally important that they develop confidence in addressing the client's spiritual needs as well.

CULTURE AND THE HEALING PROCESS

Spirituality is experienced and guided by cultural traditions and religious doctrine (DuBray, 2001). Like spirituality, culture has a significant impact on health behaviors; health problems; and the actions taken to promote, maintain, or restore health (Young & Koopsen, 2005). If healthcare providers are to attend to the spiritual needs of their clients, they must understand the vast array of cultures and their belief systems.

The United States is a unique nation, created from a blending of many native and nonnative peoples. The growth of its culturally diverse populations has been dramatic (Luckmann, 1999). Individuals of diverse cultural backgrounds now create a rainbow of color and culture that impacts the delivery of healthcare services, the understanding of disease and illness, and the challenge they present to healthcare providers. Today's healthcare professionals must provide a level of care that meets the guidelines of cultural competence and respects different cultural values and belief systems.

The advancement of technology, travel, and communication systems has allowed increased contact between people of many different cultures. With immigration, international travel, and globalization, spiritual journeys can take today's people down paths that were not available to previous generations and expose them to many different religious and spiritual practices. The traditional healthcare system in the United States (biomedicine) now accommodates other diverse systems of care rather than requiring them to assimilate into its culture. This fundamental shift calls for all healthcare providers to become culturally competent. This obligation is even more important when healthcare providers and clients use complementary, alternative, or integrative modalities.

SPIRITUALITY, RELIGION, AND HEALTH CONDITIONS

Micozzi (2006) notes that "research in the last 10 years has made an indelible mark on the way health care professionals think about the role of spirituality and religion in physical, mental, and social health. Hundreds of studies have explored the relationship between body and spirit" (p. 305). Spirituality, faith, belief, and religion are now well known to be associated with fewer medical symptoms and better outcomes when integrative medical interventions are used (Rakel, 2007). Living a spiritual life and/or having a strong faith can positively impact not only the course of a chronic disease or terminal illness but also how that disease or illness is perceived. There is more to healing or being well than just curing disease. Individuals with a life-threatening disease or those who are dying can still find beauty and meaning in life, and the importance of the role of healthcare professionals in providing spiritual support cannot be overemphasized (Sorajjakool & Lamberton, 2004). This section explores the effects of spirituality and religion on several health conditions.

Spirituality, Religion, and Depression

According to Baetz, Griffin, Bowen, Koenig, and Marcoux (2004), individuals who were involved in a religious group and who highly valued their religious faith had a decreased risk of developing depression, while individuals with no religious link raised their risk of major depression. Valuing one's religious faith is centrally important, and actively belonging to a religious group and a strong support system may provide personal spiritual meaning to difficult life experiences or personal crises. Religion and spirituality play a pivotal role in decreasing depression by fostering positive beliefs and behaviors while lessening the impact of negative situations.

Spirituality, Religion, and Chronic Disease

Due to rapid advances in healthcare technology, individuals with heart disease, Parkinson's disease, diabetes, multiple sclerosis, and other chronic diseases can now live into old age. As the burden of chronic illness grows, so does the importance of addressing how to care for individuals with these illnesses. Clinical studies are beginning to clarify how spirituality and religion contribute to the coping strategies of many clients with severe, chronic, and terminal conditions. Spirituality may provide individuals with an ability to cope with their condition, thereby improving their physical and mental health.

Spirituality, Religion, and Cancer

Spirituality and religious beliefs are central to coping with cancer and to helping individuals find meaning in their disease. Individuals with cancer often experience guilt, fear, anxiety, and resentment. Having faith in a supreme being often helps them reaffirm the value and meaning of life.

Healthcare professionals can play a major role in providing spiritual care. Although many institutions provide clergy visits, nurses in particular spend a great deal of time with their clients. Ministers, priests, or other religious advisers should be included in a client's healthcare program. At such times, privacy should be afforded and respected so the client can discuss confidential matters (Leuckenotte, 2000). All of these professions must care for clients in a way that preserves their uniqueness and their religious or spiritual beliefs.

Spirituality, Religion, and Surgery

The most important and commonly used coping strategy in the acute care setting is prayer. Religious beliefs and practices have been linked to the survival rate among surgical clients.

SPIRITUAL RITUALS

B. M. Dossey (1997) defines *rituals* as the enactments of cultural beliefs and values. Rituals involve repetition and patterns of form and behaviors that have personal, healing worth. They are spiritual acts and sacred spaces of the mind that honor the core of human experience and the power of the Invisible Force. They are also a rite of separation.

Rituals are significant aspects of many religious traditions and cultures, but any activity done with awareness can be considered a ritual. Traditional rituals are handed down from one generation to another; self-generated rituals are begun by individuals or groups and have no cultural history or tradition.

Rituals are a rich resource in caring for the spirit. They contain steps for recovery, they reduce anxiety and fear, and they reduce feelings of helplessness. Healthcare professionals can support the power of rituals by providing opportunities for individuals to consider and experience their use in their lives.

This section discusses several spiritual rituals, including prayer, gratitude, spending time in nature, rest and leisure, and art.

Prayer

Simply put, prayer represents a desire to communicate with a supreme being. Burkhardt and Nagai-Jacobson (2005) write, "An expression of the spirit, prayer is a deep human instinct that flows from the core of one's being where the longing for and awareness of one's connectedness with the source of life are blended" (p. 147).

Micozzi (2006) notes that "the use of prayer in healing may have begun in human prehistory and continues to this day as an underlying tenet in almost all religions" (p. 306). According to Micozzi, the word *prayer* comes from the Latin words *precarius* ("obtained by begging") and *precari* ("to entreat" or "to ask earnestly").

Prayer can profoundly affect the healing process. Research demonstrates that religious practices such as worship attendance and prayer may contribute to physical and emotional health. Although the studies have not demonstrated a cause-and-effect relationship, there is strong evidence of an important connection between religious practice and good health (Fontaine, 2000; Taylor, 2002). As Taylor (2002) states, "Although experimental evidence of prayer's curative effect is inconclusive, there have been several correlational studies that demonstrate relationships between prayer and psychological health benefits" (p. 207).

In addition to turning to medical care for their healing, people also turn to prayer. According to Matthews and Clark (1998):

- *People cope with illness*, when they are not completely cured of it, through a learned process by using prayer and other forms of spiritual involvement.
- *Individuals may experience the arrest of the progression of illnesses* such as cancer and heart disease.
- *Individuals may experience remission or complete healing of illnesses* through the combination of prayer and medical care.

Matthews and Clark explain the impact of prayer in this way: "Of course, we know that the faith factor is not a panacea—the mortality rate for human beings still remains 100%. But even when physical healing does not occur, some degree of improvement almost always takes place, most often a sense of peace in facing a serious illness or disability" (p. 61).

With a wide variety of forms and expressions, prayer is part of many religious traditions and rituals. In fact, prayer is the most common form of spiritual practice (Trivieri & Anderson, 2002). It may be individual or communal, public or private. Sometimes prayer is a conscious activity, and at other times it is less conscious. The elements of prayer include speaking (often silently), listening, waiting, and being silent. L. Dossey (1993) and B. M. Dossey (1997) note that prayer also includes adoration, confession, invocation, intercession, lamentation, and thanksgiving.

There are many ways to develop a daily spiritual practice of prayer and to pray for oneself and others. The types of prayer may include petitionary, intercessory, adoration, ritual, meditative or contemplative, and colloquial (Burkhardt & Nagai-Jacobson, 2005; Dossey, 2001; Holt-Ashley, 2000; Levin, 1996; Macrae, 2001; Micozzi, 2006; Taylor, 2002).

- *Petitionary prayer* involves asking a supreme being to respond to a specific request, usually for personal healing.
- *Intercessory prayer*, often called distant prayer, is petitionary prayer on behalf of others, with or without their knowledge. It occurs when one person prays for someone else to receive something. Usually this involves praying for someone else's health.
- *Adoration prayer* involves praising and glorifying a supreme being. This type of prayer is an affirmation of the loving energy within and outside oneself. It transcends the ego and involves turning one's life over to a higher power. It is not an avoidance of responsibility but rather a positive surrender to a supreme being and a willingness to do what must be done for healing to take place.
- *Ritual prayer* involves the use of spiritual readings, repetition, or formal prayers or rites such as a rosary or a prayer book. Ritual prayer involves the repetition of prayers created by another and often found in religious literature.
- *Meditative*, or *contemplative*, *prayer* involves listening for the still, small voice within and having a sense of openness toward the divine, independent of thoughts and words. The purpose is to objectively observe oneself becoming absorbed in the unity of being, to experience one's unity with a supreme being, and to experience life as it unfolds. Meditative or contemplative prayer involves the opening of the mind and heart to a supreme being who transcends words or thoughts. This type of prayer exists in all the great religious traditions of the world.
- *Colloquial prayer* involves communicating with the divine in an informal, honest, and self-revealing manner, as if talking to a friend. This type of prayer is used to seek direction and guidance in making a decision.

Many techniques are used in praying, including the following (Dossey, 1993; Fontaine, 2000; Taylor, 2002):

- Relaxation, quieting, and breath awareness
- Attention training and focusing
- Imagery and visualization
- Intentionality
- Movement, such as dancing, walking, or drumming
- Inspirational or sacred readings

- Music
- Chanting
- Anointing with oil
- Singing
- Meditation

Gratitude

The spiritual practice of gratitude is a powerful force that can be a state of mind as well as a way of life. Being grateful for what you have, instead of worrying about what you lack, enables you to let go of negative thoughts and attitudes and to reduce stress, anxiety, and depression. Being grateful increases feelings of love, knowingness, and awareness (Eliopoulos, 2004). Burkhardt and Nagai-Jacobson (2002) describe the origin of gratitude this way: "Our experience of grace as a blessing that comes into our lives unearned, without merit, calls forth the response of gratitude" (p. 71).

One way to practice gratitude is to focus on the positive aspects of life, perhaps by keeping a gratitude journal—an inventory of all the positive things that occur each day, week, and month. Keeping such a journal can set the stage for living a more spiritual life (Fontaine, 2000).

Engaging in an act of gratitude may often restore balance and perspective (Burkhardt & Nagai-Jacobson, 2002; Fontaine, 2000). Grateful acts might include any or all of the following:

- Making a list of things in your life for which you are grateful
- Creating opportunities to help others
- Calling a special friend
- Being aware that life is a gift
- Saying grace before meals
- Engaging in daily prayers
- Always remembering to say thank you when someone helps you, compliments you, or gives you a gift

Spending Time in Nature

Throughout history, most religious, spiritual, and cultural traditions have had strong connections and relationships with nature. According to Taylor (2002), "Many religious traditions consider nature, or the outdoors and its world of living things, to be the handiwork or a literal illustration of God" (p. 262). For example, the Native American religious tradition expresses a positive relationship with nature that is called nature-centered spirituality and is found in many other religious traditions worldwide (Dossey, 1997).

In today's technological society, many people have become alienated from nature. Experiencing the pleasure of the natural environment (a deserted beach, a shimmering wheat field, a majestic mountain, a lush forest, or a quiet stream) may be considered a spiritual experience. Even the act of contemplating nature may aid in a person's spiritual health, and the act of viewing nature may contribute to better health outcomes (Taylor, 2002).

Being in natural environments and viewing or experiencing nature can foster reconnection with the self physically, emotionally, and spiritually. In nature, individuals interact with primal energies in the forms of earth, water, fire, and air (Ruffing, 1997; Taylor, 2002).

- *Earth:* Spending time in nature helps to restore balance and deepen the spiritual connection. To connect with nature and the earth, individuals can take a walk in a park, hike through the woods, do gardening, ride a bike, camp out, or take a sailing trip.
- *Water:* Spending time near or in the water can contribute to feelings of well-being. Swimming in the ocean, a lake, or a river and soaking in a mineral hot spring are excellent ways to benefit from this life-enhancing energy.
- *Fire:* Exposure to fire in a campground or fireplace may have health benefits. To Native Americans, fire is an important part of the vision quest ritual used to connect with the Great Spirit.
- *Air:* Of all of nature's elements, air may be the purest manifestation of Spirit. Air is essential to life and health on all levels.

In the healthcare setting, helping clients experience a positive connection with nature promotes spiritual as well as physical health. Approaches to using nature as a resource in providing spiritual care may include the following (Taylor, 2002):

- Providing a window view of natural surroundings
- Displaying an aquarium of beautiful fish
- Providing access to animals or an animal-assisted therapy program
- Putting flower boxes in a client's room
- Displaying photographs, pictures, or illustrations of natural settings

Rest and Leisure

Rest and leisure are integral aspects of spiritual care for both healthcare providers and clients. Engaging in exercise, listening to music, using imagery, and creating a specific time for rest and quiet—and making the commitment to incorporate these experiences into one's daily life—encourage rest and leisure (Burkhardt & Nagai-Jacobson, 2005).

Art

Art is an important aspect of the spirit. Many individuals find that the many forms of art are doors to, and expressions of, the spirit. Art can nurture the spirit and take the following forms (Burkhardt & Nagai-Jacobson, 2005; Rollins & Riccio, 2002; Taylor, 2002):

- Drawing
- Painting
- Sculpting
- Cooking
- Sewing
- Designing and building
- Conducting a symphony
- Listening to or creating music
- Writing or reading literature
- Writing or reading poetry
- Dancing
- Drumming
- Gardening

Engaging in these activities may provide a sense of accomplishment, the opportunity to be creative (which is, in itself, an expression of spirituality), a connection with other cultures, or a transcendence to another state of mind. Artists can play an important role on the interdisciplinary team in providing spiritual care in the healthcare setting.

SPIRITUALITY AND THE AGING POPULATION

Today, two related trends are converging. First, people are living longer into old age. Second, society is increasingly concerned about extended life, ethics, and aging. Together these trends generate interest in the meaning of living longer and the aging process.

Even though physical functioning may decline as an individual ages, spiritual functioning does not necessarily do the same. Isaia, Parker, and Murrow (1999) report that there is "no evidence that the spirit succumbs to the aging process, even in the presence of debilitating illness" (p. 16). Spiritual awakening and development with aging can provide the individual with wonderful opportunities for growth and for the release of old patterns and beliefs that are no longer relevant. Faith provides the aging individual with the inner strength needed to transcend the physical disabilities associated with aging and to develop the emotional resilience needed to achieve longevity (Koenig, 1999). Many older adults turn to spirituality and religion to cope with illness, the death of loved ones, or the anticipation of their own deaths. Many Americans believe their spirituality helps promote healing, especially when medications and other treatments cannot provide a cure for their conditions.

Religion also provides individuals, especially the elderly, with effective strategies for coping with personal difficulties and stress. Religious coping strategies include personal strength or support from God, the use of prayer to help cope with difficulties and stress, and seeking God's guidance when making important decisions (Krause, 1998).

As people age, feelings of self-worth may diminish. Which factor prevents older adults from experiencing these feelings when dealing with declining health or retirement? Krause (1995) found that religious coping strategies were the most important factors linked to healthy self-esteem in seniors in the United States. Feelings of self-worth tended to be lowest for those with very little religious commitment and highest in those with a strong religious commitment.

For the older adult, spirituality can provide several elements essential to a healthy life (Fischer, 1998):

- Spirituality promotes acceptance of the past, contributes to enjoyment of the present, and provides hope for the future.
- Spirituality meets a basic human need.
- Spirituality helps during stressful life events, increases an individual's understanding of the meaning of life, and helps in preparing for death.
- Spirituality provides support during phases of multiple losses and during the grieving process.

Spirituality becomes important for most older adults during the stress of hospitalization, healthcare procedures, or surgery. At such times, individuals reflect on suffering, death, and their relationships with self, others, and a supreme intelligence in order to make meaning of their lives.

The aging process is an important step in an individual's spiritual journey and spiritual growth. Spiritual individuals strive to transcend the many changes and losses that accompany aging and to achieve a higher understanding of life and its meaning. Spirituality is a critical component of health and well-being for the aging individual, and it becomes increasingly important as a person grows older. A key element of that spirituality is a realistic perspective of what is involved in the aging process so the realities are neither over- nor undervalued (Young & Koopsen, 2005).

SPIRITUALITY AND THE HEALTHCARE SYSTEM

The level to which healthcare professionals nurture and care for themselves influences their ability to function effectively in a healing role with another person. Attentiveness to one's own spirit is a key factor of living in a healing way and provides the foundation for integrating spirituality into health care. Healthcare professionals must also become confident and competent with spiritual caregiving, expand their skills in assessing the spiritual domain, and develop and implement appropriate spiritual interventions.

According to Shea (2000), there are six spiritual interests in health care: spiritual interest of clients, of medical caregivers in clients, of medical caregivers in themselves, of chaplains, in organizational life, and in ethics.

Spiritual Interest of Clients

How do clients, their friends, and their families handle suffering and loss? People resist sickness because it reminds them of their own mortality and causes them to face questions of loss and limits. However, as they face these crucial questions, clients become interested in the spiritual. The entire healthcare environment suggests the precariousness of physical life and the presence of limits everywhere (Shea, 2000). Healthcare professionals need to be aware of this situation because clients want a trusting and caring relationship with their healthcare provider in order to feel spiritually supported and nurtured.

In delivering spiritual care and addressing the spiritual interests of clients, healthcare providers face many choices. They must decide whether to pray with clients, how to create a healing environment, how to address difficult questions, and how to help clients and their families find meaning in the face of pain and suffering (Sierpina & Sierpina, 2004).

Spiritual Interest of Medical Caregivers in Clients

The interests of physicians, nurses, social workers, family, friends, and other caregivers overlap with those of the client. All of these caregivers want to know how to integrate spirituality into client care. Since studies have shown that religion and spirituality have positive effects on physical and mental health, caring for clients in a holistic manner means addressing all of their health concerns. When clients discuss their religious or spiritual concerns, it is important for caregivers to assess those concerns and develop appropriate interventions (Shea, 2000).

Regardless of their belief systems, healthcare professionals must not allow their own biases to prevent them from appreciating the fact that religious and spiritual beliefs play an important role for many of their clients.

Spiritual Interest of Medical Caregivers in Themselves

Healthcare professionals sometimes see themselves as heeding a call that arises out of their own talents and desires and also out of a transcendent source (Shea, 2000). As they care for others, medical caregivers begin to walk their own spiritual path, personally developing their own spirituality.

Medical caregivers who are not religious or spiritual must take care not to underestimate the importance of the client's belief system. Respect for the client's spiritual or religious perspective must transcend the medical caregiver's ideology. Because the beliefs of the client and healthcare providers may not coincide, caregivers must understand their own belief system and how it gives meaning and purpose to their lives (Sierpina & Sierpina, 2004).

Spiritual Interest of Chaplains

The responsibility of helping clients spiritually, especially during times of crisis, has traditionally belonged to the chaplain or pastoral care provider. However, tending to the spiritual needs of clients is meant to enhance well-being and should not be reserved for times of crisis. Chaplains and pastoral care providers are the most accessible resource in the healthcare organization and they usually provide care to an expanding interfaith population (Shea, 2000).

Chaplains usually have specialized knowledge of how medical procedures are viewed by various religious groups and, in many cases, they are the first to elicit the client's current understanding or belief about getting permission for a procedure. They are a valuable spiritual resource in healthcare organizations.

Spiritual Interest in Organizational Life

If a healthcare organization encourages spiritual interests, it must have policies and structures that are friendly to those spiritual interests, and the policies and structures must address the interests of clients, caregivers, employees, and associates. Spiritually developed people have the qualities to survive and to thrive in a changing work environment (Shea, 2000).

Spiritual Interest in Ethics

The incorporation of spirituality into the healthcare setting must involve the consideration of ethics. Ethical standards and guidelines focus on medical procedures, clients' rights, business conduct, and an array of organizational issues from hiring to severance. Thinking ethically about new initiatives in the area of spirituality is therefore essential, and it involves an array of questions. For example:

- Should spiritual care include advocating prayer to clients?
- Are spiritual assessments an invasion of privacy?
- How does the healthcare or spiritual care provider deliver spiritual care to nonreligious clients?
- What role does culture play in ethical decision making?

When changes are introduced, healthcare practices and everyday organizational procedures must be evaluated in terms of their ethical consequences (Shea, 2000).

SPIRITUAL CARE PROVIDERS

Individuals often believe that their identity is tied to success, wealth, prestige, family, or accomplishments. When individuals experience a crisis they sometimes find themselves in the hospital, waiting for the results of medical tests. In these vulnerable moments, things that seemed so important and brought comfort in the past suddenly lose their power. They need help from outside themselves, and this need can take the form of spiritual care (Sorajjakool & Lamberton, 2004).

Several types of care providers can be called upon as resources for providing spiritual care. Physicians, nurses, and social workers are described as spiritual care generalists, while chaplains, clergy, parish nurses, spiritual mentors, folk healers, friends, and family are considered spiritual care specialists (Taylor, 2002). Each type of care provider is briefly described in the following paragraphs.

Physicians

Many physicians have not received training in the area of spiritual care and thus may make referrals to the appropriate spiritual care provider. As more physicians receive training in this area, they will assume a more active role in the spiritual care process.

Nurses

Most nurses consider themselves to be religious, and many consider their personal religious training to be adequate training for spiritual caregiving. In reality, this misconception may influence the practice of many nurses and result in the provision of inadequate spiritual care. Most nurses have had no formal training in spiritual care skills except for some basic information during their training. However, more and more nurses are acquiring education in this area through various informal and formal programs, chaplaincy training, or graduate programs in pastoral counseling or ministry. Trained nurses can provide excellent spiritual care and referrals to other spiritual care providers.

Social Workers

Social workers may assist in the spiritual care process in many ways, from helping families organize their care support system to guiding the client and family in meeting their emotional, spiritual, psychological, and bereavement needs.

Chaplains

The nonprofit, independent Joint Commission, which is widely recognized for certifying and accrediting healthcare organizations in the United States, requires that institutions make formal arrangements for chaplain services. Taylor (2002) describes these professionals as representing "a merger of theology and psychology" (p. 181). An estimated 9,000 chaplains in the United States help people with health-related transitions. Some institutions use professional chaplains, and others use volunteer clergy and chaplains.

Chaplains have four broad roles:

- Conducting spiritual assessments
- Responding to clients' religious concerns and helping them with religious coping strategies
- Supporting professional staff
- Functioning as liaisons with religious communities

Nurses consult with chaplains for many reasons, including:

- Helping with family support in times of death, emergencies, or difficult decision making
- Arranging bedside religious rites
- Helping with cessation of life support
- Assisting with an anxious or fearful client

Chaplains are also a tremendous staff resource since they can assist staff members in coping with their own grief and provide education in the areas of ethics, spirituality, and coping strategies.

Clergy

These professionals have been trained in religious ministry, but their training can vary greatly. Although some have no college diplomas at all, others have earned master's degrees. Some may not have received any training in how to help clients through healthcare crises while others may be very qualified in this area. According to the institution's policies, chaplains often make referrals to clergy, and nurses need to be sensitive to this practice. In some organizations, nurses can initiate referrals to clergy.

Parish Nurses

These registered nurses have specialized training to provide holistic care to members of a religious congregation. Parish nurses know their parishioners intimately, they collaborate with ministers and staff, and they promote health and prevent disease. They act as health educators, role models, personal health counselors, volunteer coordinators, advocates and facilitators, and referral agents or community liaisons. They do not perform the services unique to home care nurses or public health nurses, nor do they perform invasive procedures or administer medications. While their educational backgrounds may vary, all have received training in spiritual caregiving. Referrals to parish nurses are especially relevant when the clients' health concerns relate to their religious practices.

Spiritual Mentors

Mentors are spiritual directors who help others develop spiritually. They can be of any religious denomination and they often meet regularly with their clients. They have received special training and may be religious professionals. They can provide encouragement and comfort as well as challenge individuals to increase their spiritual awareness and discipline.

Folk Healers

These lay healers use techniques that are unique to their culture and usually quite different from traditional Western medicine. They may use special rituals, herbs, or other natural materials to promote health. They usually receive their education as a result of an apprenticeship, personal study, or experience.

Friends and Family

Although they may or may not have spiritual training, friends and family are often the ones clients say they need when they require spiritual nurturing. Family and friends can function as supportive companions by providing assistance with prayer, reading, or singing; by providing comforting thoughts; by sharing a healing ritual; or by providing much-needed empathy. Because friends and family share an intimate history with the client, they can provide a type of support that no other individuals can.

SPIRITUAL ASSESSMENT AND INTERVENTIONS

An important component in the holistic care of clients, the spiritual assessment helps determine spiritual needs and resources, evaluate the impact of beliefs on healthcare outcomes and decisions, and uncover barriers to using spiritual resources. The spiritual assessment includes questions on religious background, spiritual values, prayer experiences, and faith and beliefs. Example questions include (Benedict, 2002):

- How does your spiritual side affect your health?
- Would you describe yourself as a religious person?
- What does spirituality mean to you?
- Do you use prayer in your life? How often?
- How would you describe your God?
- What gives you meaning and purpose in life?
- How do you express your spiritual or religious side?
- What types of spiritual activities or experiences do you enjoy?
- What does dying mean to you?
- How can I, as a healthcare provider, assist you in maintaining the religious and/or spiritual resources in your life?
- What gives you peace?
- How do you perceive that you are loved by others?
- What do you do when you need help?
- Have you ever experienced feelings of guilt, anger, resentment, and/or bitterness?
- How do you handle these feelings?
- Whom do you need to forgive?
- What prompts you to forgive others?

- What resources do you use to help you accept forgiveness?
- What are your spiritual issues or concerns?
- What resources do you use to obtain or maintain a sense of hope?

When performing a spiritual assessment, the following guidelines are helpful (Benedict, 2002):

- Sit down with the person and plan a time for the assessment.
- Listen with your heart as well as your head.
- Remain nonjudgmental about the other person's beliefs and practices.
- Respect the person and his or her religious or spiritual behaviors.
- Perform the assessment in an environment of trust, dignity, and safety.
- Focus on living rather than on illnesses or death and dying.
- Integrate the spiritual aspect of the individual into holistic care.

Spiritual Distress

Benedict (2002) defines *spiritual distress* as "the disruption in the life principle that pervades a person's entire being and that transcends one's biological and psychological nature. In other words, it means the person's self is disintegrating" (p. 7). Benedict lists the following symptoms of spiritual distress:

- Fear
- Guilt
- Denial
- Grief/loss
- Anger/bitterness
- Crying
- Withdrawal
- Anorexia
- Insomnia
- Despair/depression
- Sleep disturbances/disturbing dreams
- Anxiety/restlessness
- Lack of responsibility for problems
- Cynicism
- Loneliness

Spiritual Interventions

Spiritual interventions are easily remembered by using the acronym REST (Benedict, 2002):

- *Respect* what the individuals are going through and how they express their distress.
- *Encourage* individuals to discuss their concerns and beliefs by listening, touching (appropriately), being silent, being near, and responding immediately to their needs.
- *Support* the process they are undergoing by allowing the presence of spiritual symbols, praying with them, or arranging for healing services as requested.
- *Trust* your own intuition and build trust with individuals through honesty, caring behavior, being genuine, and following through on commitments.

KEY CONCEPTS

1. To effectively address the special concerns and health issues of their clients, healthcare professionals must become familiar with and understand the spiritual and religious values, beliefs, and practices of the diverse cultures and spiritual expressions in today's society.
2. Current research is beginning to define the complex connections between religious and spiritual beliefs and practices and an individual's physical and psychological health.
3. As research reveals new relationships and connections, healthcare practices must be modified to best meet the needs of clients and to provide optimal, quality, integrative health care.

QUESTIONS FOR REFLECTION

1. Why should healthcare professionals concern themselves with issues of religious and spiritual practices in the healing process?
2. Based on current research, how do you see the fields of spirituality and health integrating and evolving in the future?
3. While no one has been able to provide a universally accepted definition of spirituality, how would you define spirituality?

REFERENCES

Altea, R. (2006). *You own the power: Stories and exercises to inspire and unleash the force within.* New York: Harper.

Baetz, M., Griffin, R., Bowen, R., Koenig, H. G., & Marcoux, E. (2004, December). The association between spiritual and religious involvement and depressive symptoms in a Canadian population. *Journal of Nervous and Mental Disease, 192*(12), 818–822.

Benedict, L. M. (2002). *Spiritual assessment.* EDA 318-0479. Carrollton, TX: PRIMEDIA Healthcare: Long Term Care Network.

Benor, D. J. (2006). *Personal spirituality: Science, spirit, and the eternal soul.* Medford, NJ: Wholistic Healing.

Bergquist, S., & King, J. (1994). Parish nursing: A conceptual framework. *Journal of Holistic Nursing, 12*(2), 155–170.

Burkhardt, M. A. (2007). Commentary on spirituality in nursing and health-related literature: A concept analysis. *Journal of Holistic Nursing, 25*(4), 263–274.

Burkhardt, M. A., & Nagai-Jacobson, M. G. (2002). *Spirituality: Living our connectedness.* Albany, NY: Delmar Thomson Learning.

Burkhardt, M. A., & Nagai-Jacobson, M. G. (2005). Spirituality and health. Sudbury, MA: Jones and Bartlett.

Chandler, E. (1999). Spirituality. *Hospice Journal, 14*(34), 63–74.

Daniels, R., Nosek, L. J., & Nicoll, L. H. (2007). *Contemporary medical-surgical nursing.* Clifton Park, NY: Thomson Delmar Learning.

DeLaune, S. C., & Ladner, P. K. (2006). *Fundamentals of nursing: Standards and practice* (3rd ed.). Clifton Park, NY: Thomson Delmar Learning.

Dossey, B. M. (1997). *Core curriculum for holistic nursing.* Gaithersburg, MD: Aspen.

Dossey, B. M., Keegan, L. & Guzzetta, C. E. (2005) *Holistic nursing: A handbook for practice* (4th ed.). Sudbury, MA: Jones and Bartlett.

Dossey, L. (1993). *Healing words: The power of prayer and the practice of medicine.* San Francisco: HarperCollins.

Dossey, L. (2001). *Healing beyond the body: Medicine and the infinite reach of the mind.* Boston: Shambhala.

Dossey, L. (2002). How healing happens: Exploring the nonlocal gap. *Alternative Therapies in Health and Medicine, 8*(2), 12–16, 103–110.

DuBray, W. (Ed.). (2001). *Spirituality and healing: A multicultural perspective.* New York: Writers Club Press.

Ebersole, P., & Hess, P. (1997). *Toward healthy aging: Human needs and nursing response* (5th ed.). St. Louis, MO: Mosby-Year Book.

Eliopoulos, C. (2004). *Invitation to holistic health: A guide to living a balanced life.* Sudbury, MA: Jones and Bartlett.

Falk-Rafael, A. R. (2000). Watson's philosophy, science, and theory of human caring as a conceptual framework for guiding community health nursing practice. *Advances in Nursing Practice, 23*(2), 34–49.

Fischer, K. (1998). *Winter grace: Spirituality and aging.* Nashville: Upper Room Books.

Fontaine, K. L. (2000). *Healing practices: Alternative therapies for nursing.* Upper Saddle River, NJ: Prentice Hall.

Freeman, L. (2004). *Mosby's complementary and alternative medicine: A research-based approach* (2nd ed.). St. Louis, MO: Mosby.

Frisch, N. C. (2005). Nursing theory in holistic nursing practice. In B. M. Dossey, L. Keegan, & C. E. Guzzetta, *Holistic nursing: A handbook for practice* (4th ed., pp. 79–90). Sudbury, MA: Jones and Bartlett.

Hatch, R. L., Burg, M. A., Naberhaus, D. S., & Hellmich, L. K. (1998). The spiritual involvement and beliefs scale: Development and testing of a new instrument. *Journal of Family Practice, 46*(6), 476–486.

Hiatt, J. F. (1986). Spirituality, medicine, and healing. *Southern Medical Journal, 79*(6), 736–743.

Holt-Ashley, M. (2000). Nurses pray: Use of prayer and spirituality as a complementary therapy in the intensive care setting. *AACN Clinical Issues: Advance Practice in Acute Critical Care, 11*(1), 60–67.

Isaia, D., Parker, V., & Murrow, E. (1999). Spiritual well-being among older adults. *Journal of Gerontological Nursing, 25*(8), 16–21.

Kligler, B., & Lee, R. (2004). *Integrative medicine: Principles for practice.* New York: McGraw-Hill.

Koenig, H. G. (1999). *The healing power of faith.* New York: Simon & Schuster.

Koenig, H. G., Idler, E., Kasl, S., Hays, J., George, L. K., Musick, M., et al. (1999). Religion, spirituality, and medicine: A rebuttal to skeptics. *International Journal of Psychiatry in Medicine, 29*(2), 123–131.

Krause, N. (1995). Religiosity and self-esteem among older adults. *Journal of Gerontology: Psychological Sciences, 50B*(5), 236–246.

Krause, N. (1998). Neighborhood deterioration, religious coping, and changes in health during late life. *Gerontologist, 38*(6), 653–664.

Larson, D. B., Swyers, J. P., & McCullough, M. E. (1998). *Scientific research on spirituality and health.* Rockville, MD: National Institute for Healthcare Research.

Lemmer, C. (2005). Recognizing and caring for spiritual needs of clients. *Journal of Holistic Nursing, 23*(3), 310–321.

Leuckenotte, A. G. (2000). *Gerontologic nursing.* St. Louis, MO: Mosby.

Levin, J. S. (1996). How prayer heals: A theoretical model. *Alternative Therapies, 2*(1), 66–73.

Luckmann, J. (1999). *Transcultural communication in nursing.* Albany, NY: Delmar Thomson Learning.

Macrae, J. A. (2001). *Nursing as a spiritual practice: A contemporary application of Florence Nightingale's views.* New York: Springer.

Mahoney, M. J., & Graci, G. M. (1999). The meanings and correlates of spirituality: Suggestions from an exploratory survey of experts. *Death Studies, 23*(6), 521–529.

Martsolf, D. S., & Mickley, J. R. (1998). The concept of spirituality in nursing theories: Differing world-views and extent of focus. *Journal of Advanced Nursing, 27*(2), 294–303.

Matthews, D. A., & Clark, C. (1998). *The faith factor: Proof of the healing power of prayer.* New York: Penguin Books.

McSherry, W., & Draper, P. (1998). The debates emerging from the literature surrounding the concept of spirituality as applied to nursing. *Journal of Advanced Nursing, 27*(4), 683–691.

Meraviglia, M. G. (1999). Critical analysis of spirituality and its empirical indicators. *Journal of Holistic Nursing, 17*(1), 18–33.

Micozzi, M. S. (2006). *Fundamentals of complementary and integrative medicine* (3rd ed.). St. Louis, MO: Saunders Elsevier.

Neuman, B., & Fawcett, J. (2002). *The Neuman systems model* (4th ed.). Upper Saddle River, NJ: Prentice Hall.

Newman, M. (1994). *Health as expanding consciousness* (2nd ed.). Sudbury, MA: Jones and Bartlett.

Parse, R. R. (1999). *Illuminations: The human becoming theory in practice and research.* Sudbury, MA: Jones and Bartlett.

Rakel, D. (2007). *Integrative medicine* (2nd ed.). Philadelphia: Saunders Elsevier.

Reynolds, C. (2001). *Spiritual fitness.* London: Thorsons.

Rollins, J. A., & Riccio, L. (2002). ART is the heART: A palette of possibilities for hospice care. *Pediatric Nursing 28*(4), 355–362.

Ruffing, J. (1997). "To have been one with the earth . . .": Nature in contemporary Christian mystical experience. *Presence: The Journal of Spiritual Directors International, 3*(1), 40–54.

Saewyc, E. M. (2000). Nursing theories of caring: A paradigm for adolescent nursing practice. *Journal of Holistic Nursing, 18*(2), 114–128.

Seaward, B. L. (2006). *Managing stress: Principles and strategies for health and well-being* (5th ed.). Sudbury, MA: Jones and Bartlett.

Shea, J. (2000). *Spirituality and health care.* Chicago: Park Ridge Center for the Study of Health, Faith, and Ethics.

Sierpina, V., & Sierpina, M. (2004). Spirituality and health. In B. Kligler & R. Lee, *Integrative medicine: Principles for practice* (pp. 301–310). New York: McGraw-Hill.

Sorajjakool, S., & Lamberton, H. (Eds.). (2004). *Spirituality, health, and wholeness: An introductory guide for health care professionals.* Binghamton, NY: Haworth Press.

Stanley, M. E., & Beare, P. G. (1995). *Gerontological nursing*. Philadelphia: F. A. Davis.

Taylor, E. J. (2002). *Spiritual care: Nursing theory, research, and practice*. Upper Saddle River, NJ: Prentice Hall.

Trivieri, L., Jr., & Anderson, J. W. (Eds.). (2002). *Alternative medicine: The definitive guide* (2nd ed.). Berkeley, CA: Celestial Arts.

Tuck, I., Wallace, D., & Pullen, L. (2001). Spirituality and spiritual care provided by parish nurses. *Western Journal of Nursing Research, 23*(5), 441–453.

Watson, J. (2005). *Caring science as sacred science*. Philadelphia: F. A. Davis.

Weil, A. (1997). *Eight weeks to optimum health*. New York: Alfred A. Knopf.

Young, C., & Koopsen, C. (2005). *Spirituality, health, and healing*. Sudbury, MA: Jones and Bartlett.

CHAPTER 3

Energy Healing

Our remedies oft in ourselves do lie.
—WILLIAM SHAKESPEARE

LEARNING OBJECTIVES

1. Describe the types of energy.
2. Explain the universal energy field (UEF).
3. Explain the human energy field (HEF).
4. Describe the seven auric layers.
5. Describe the seven chakras.
6. Define the concept of energy healing.
7. Describe various types of energy healing.

INTRODUCTION

For centuries, traditional healers worldwide have practiced methods of energy healing, viewing the body as a complex energy system with energy flowing through or over its surface (Rakel, 2007). Until recently, the Western world largely ignored the Eastern interpretation of humans as energy beings. However, times have changed dramatically and an exciting and promising new branch of academic inquiry and clinical research is opening in the area of energy healing (Oschman, 2000; Trivieri & Anderson, 2002).

Scientists and energy therapists around the world have made discoveries that will forever alter our picture of human energetics. The National Institutes of Health (NIH) is conducting research in areas such as energy healing and prayer, and major U.S. academic institutions are conducting large clinical trials in these areas. Approaches in exploring the concepts of life force and healing energy that previously appeared to compete or conflict have now been found to support each other. Conner and Koithan (2006) note that "with increased recognition and federal funding for energetic healing, there is a growing body of research that supports the use of energetic healing interventions with patients" (p. 26).

With mounting scientific evidence now supporting the efficacy of ancient healing systems, the old paradigms of health care are shifting and a growing number of researchers, physicians, nurses, and other health practitioners are embracing a new view of healing that includes energy healing. The healthcare community is combining traditional methods of energy healing with modern medicine. Energy medicine is the medicine of the future (Trivieri & Anderson, 2002).

WHAT IS ENERGY?

Conventional descriptions refer to energy at the physical level and define it as the capacity to do work and overcome resistance. Conventional science recognizes four types of energy or forces (Benor, 2004; Tiller, 1999):

- *Strong nuclear force*: The strong nuclear force binds neutrons and protons in the atomic nucleus that acts over short distances.
- *Weak nuclear force:* The weak nuclear force also contributes to nuclear structure and radioactive decay. Both strong and weak nuclear forces have little effect outside the nucleus.
- *Electromagnetic (EM) force:* This force pervades the cosmos, from atomic structures to chemical molecular interactions and electrical power.
- *Gravity:* This force is weaker than the others over short distances and is active in proportion to the mass of an object. Gravity is the dominant force. Although its effects are measurable, its nature is the least understood and there are no clear theories to explain how it works.

Until recently, Western science assumed that there were no other energies than these four. However, a substantial body of evidence suggests the existence of bioenergies that are not recognized in conventional science. Schwartz (2007) offers a higher, more comprehensive description of energy as being the capacity to do anything, whether at the physical, psychological, or spiritual level. Trivieri and Anderson (2002) state that "the term *energy* can refer to familiar and easily measurable frequencies of the electromagnetic spectrum, such as light (including color) and sound, or to less familiar influences of living systems for when measurement is currently more difficult" (p. 203). There is also growing acknowledgment among quantum physicists of the role of consciousness in selecting processes that determine which of several quantum pathways are followed (Benor, 2004). Pressman (2006) notes that "more and more we become aware of the fact that the 'word' (consciousness) is the source of all energy" (p. 313).

These newer definitions recognize two types of energy:

- *Veritable energies* can be measured and they include vibrations (e.g., sound) and electromagnetic forces, including visible light, magnetism, monochromatic radiation (e.g., laser beams), and rays from other parts of the electromagnetic spectrum.
- *Putative energies*, also referred to as biofields, are difficult or impossible to measure.

Therapies involving veritable energies use specific, measurable wavelength frequencies to treat clients. Therapies involving putative energy fields are based on the concept that human beings are infused with a subtle form of energy. This vital energy is known under different names in different cultures, such as:

- Chi or qi (pronounced *chee*) in traditional Chinese medicine.
- Ki in the Japanese Kampo system.
- Doshas in Ayurvedic medicine.
- Prana, etheric energy, fohat, orgone, odic force, mana, and homeopathic resonance elsewhere in the world.

The concept that sickness and disease arise from imbalances in the body's vital energy field has led to many forms of therapy. For example, traditional Chinese medicine balances the flow of qi through a series of approaches, such as herbal medicine, acupuncture, Qigong (pronounced *chee gong*), diet, and behavior changes.

The Universal Energy Field (UEF)

Physicist and healer Barbara Brennan defines the *universal energy field* (*UEF*) as the life energy that surrounds and interpenetrates everything. The UEF may exist between matter and energy. Some scientists refer to the phenomenon of UEF as bioplasma (Brennan, 1988, 1993).

Drs. John White and Stanley Krippner list many of the properties of the UEF (Brennan, 1988):

- The UEF permeates all space, as well as animate and inanimate objects. It connects all objects to each other.
- It flows from one object to another.
- Its density varies inversely with the distance from its source.

- It follows the laws of harmonic inductance and sympathetic resonance (the phenomenon that occurs when you strike a tuning fork and another one near it begins to vibrate at the same frequency, giving off the same sound).

Brennan (1988) states, "Visual observations reveal the field to be highly organized in a series of geometric points, isolated pulsating points of light, spirals, webs of lines, sparks and clouds. It pulsates and can be sensed by touch, taste, smell and with sound and luminosity perceivable by the higher senses" (p. 40).

The UEF is the source of energy absorbed through the seven energy centers (chakras) of the human etheric body, an invisible duplicate of the physical body. Invisible to the naked eye, this highly structured energy field vibrates at a higher energy frequency than the physical body (Gerber, 2000). From the UEF, an attuned healer can direct healing energy to a client. The UEF is also the information storage hologram, the energetic imprint of everything that has happened or has ever been known; therefore, it is the medium by which an attuned healer can access past and future time dimensions and knowledge and perform distant diagnostics.

Benor (2004) notes, "Heat and other measurable energies emanate from the human body" (p. 394). Healers may sense this energy when they pass their hands around the body, and the laying on of hands may work through these known energies.

The Human Energy Field (HEF)

In this era of rapid scientific progress, many of the concepts we were absolutely certain about are no longer true. Of all the stories of exploration and discovery that could be told, none is more fascinating than that of the *human energy field (HEF)*. Scientists have gone from a conviction that there is no such thing to believing with absolute certainty that one exists (Oschman, 2000).

The physical body has an energy counterpart referred to by many names: ethereal body, aura, energy field, bioenergy field, and human energy field. The HEF and the physical body interact with each other, and an understanding of their interrelationship is invaluable for successful therapeutic treatment.

Many people can sense the bioenergy fields of heat and other measurable energies that emanate from the human body. Healers interpret these sensations as indications of specific energy blocks, illnesses, and psychological states. Some of the fields that healers sense appear to involve energies that conventional science has difficulty assessing; auras are just one example. Healers can diagnose an individual's physical, mental, emotional, and spiritual conditions by examining his or her aura (Benor, 2004).

The work of William A. Tiller, PhD, one of the world's leading scientists on solid-state physics and psychoenergetics, supports these observations. According to Tiller our eyes detect only a small fraction of the total electromagnetic spectrum and our ears detect only a small fraction of the total available sound spectrum. It can be suggested, therefore, that most of us detect only one band in the total spectrum of reality but that some individuals are cognitively aware of the normally unseen bands (Tiller, 2002).

As McTaggart (2002) states, "Human beings and all living things are a coalescence of energy in a field of energy connected to every other living thing in the world. This pulsating energy field is the central engine of our being and our consciousness, the alpha and the omega of our existence" (p. xiii). The energy field must be tapped for healing to take place. The field is the force responsible for our mind's highest functions. It is our brain, our heart, our memory, a blueprint of the world for all time. Einstein once said that the "field is the only reality."

The Seven Auric Layers of the Human Energy Field

According to Brennan (1988), the human energy field has several components and can be divided into at least seven layers encompassing the body. Each layer has its own frequency and hence its own color. Each is connected through the chakras to the physical body.

First Layer: Ethereal Body

The ethereal layer lies closest to the body and is the energy matrix within which bodily tissues are formed prior to manifesting into physical form. This layer has the same structure as the physical body, including all the anatomical parts and organs. This energy field sets up the matrix in the shape of the body parts prior to their cellular growth in their ultimate physical form, and it does so before the cells materialize physically.

Just 0.25–2 inches in width, light blue to gray in color, the ethereal layer is composed of a sparkling web of energy lines upon which the physical matter of the body tissues is shaped and anchored (Brennan, 1988; Govinda, 2002).

Second Layer: Emotional Body

This layer, which is associated with emotions and feelings, follows the outline of the physical body and penetrates the ethereal field. Extending about 3 inches beyond the physical body (Govinda, 2002), the emotional body comprises all the colors of the rainbow in constant fluid motion. The colors become clearer and more vivid when they are influenced by highly energized feelings such as love, excitement, joy, or anger. Confused and depressive feelings tend to muddy and darken the hue (Brennan, 1988).

Third Layer: Mental Body

The third aura body is associated with thoughts and mental processes. Appearing predominantly as a bright yellow light radiating about the head and shoulders, the third layer extends about 3–8 inches from the body (Govinda, 2002). It extends and brightens as the owner concentrates on mental processes. Thought forms appear as blobs of bright yellow with additional colored hues emanating from the emotional layer (Brennan, 1988).

Fourth Layer: Astral Body

Through this layer and its associated chakra filter all the energies, thoughts, and experiences that ultimately affect us emotionally, physically, and spiritually. The fourth layer is infused with the rose color of love. This dividing band between the lower and upper groups is associated with the heart chakra through which all energies must pass in transit from one group of layers and from one reality to another. In other words, spiritual energy must pass through the heart process to be transformed into physical energy. Conversely, physical energy transforms to spiritual as it exits through the heart chakra. It extends 6–12 inches beyond the body (Govinda, 2002).

A great deal of interaction takes place between people on this astral level. Brennan (1988) claims she can observe energy forms exchanging between a man and a woman fantasizing about lovemaking. She claims there is an actual testing in the energy fields to see whether the fields are synchronous and whether the people are compatible. She adds that when people form relationships, they grow cords out of the aura fields, through the chakras that connect them. The longer the relationship, the more cords there are and the stronger they are. When the relationship ends, the cords are torn, often causing a great deal of pain (heartache) until they disconnect and reroute within the self.

Fifth Layer: Template Body

This layer contains all the forms that exist on the physical plane in a template or blueprint form, like a negative; hence it is known as the template body. This template of the body is projected to the etheric layer (first layer) where body tissues are materialized on the grid matrix upon which the physical body grows. It extends 1.5–2 feet from the body (Brennan, 1988; Govinda, 2002). When distortion in the etheric layer is detected, work is necessary in the template layer to provide support for the etheric layer in its original template form.

To the attuned healer, the template form contains the entire structure of the auric field, including chakras, body organs, and body forms in a negative blueprint format. This layer connects physical reality with other realities.

Sixth Layer: Celestial Body

The sixth layer, or celestial body, is the emotional level of the spiritual plane, through which we experience spiritual ecstasy. We can achieve this experience through meditation and other forms of transformation. From here we can reach a point of "being," where we know our connection with all the universe—we immerse in the Light and feel we are of it and it of us—and we are at one with God (Brennan, 1988).

When the open celestial chakra connects with the open heart chakra, we experience unconditional love of all humanity, of humans in the flesh, and of spiritual love that goes beyond the physical to all realms of reality.

The sixth layer extends 2–3.25 feet from the body in a shimmering opalescent pastel light (Govinda, 2002). It appears to radiate from the body like the glow around a candle.

Seventh Layer: Ketheric Template or Causal Body

The causal body is sometimes considered the closest thing to the soul. The record of all that a soul has experienced on the physical earth plane (during current as well as past lives) is said to be contained in an individual's causal body (Gerber, 2000).

This mental level of the spiritual plane extends about 2.5–3.5 feet in an oval shape around the body. It comprises a shimmering light of golden-silver threads, pulsating at a very high frequency and holding the whole auric form together. It has a thin protective layer on the outside, rather like an eggshell, which protects the enclosed fields (Brennan, 1988).

This golden field supplies the main power current that runs up and down the spine and nourishes the entire body. As this current pulsates up and down the spine, it carries energy through the roots of each chakra and connects them to the energies that the chakras carry into the body.

The seventh layer can be perceived only through the experience of enlightenment—the level of one's divine self (Govinda, 2002).

Meridians: Energy Pathways

Donna Eden (1998) defines *meridians* as "energy pathways that 'connect the dots,' hundreds of tiny reservoirs of heat, electromagnetic, and more subtle energies along the surface of the skin. Known in Chinese medicine as

Kirlian Photography

The aura is traditionally described as a multilayer field of energy surrounding the physical body. The dedicated work of two Russians demonstrated that the aura could be caught on film. Semyon and Valentina Kirlian's experiments with photographing the human energy field resulted in what is now known as Kirlian photography. In 1939, they accidentally discovered that if an object on a photographic plate is subjected to a strong electric field, an image is created on the plate. Unlike a traditional camera that captures light through a glass lens, Kirlian photography is a form of contact photography that captures an image of the electromagnetic energy emitted by any living matter, including human (Gerber, 2000). It may be used in the diagnosis of disease, past or present, in the host body.

Kirlian photography is a new field of research for Western medical science; however, numerous practitioners in eastern Europe use this diagnostic technique (which they term bioelectrography). Physical and emotional health and disease can be identified in plants, animals, and humans using this method (Benor, 2004).

acupuncture points, these energy dots or 'hot spots' can be stimulated with needles or physical pressure to release or redistribute energy" (p. 96).

The meridians affect every organ and every physiological system, including the immune, nervous, endocrine, circulatory, respiratory, digestive, skeletal, muscular, and lymphatic systems. There are 12 main meridians and each is a segment of a single energy pathway that runs throughout the body. Each segment is named for the primary organ or system it services:

- Lung
- Kidney
- Gallbladder
- Liver
- Stomach
- Spleen
- Heart
- Small intestine
- Large intestine
- Urinary bladder
- San jiao (three heater or triple warmer)
- Pericardium (heart protector or circulation sex meridian)

In 1971, medical scientist Robert Becker conducted a series of experiments to test the theory that acupuncture meridians "were electrical conductors that carried an injury message to the brain, which responded by sending back the appropriate level of direct current to stimulate healing in the troubled area" (Becker & Selden, 1985, p. 234). The tests measured the flow of electrical current in the perineural cells just under the skin. The results indicated that each acupuncture point along the way was electrically positive compared to its environs and that each was surrounded by a field with its own characteristic pattern. Later tests isolated the interfering reaction of the nerves along the route, indicating that the response was carried not by the nerves themselves but by the underlying perineurial sleeve.

The Chakras

Chakra is Sanskrit for "wheel." Eden (1998) notes that "while the term *chakra* has its origins in India, many cultures have identified and work with these spiraling centers, and any healer who is sensitive to the body's subtle energies will eventually stumble upon them" (p. 137). Chakras are centers of awareness in the human body. They are neither physical nor anatomical and are found in the subtle energy system (Govinda, 2002). Subtle energies are the energies that exist in the field beyond those defined by the five-sense field, in an energetic spectrum, and in the thought realms, known as the spiritual realm (Micozzi, 2006). Whereas meridians are an energy transportation system, chakras are energy stations (Eden, 1998). Most traditions identify seven major chakras, and each influences organs, muscles, ligaments, veins, and all other systems, especially the endocrine system, within its energy field. Chakras are energy centers traversing the length of the spine, each accounting for a different mode of perception (Smith, 2006).

Chakra work is one of the subtlest methods of healing. Hiroshi Motoyama theorized that if an enlightened individual could influence the chakras, the energy output could be measured. Using a lead-lined recording booth, Motoyama measured the energy fields opposite various chakras that subjects claimed to have awakened, usually through years of meditation. His findings demonstrated significantly greater energy levels at those areas than over the same areas on controlled subjects (Guiley, 1991).

The First (Root) Chakra

The root or base chakra is located at the base of the spine at the perineum (Gerber, 2000; Redmond, 2004). It carries life energies up into the body, through the other chakras, as well as down the legs. This chakra is the grounding connection to the earth's subtle energies; through it we are connected with the earth and our origins (Eden, 1998; Govinda, 2002). Kundalini energy, the power of creativity, resides in the root chakra. The root chakra is as spiritually relevant as the higher chakras, and it is the chakra in which the desire to satisfy sexual needs arises.

The root chakra, linked to the physical body, is most often associated with the color red, but this is not always the case because other colors can be seen in the chakra in response to various influences (Leadbeater, 2001; White, 2004).

The Second (Sacral) Chakra

Known as the sacral or abdominal chakra because of its location over the lower abdominal area, this chakra is the container of imagination and creative impulse (Eden, 1998). It is located directly over the ovaries in women and over the testes in men. The sacral chakra is the center of sensuality, procreation, and sexuality (Gerber, 2000; Govinda, 2002; Redmond, 2004). The second chakra reveals the affection and compassion of the soul—the essence within. Hence most caring and dedicated healers have a strong and active second chakra.

Linked to the etheric body, the sacral chakra is associated with the color orange (White, 2004).

The Third (Solar Plexus) Chakra

The solar plexus chakra, located over the pit of the stomach, is linked with the pancreas and adrenal glands. It contributes to digestive functioning and the body's acute response to stress (Gerber, 2000). To its left side are the spleen, pancreas, and stomach; to its right are the liver and gallbladder; and to the rear, the kidneys and adrenals (Govinda, 2002).

Eden (1998) describes the relationship between the third chakra and the body's organs as follows:

> Each organ's function in your body parallels its role in your emotional life. Consider the organs within the third chakra. As the filtering system that detects toxins in your bloodstream, the kidneys are your prototype for fear and caution, for detecting and eliminating that which is dangerous. As a factory that breaks down whatever is harmful to your system, your liver is your prototype for self-protective anger. As the alarm system that triggers great rushes of energy for emergencies, the adrenals are the prototype for the panic response that mobilizes you in a crisis. As the body's producer of metabolic juices, the pancreas is the prototype for assimilating what you can embrace. As the organ that sends stale air out of your body, the diaphragm is the prototype for grieving and finding closure with whatever is passing out of your life. (p. 152)

Linked to the astral body and plane, the third chakra is associated with the color yellow (White, 2004).

The Fourth (Heart) Chakra

The heart chakra has within its area of influence the heart, lungs, thymus, and pericardium (a protective sac that surrounds the heart). This chakra lies at the center of the chakra system, and in most cultures the heart is linked to the power of love (Govinda, 2002).

As the middle chakra, it has the middle color of the spectrum—green—but other colors may be evident. When the heart chakra emits a golden hue, it usually indicates that the person has a universal love that attracts people to him or her. A soft pink hue is evident in those who are loving, kind, and soft.

Many heart chakras are underdeveloped because people are guided more by their heads than by their hearts. Conversely, disturbances in the heart chakra can cause one to feel easily overwhelmed by others (Govinda, 2002), and people with such disturbances tend to take on everyone's pain and problems to their own detriment. In this case, they should build up the other chakras to create more balance in the entire energy system.

The heart chakra is the center through which all energies must pass in transit from one group of layers and from one reality to another. This chakra and its associated layer filter all energies, thoughts, and experiences, which ultimately affect us emotionally, physically, and spiritually. Linked to the feeling body, the heart chakra is the central focus between the lower and upper groups (White, 2004).

The Fifth (Throat) Chakra

Expression is the product of the throat chakra. Through it, all energies and information are disseminated as they pass to and from the higher seventh and sixth chakras to the lower heart, third, second, and base chakras. This is the filtering point for all data that is sorted, systematized, and then disseminated as our personal expression. The throat chakra is the center of sound and responsible for speech and communication, as well as for hearing (Govinda, 2002).

The throat chakra's areas of influence include the thyroid and parathyroid glands. Just as the thyroid breaks down food for the body, it also breaks down the energies that pass through it to maintain the energy body. All energies that flow up and down the meridians of the body pass through this area. Linked to the lower mental body or plane, the throat chakra is normally associated with the color blue (White, 2004).

The Sixth (Forehead) Chakra

The forehead chakra is the spiritual center of awareness, intelligence, concentration, and intuition (Govinda, 2002; Redmond, 2004). The forehead chakra, or third eye, influences the eyes, ears, lower area of the brain cortex, pituitary gland, and the director of bodily operations, the hypothalamus. Through the sixth chakra, we are able to access the psychic plane and traverse the dimensions of time and space (White, 2004).

Modern thinking, intellect, and busy minds tend to dominate the more subtle but powerful connections to the psychic, which are the channels we use to receive guidance and subtle energies beyond our ordinary perception. This chakra—the third eye—is the portal through which we gain entrance to the spiritual world. Many cultures associate it with psychic development (Govinda, 2002).

The color associated with this chakra is indigo.

The Seventh (Crown) Chakra

The crown chakra, linked with the activity of the pineal gland (Gerber, 2000), is associated with spirituality, the soul, ultimate knowledge, bliss, and the integration of personality with life, which gives us a sense of purpose to our existence (Redmond, 2004). The crown chakra relates to the whole being—physical, mental, spiritual, and emotional—in a holistic state of balance. The central themes of this chakra are spirituality, self-realization, and enlightenment (Govinda, 2002). Meditation, prayer, energy work, and rituals are safe but potent ways of opening the crown chakra and deepening our spiritual awareness and connection (Eden, 1998).

Linked to soul and the causal body (mental level), the crown chakra is associated with the color violet (White, 2004).

ENERGY HEALING DEFINED

Every culture includes the concept that energy can be sensed around people, animals, and plants (Slater, 2005). The ability of humans to tap into and deliver these unseen energies is the fundamental basis of all energy healing.

Dossey, Keegan, and Guzetta (2005) explain energy healing as follows:

> The philosophy underpinning energetic healing is that the soul/mind precedes energy and that energy precedes biology. Radical, yes. It changes everything. If the soul/mind somehow determines the form energy will take, it is ultimately the builder of biology, chemistry, emotions, relationships—everything a person experiences. The body, mind, emotions, and spirit are integrated; in other words, they are different reflections of the same energy and of the same consciousness, not

> separate phenomena. This philosophy enables us to chart our own healing, rather than rely just on outside forces to help us heal. (p. 173)

Slater (2005) defines energetic healing as "the process of using a coherent energy field to induce a change in one's own or another's field" (p. 176). Energy healing alters the subtle flow of energy within and around a person or organism. It is based on the belief that our life force creates energy fields that become unbalanced during emotional or physical disease. Because our energy fields are part of an interconnected whole, an individual's use of focused intention can aid in the health and well-being of another.

As a result of their diverse educational and experiential backgrounds, researchers and practitioners in the field of complementary and alternative medicine (CAM) have different intuitive understandings of the concept of energy healing (Hintz et al., 2003). Although the term suggests an exchange of energy during healing treatments, consistent findings of energies have not been identified across different healing modalities (Benor, 2004). Therefore, the term *energy healing* is broadly meant to describe the basis of healing in various practices, such as Qigong, Reiki (pronounced *ray kee*), Therapeutic Touch, acupuncture, pranic healing, spiritual healing, and distant healing.

Energy healing does not identify a particular type of energy. For instance, distant healing appears to act in a nonlocal, nontemporal, and nonmediated manner and does not conform to the commonly accepted definitions of energy (Dossey, 2002a). In another form of energy healing, the healer acts as a channel, allowing positive energy to pass to the healee through one hand and extracting negative energy with the other hand. In a third form, the healer sends energy out through the palms of both hands to the healee.

According to holistic psychiatric psychotherapist Daniel Benor, MD, ABHM (2004), "Many healers suggest that it is a biological energy *(bioenergy)* interaction between the healer and healee which produces the healing effects. Healers report that they harmonize healees' bioenergies that have become disorganized through trauma, toxins, disease or degenerative processes" (p. 1). Benor (2004) continues:

> While skeptics theorize that healing is no more than a placebo ("sugar pill") effect, produced by healers' suggestions and healees' expectations, this theory is clearly contradicted by the research evidence of healing effects on animals, plants and other living things. The fact that healers can improve the health of animals and plants supports the healers' claims that healing is definitely more than a placebo. The skeptics may not be entirely wrong, however. The placebo effect is actually a manifestation of the enormous self-healing capacities of people to alter their own states of health and illness. (p. 2)

Research demonstrates that energy healing helps relieve pain, reduce anxiety and stress, accelerate wound healing, and promote well-being (Eliopoulos, 2004). Energy treatment modalities have been used for stress reduction; reduction of inflammation, edema, and pain; improvement of appetite, digestion, and sleep patterns; and reduction of anxiety, panic attacks, depression (Leddy, 2006).

Energetic healing ability varies among individuals. In *A Practical Guide to Vibrational Medicine*, Dr. Richard Gerber (2000) says, "Learning to channel healing energy is actually fairly simple. But the degree to which we may each become successful healers will vary from person to person. For instance, most people can play a game of checkers or chess, but not everyone will graduate to the proficiency level of chess master" (p. 398).

TYPES OF ENERGY HEALING

Energy healing programs emerged from both a spiritual tradition and a scientific approach. Despite their dual theoretical foundation, these programs have more similarities than differences. Most programs recognize the spiritual layers of the energy field. Even those that evolved within the nursing profession with a strong scientific base, such as Healing Touch and Therapeutic Touch, include reference to the spiritual levels of life. Energy healing provides an arena where science and spirituality clearly meet.

Today, energy healing courses are available under a myriad of names, including Reiki, pranic healing, Qigong, distant healing, Therapeutic Touch, and Healing Touch. All of these can be assumed to be some form of energy healing.

Reiki

Reiki is a combination of two Japanese words, *rei* and *ki*, meaning universal life energy. This ancient healing technique involves the transference of energy between practitioners and their clients to restore harmony to the biofield, increase the client's energy to heal, and balance the body's subtle energies (physical, emotional, mental, and spiritual) (Trivieri & Anderson, 2002).

Reiki principles evolved from ancient Tibetan Buddhist healing practices and were handed down from teacher to disciple (Trivieri & Anderson, 2002). There are many varieties of Reiki, depending on the beliefs and experience of the teachers. Considered to be a spiritual system, Reiki has been used by practitioners of Christianity, Buddhism, Shintoism, Hinduism, and Islam.

Reiki is used for treating a variety of health conditions, including the effects of stress, chronic pain, and the side effects of chemotherapy and radiation therapy. It is also used to improve immunity, a sense of well-being, and recovery from surgery and anesthesia. Reiki has been demonstrated to decrease anxiety and promote relaxation, support the healing process, and ease distress (Potter, 2007). Clients usually experience a deep feeling of relaxation after a Reiki session. Other experiences include a feeling of warmth, tingling, sleepiness, and being refreshed.

Reiki practitioners undergo a number of training levels. Although Reiki has not received the same degree of scientific study in the United States as Therapeutic Touch and Healing Touch, evidence of its efficacy does exist (Trivieri & Anderson, 2002).

Pranic Healing

Over 5,000 years old, the ancient Indian spiritual tradition talks of a universal energy called prana (Brennan, 1988). *Prana* is a Sanskrit word that means "life-force." The Chinese refer to this subtle energy as qi, and the Old Testament refers to it as ruah ("breath of life"). Yogis practice manipulating this energy through breathing techniques, meditation, and physical exercise to maintain altered states of consciousness (Brennan, 1988).

Pranic healing is a highly developed system of energy-based healing techniques that utilizes prana to balance and harmonize the body's energy processes. The method is a simple yet powerful and effective form of no-touch energy healing. It is based on the principle that the body is a self-repairing living entity that possesses the innate ability to heal itself. Pranic healing therefore accelerates the healing process by increasing the life force, or vital energy, on the affected part of the physical body. Diseases appear as energetic disruptions in the energy field before manifesting as ailments in the physical body. Pranic healing is applied on the bioelectromagnetic field known as the aura. The aura contains the blueprint of the physical body; this bioplasmic body absorbs life energy and distributes it to the organs and glands.

Qigong

Qigong is a combination of two ideas: qi, the vital energy of the body, and gong, the practice of working with qi (Kligler & Lee, 2004). The original concept of qi came from the ancient Chinese philosophical theory of primordial energy, which states that all things in the universe (with or without life) are formed by an invisible yet ever-existing qi.

Qigong stems from an ancient Chinese self-healing energy medicine method that combines movement and meditation. The term *Qigong* was first used in modern China in the 1950s to define a type of health-promoting exercise that emphasized breathing regulation (Schlitz & Amorok, 2005). This self-healing modality stimulates and balances the flow of qi (vital life energy) along the acupuncture meridians (energy pathways in the body). In China, Qigong is a national self-care system of health maintenance and personal development that cultivates inner strength, calms the mind, and restores the body to its natural state of health (Trivieri & Anderson, 2002). Qualified instructors now teach it in the United States in innovative hospital programs, churches, adult education centers, and community fitness programs.

Qigong practitioners develop an awareness of qi sensations (energy) in their bodies and use their minds to guide the qi. Visualizations are used to enhance the mind-body connection and assist healing. Benefits include enhanced vital energy flow, improved circulation, improved resistance to disease and infection, and enhanced immune function (Trivieri & Anderson, 2002).

Distant Healing

Throughout the history of the human race, people have believed that healing can be done at a distance (Dossey, 2002b). *Distant healing*, a term now used at the National Institutes of Health and at an increasing number of hospitals, may be defined as a conscious act of the mind, intended to benefit the physical and/or emotional well-being of another person. Distant healing includes deliberate thoughts, wishes, feelings, images, intentions, meditation, rituals, or prayers.

Terms such as intercessory prayer, nondirected prayer, energy healing, shamanic healing, noncontact therapeutic touch, and spiritual healing have been used to describe interventions that fall into the category of distant healing. Each term describes a particular theoretical, cultural, and pragmatic approach to attempt to mediate a healing or biological change through mental intentions (Targ, 2002).

Studies have provided evidence that certain individuals, operating at a distance under controlled conditions, can positively affect a wide range of living systems, including plants, microbes, animals, and human beings. Distance, even thousands of miles, does not appear to limit the effects of healing (Schlitz & Braud, 1997).

Therapeutic Touch

Derived from the ancient technique of the laying on of hands, Therapeutic Touch is a contemporary interpretation of several ancient healing practices that consist of a learned skill for consciously directing or sensitively modulating human energies (Krieger, 1993). Therapeutic Touch was developed in the early 1970s by Dolores Krieger, PhD, RN, and Dora Kunz, a gifted and respected healer. Both were contemporary pioneers in integrating the spiritual dimension of healing with mainstream professional nursing practices. According to Krieger (1993), several basic scientific assumptions guided the development of Therapeutic Touch:

- All the life sciences agree that, physically, a human being is an open energy system. This implies that the transfer of energy between people is a natural, continuous event.
- Anatomically, a human being is bilaterally symmetrical.
- Illness is the result of an imbalance in the individual's energy field.
- Human beings have the ability to transform and transcend their conditions of living.

Therapeutic Touch is based on the theory that the body, mind, and emotions form a complex energy field (Krieger, 1993). In this form of healing, there may or may not be contact with the client's physical body, but contact is always made with the client's energy field. Practitioners move their hands over the client's body to become attuned to his or her condition, with the intent of strengthening and reorienting the client's energies. Practitioners use the subtle energy fields in and around the body to identify energy imbalances. A typical session lasts 20–30 minutes, while the fully clothed client sits or lies down. Practitioners first center themselves to become harmonious and more deeply connected with the client. Then the practitioner performs an assessment and utilizes his or her energy to effect the client's recovery. Healing is promoted when the body's energies are in balance (Freeman, 2004; Moore & Schmais, 2000; Rankin-Box, 1996).

Clients report a variety of benefits, including feelings of relaxation, improved energy levels, pain reduction, reduced stress, and a general sense of well-being (Trivieri & Anderson, 2002). Studies have demonstrated the effectiveness of Therapeutic Touch in a wide range of conditions, including wound healing, pain, depression, immune function, hypertension, osteoarthritis, migraine headaches, and anxiety in burn clients, among others (Benor, 2004).

Therapeutic Touch is taught mainly by nurses but also by laypersons, and it is currently used by doctors, nurses, and other health professionals in the United States and throughout the world (Seaward, 2006). The most important aspect in healing is the compassionate, focused intentionality of the practitioner toward the client. Hundreds of research studies have been conducted documenting its efficacy for both mental and physical illnesses (Freeman, 2004; Trivieri & Anderson, 2002).

Therapeutic Touch has been associated with relativity theory, quantum theory, and nursing theory.

Healing Touch

Developed by Janet Mentgen, RN, in 1981, Healing Touch is a variation of Therapeutic Touch. Using their hands with light or near-body touch, Healing Touch practitioners help to clear, balance, and energize the human energy system, thus promoting healing for the mind, body, and spirit.

Healing Touch skills are becoming increasingly validated in healthcare systems around the country, and the method is now part of client care systems in many U.S. hospitals. This form of energy healing hastens the healing process, helps to relieve pain, reduces anxiety, and improves one's overall sense of well-being (Trivieri & Anderson, 2002). It has been demonstrated to provide comfort in end-of-life care by providing increased calmness, improved breathing, increased relief of pain, and increased relaxation (Wardell, 2007). Hospitals that support the practice of Healing Touch as part of their integrative healthcare system have found that it facilitates the return of compassion to the forefront of client care.

KEY CONCEPTS

1. Scientists and energy healers around the world have made discoveries that have changed our views about energy healing.
2. The types of energy healing modalities include Reiki, pranic healing, Qigong, distant healing, Therapeutic Touch, and Healing Touch.
3. In these times when natural therapies are increasingly accepted by a wider proportion of the population, healthcare providers can derive profound benefits by adding this extra dimension to their practices and using the unseen energy of the human body—where a large proportion of disease begins—to treat the core of the problem.

QUESTIONS FOR REFLECTION

1. What types of energy healing methods have you experienced and how have they affected your health and well-being?
2. How would you define energy healing?
3. What are the characteristics, locations, and purposes of the seven chakras?

Both Therapeutic Touch and Healing Touch have been sanctioned by the American Holistic Nurses Association since 1989.

REFERENCES

Becker, R. O., & Selden, G. (1985). *The body electric*. New York: Quill.

Benor, D. J. (2004). *Consciousness, bioenergy, and healing*. Medford, NJ: Wholistic Healing.

Brennan, B. A. (1988). *Hands of light: A guide to healing through the human energy field*. New York: Bantam.

Brennan, B. A. (1993). *Light emerging: The journey of personal healing*. New York: Bantam.

Conner, M., & Koithan, M. (2006). The emerging science of energy healing. *AHNA Beginnings*, *26*(1), 1, 26–27.

Dossey, B. M., Keegan, L., & Guzzetta, C. E. (2005). *Holistic nursing: A handbook for practice* (4th ed.). Sudbury, MA: Jones and Bartlett.

Dossey, L. (2002a). But is it energy: Reflections on consciousness, healing, and the new paradigm. *Subtle Energies*, *3*(3), 69–82.

Dossey, L. (2002b). How healing happens: Exploring the nonlocal gap. *Alternative Therapies in Health and Medicine*, *8*(2), 12–16, 103–110.

Eden, D. (1998). *Energy medicine*. New York: Penguin Putnam.

Eliopoulos, C. (2004). *Invitation to holistic health: A guide to living a balanced life*. Sudbury, MA: Jones and Bartlett.

Freeman, L. (2004). *Mosby's complementary and alternative medicine: A research-based approach* (2nd ed.). St. Louis, MO: Mosby.

Gerber, R. (2000). *A practical guide to vibrational medicine*. New York: Quill.

Govinda, K. (2002). *A handbook of chakra healing: Spiritual practice for health, harmony, and inner peace*. Old Saybrook, CT: Konecky and Konecky.

Guiley, R. (1991). *Harper's encyclopedia of mystical and paranormal experience*. New York: HarperCollins.

Hintz, K. J., Yount, G. L., Kadar, I., Schwartz, G., Hammerschlag, R., & Lin, S. (2003). Bioenergy definitions and research guidelines. *Alternative Therapies in Health and Medicine*, *9*, 13–30.

Kligler, B., & Lee, R. (2004). *Integrative medicine: Principles for practice*. New York: McGraw-Hill.

Krieger, D. (1993). *Accepting your power to heal: The personal practice of Therapeutic Touch*. Santa Fe: Bear.

Leadbeater, C. W. (2001). *The chakras*. Wheaton, IL: Quest Books.

Leddy, S. K. (2006). *Integrative health promotion: Conceptual bases for nursing practice* (2nd ed.). Sudbury, MA: Jones and Bartlett.

McTaggart, L. (2002). *The field: The quest for the secret force of the universe.* New York: HarperCollins.

Micozzi, M. S. (2006). *Fundamentals of complementary and integrative medicine* (3rd ed.). St. Louis, MO: Saunders Elsevier.

Moore, K., & Schmais, L. (2000). The ABCs of complementary and alternative therapies and cancer treatment. *Oncology Issues, 15*(6), 20–22.

Oschman, J. L. (2000). *Energy medicine: The scientific basis.* New York: Churchill Livingstone.

Potter, P. (2007). Breast biopsy and distress: Feasibility of testing a Reiki intervention. *Journal of Holistic Nursing, 25*(4), 238–248.

Pressman, M. (2006). Energetic healing. In M. S. Micozzi, *Fundamentals of complementary and integrative medicine* (3rd ed., pp. 313–325). St. Louis, MO: Saunders Elsevier.

Rakel, D. (2007). *Integrative medicine* (2nd ed.). Philadelphia: Saunders Elsevier.

Rankin-Box, D. F. (Ed.). (1996). *The nurses' handbook of complementary therapies.* Edinburgh: Churchill Livingstone.

Redmond, L. (2004). *Chakra meditation: Transformation through the seven energy centers of the body.* Boulder, CO: Sounds True.

Schlitz, M., & Amorok, R. (2005). *Consciousness and healing: Integral approaches to mind-body medicine.* St. Louis, MO: Saunders Elsevier.

Schlitz, M., & Braud, W. (1997). Distant intentionality and healing: Assessing the evidence. *Alternative Therapies in Health and Medicine, 3*(6), 62–73.

Schwartz, G. E. (2007). *The energy healing experiments: Science reveals our natural power to heal.* New York: Atria Books.

Seaward, B. L. (2006). *Managing stress: Principles and strategies for health and well-being* (5th ed.). Sudbury, MA: Jones and Bartlett.

Slater, V. (2005). Energetic healing. In B. M. Dossey, L. Keegan, & C. E. Guzzetta, *Holistic nursing: A handbook for practice* (4th ed., pp. 175–207). Sudbury, MA: Jones and Bartlett.

Smith, K. (2006, March–May). Bioenergetics: A new science of healing. *Shift: At the Frontiers of Consciousness, 10*, 11–13, 34.

Targ, E. (2002). Research methodology for studies of prayer and distant healing. *Complementary Therapies in Nursing and Midwifery, 8*, 29–41.

Tiller, W. A. (1999, May–June). Subtle energies. *Science and Medicine, 6*(3), 28.

Tiller, W. A. (2002). The real world of modern science, medicine, and Qi Gong. *Bulletin of Science, Technology, and Society, 22*(5), 352.

Trivieri, L., Jr., & Anderson, J. W. (Eds.). (2002). *Alternative medicine: The definitive guide* (2nd ed.). Berkeley, CA: Celestial Arts.

Wardell, D. (2007). Using healing touch for end of life care. *AHNA Beginnings, (27)*4, 28–29.

White, R. (2004). *Using your chakras: A new approach to healing your life.* New York: Barnes and Noble Books.

CHAPTER 4

Healing Elements of Meditation

What joy awaits discovery in the silence behind the portals of your mind no human tongue can tell. But you must convince yourself; you must meditate and create that environment.

—Paramahansa Yogananda

LEARNING OBJECTIVES

1. Describe the practice of meditation.
2. Discuss the various meditation traditions.
3. Describe meditation techniques, including breathing meditation, Transcendental Meditation, mindfulness meditation, and concentration meditation.
4. Describe walking and moving meditation, medical meditation, and meditating using visualization.
5. Describe meditating with sound and receptive and creative meditation.
6. List the physiological benefits of meditation.
7. List the psychological benefits of meditation.

INTRODUCTION

Meditation originated in ancient India about 3,000 years ago and has existed in some form in most major religions and in many secular organizations. Because many individuals regularly practice meditation in a prescribed manner, it can also be considered a ritual and a process to spiritual transformation (Taylor, 2002). Meditation is practiced in almost every religion as a way to reach union with the Divine; however, you don't have to be religious to meditate (Borysenko, 2001).

The reasons people meditate vary almost as much as the types of practices. When practiced in a disciplined manner, meditation provides many physiological benefits, such as stress reduction, improved immune and cardiovascular function, relaxation, and decreased pain. Through the learned skill of meditation, people can train their minds to abandon negative qualities and to generate and enhance positive qualities (Dalai Lama, 2003). The regular practice of meditation may also lead to new insights about life issues, heightened creativity, inspiration, greater compassion for others, and a greater connection to one's own inner guidance.

Only over the past few decades has meditation been researched as a medical intervention in Western culture (Freeman, 2004). Fortney and Bonus (2007) note that "meditation is one of the most important components of any health plan. Its unique ability to elicit physical ease and mental stability provides a foundation for healing and directly influences one's ability to meet the challenges resulting from illness and chronic disease" (p. 1051).

THE PRACTICE OF MEDITATION

Individuals approach the practice of meditation from different points of view, from different levels, and for different reasons (Jou, 2000). Some view it as an intensely spiritual experience while others view it as a practice of awareness. Buddhism describes meditation as "stopping and seeing." Christianity describes it as practicing the presence of God, a practice that transforms people in Christ or unites people with God (Chilson, 2004). Another description posits that those who meditate are not trying to experience, visualize, or achieve anything; they are open to whatever is—beyond concept (Borysenko & Dveirin, 2007).

Bright (2002) explains that "the word *meditation* can be used to describe many different methods of quiet contemplation or observation" (p. 105). Both *meditate* and *medical* come from the Latin root *in mederi*, meaning "to cure." Other sources indicate that the word *meditate* comes from the Sanskrit word *medha*, meaning "wisdom" (Leddy, 2006). Still other definitions include "to ponder," "to reflect," and "to contemplate deeply."

Patience is key to achieving success in meditation. The goal of all meditation paths, whatever the method, ideology, or tradition, is to transform the meditator's consciousness (Goleman, 1988).

MEDITATION TYPES BY TRADITION

Meditation has been practiced since people first discovered the joy of sitting quietly and contemplating their inner and outer worlds (Bright, 2002). Used by diverse cultures, meditation is rooted in the traditions of the great religions and has been practiced for thousands of years to alleviate suffering and promote healing. This section explores several meditation traditions:

- Hindu
- Taoist

- Buddhist
- Jewish
- Christian
- Sufi

Hindu Meditation

Hinduism is the oldest religion to practice meditation. Types of meditation in Hinduism include (Goleman, 1988):

- Patanjali's ashtanga yoga (stills the mind)
- Japa yoga (a mantra is repeated aloud or silently)
- Bhakti yoga (the yoga of love and devotion focused on a divine being such as Krishna)
- Indian tantra (alters consciousness by arousing normally latent energies)
- Kundalini yoga (a tantric teaching that a huge spiritual energy reserve is located at the base of the spine and, when activated, travels upward to the higher chakras)
- Surat shabd yoga (sound and light meditation)

Though the means may differ in each method, Goleman (1998) states that "all yogic paths seek to transcend duality in union." Goleman adds that "all these paths see the locus of duality as within the mind, in the separation between the mechanisms of awareness and their object. To transcend duality, the seeker must enter a state in which this gap is bridged, the experiencer and the object merging" (p. 72).

Taoist Meditation

One of the most ancient of the Eastern traditions, Taoism is becoming increasingly popular in the modern West, partly because Taoism is scientific yet also humanistic and spiritual. As Cleary (2000) explains, "Meditation is one element of Taoism that interests a broad spectrum of people, because the state of mind is central to the well-being and efficiency of the whole organism" (p. 2).

Tao is translated in the English language as "the way." Taoism is a way of life and a path toward the ultimate truth. For some, Taoism is a religion; for others, it is a philosophy of life; and for others, it is a science that helps them understand the great cosmos. Shear (2006) defines Tao as "everything we can conceive and can't conceive with our limited mind. It is everything definable and undefinable. It is both physical and nonphysical. It has to be understood through introspection and realization of a greater consciousness" (p. 54).

Taoism can be practiced within the framework of other world religions or without any religious framework at all (Cleary, 2000).

Taoists believe that their lives are not predetermined, so they emphasize cultivating both the spirit and the physical body. They use meditation to clear what they call the mental space (an inner area of the mind for peaceful contemplation) and to allow the meditator to return to the stage known as Wu-chi, or the void. The clearing out of the mental space can be compared to cleaning out a room full of cluttered possessions (Jou, 2000).

While Taoist techniques emphasize the art of harmonizing the breath to reach states of superior ecstasy (Odier, 2003), the various schools of meditation teach different methods. The following seven techniques may be used (Jou, 2000).

- *Concentration:* Concentration can be either internal (concentrating on one point in the body about 2 inches below the navel and 1.5 inches inside the body) or external (focused on an outside object such as a picture).
- *Contemplation:* Contemplation requires a more advanced use of the imagination. An example is experiencing thoughts as individual bubbles rising through the water of the inner self, allowing the meditator to regulate the timing of thoughts and to experience each thought as an individual entity.
- *Counting the breath:* Probably the easiest technique, counting the breath can be practiced by anyone. A breath is a complete cycle of inhalation and exhalation. Any number of breaths can be counted; the important thing is to think only of the counting and the breath. If thoughts disturb this technique, begin again.
- *Meditation of self-inquiry:* A difficult type of meditation, this type involves asking the mind to ask itself who it really is. Each answer must be examined and then rejected in search of a clearer answer as the meditator continues to ask, "What is my inner self?"
- *Unstructured meditation:* This type of meditation has no structure or technique. The mind chooses an image or concept and actively examines and contemplates it. Interfering thoughts are explored and discarded.
- *Use of a sound or mantra:* This is an excellent technique for those who find it difficult to concentrate. The Taoists use a mantra of Who, Shoe, Foo, Way, Chemmy, She, which trains concentration and strengthens the body through the correspondence of each sound with an internal organ.
- *Movement:* An example is Tai Chi Chuan. During this type of meditation one must give up all thoughts and become tranquil.

Buddhist Meditation

In Buddhist practice, meditators learn to simply rest in an awareness of thoughts, feelings, and perceptions as they occur. In the Buddhist tradition, this gentle awareness is known as *mindfulness*, which is the art of becoming deeply aware of the present moment and experiencing what happens in the now. In Buddhism, loving-kindness meditation has been used for centuries to develop love and transform anger into compassion. Preliminary research demonstrates that a loving-kindness program can be beneficial in reducing pain, anger, and psychological distress in clients with chronic low back pain (Carson et al., 2005).

Tibetan Buddhism Meditation

In this practice, the meditator realizes three moral precepts—known as the triple refuge of Buddha, Dharma, and Sangha—as internal realities. The Tibetan Buddhist meditator follows three precepts:

- *Sila:* Vows of upright behavior
- *Samadhi:* Fixing the mind on one object to develop one-pointedness
- *Vipassana:* The discarding of ego beliefs

The Dalai Lama (2003) explains that "the whole purpose of meditation is to lessen the deluded afflictions of our mind and eventually eradicate them from their very roots" (p. 21). In Tibetan Buddhism, the fundamentals of the path to highest enlightenment are compassion, altruistic thought, and the perfect view. Fundamental in effecting this positive transformation is the practice of the three trainings (Dalai Lama, 2003):

- Renunciation, or the determination to be free from the prison-like three realms of existence and to transcend suffering
- The awakening mind of bodhichitta, an altruistic wish to achieve Buddhahood for the sake of all sentient beings
- Wisdom, or realizing emptiness

It is difficult to assess the true nature of Tibetan Buddhism without participating in its practices. Specific methods in Tibetan Buddhism are transmitted only from teacher (guru) to student in centuries-old teaching lineages (Goleman, 1988).

Zen Buddhism Meditation

Zen is similar to Taoism in many ways and differs from other forms of Buddhism (Chilson, 2004). Unlike other Buddhist schools of thought, Zen includes the following four characteristics (Odier, 2003):

- Transmission of information beyond what is told in the Buddhist scriptures
- Non-reliance on and detachment from the ancient texts
- Realization of the absolute purity of one's mind
- Contemplation of one's own nature in order to obtain the state of the Buddha

Zen teaches that awakening must be experienced in all of life's activities, which are symbolized by the four postures of walking, standing, sitting, and lying. Sitting is the most common posture because it is the most stable (Roshi, 2006). In Zen, seated meditation is called zazen. Roshi (2006) describes it this way:

> Zazen is an endless path, with as much to offer the beginner as to the longtime meditator. The experience only grows in depth and richness as we continue on. Where in life is there true happiness and meaning outside of this? Money can be replaced, property can be recovered, but time, once past will never come again. No one knows when death will strike, or when failing health will make practice difficult. Each moment of life is precious. While we still have life, let us do what we can to realize our true mind. (p. 21)

In zazen, the meditator's goal is to let go of all external distractions, return to the original stillness within, and discover the essence of who he or she truly is. Full lotus (cross-legged with the feet pressed into the groin) and half lotus (cross-legged with the feet pressed into the fold of the leg) are the preferred ways of sitting to create a stable foundation. Sitting cushions, known as zafu, help support the body to maintain the correct posture (Roshi, 2006). In the sitting posture, the meditator aims for a heightened state of concentrated awareness with no primary objective. The meditator sits, with open eyes, aware of whatever goes on in and around him or her, alert and mindful, free from discriminating thoughts, merely watching (Goleman, 1988). Roshi (2006) describes the accompanying breathing as follows: "Open, relaxed, and expansive breathing is essential to the practice of zazen. The exhalations should be long, extended, and without tightness in the area of the diaphragm" (p. 7).

Jewish Meditation

Although many people are surprised to hear the term *Jewish meditation*, the tradition goes back thousands of years (Kaplan, 1985). Meditation was practiced by a large portion of the Israelite people during the period when the Bible was written, and prophets led regular schools of meditation. Kaplan (1985) notes that "references to Jewish meditation are found in major Jewish texts in every period from biblical to the post modern era" (p. 40). Both the

Talmud and the Midrash state that millions of people practiced meditation (Kaplan, 1985).

Most writers focus on the mystical elements of Jewish meditation practices that are explained in Hassidic philosophy and in Kabbalah (a meditative field of study involving the hidden teachings of Judaism) (Goleman, 1988). However, there is a strong tradition of meditation and mysticism in mainstream Judaism as well (Kaplan, 1985).

Oral Conversation as a Meditative Practice

Using oral conversation as a meditative practice is an ancient Jewish tradition documented in a number of Jewish texts. Three important factors are addressed in this type of meditation (Kaplan, 1985):

- It is a verbal type of meditation that involves words in thought or speech rather than images.
- It is inner directed rather than determined by an external stimulus.
- It is unstructured and the meditator has no preconceived notion of which direction the meditation will take.

Meditation Using a Written Agenda

Another type of meditation is meditating with a written agenda, a practice favored by the Musar schools in Judaism. Used by the mystics of Safed in the 16th century, this structured type of meditation might use a biblical verse as the object of the meditation.

Action Meditation

A third type, action meditation, is most important when connected with the performance of the commandments and rituals. Many Jewish sources speak of the commandments as meditative devices that can bring a person to a high level of God consciousness.

According to Kaplan (1985), "any action can be seen as using the kinesthetic sense, even if other senses are involved" (p. 23). The most important aspect is to concentrate on the act and elevate it to an expression of divine worship. The act can be something as simple or commonplace as washing the dishes.

Christian Meditation

Christian meditation is a form of prayer that goes back to the time of Jesus and the Jewish tradition. The first Christian monks sought isolation to commune with God, free of worldly distractions. Although they used the teachings of Jesus as their inspiration, their meditative techniques were similar to those from the East: they meditated with a verbal or silent repetition of a single phrase from the Scriptures, the Christian equivalent of a mantra (Goleman, 1988).

The term *centering prayer* is new to the 20th century and is best described as a receptive method of meditation. Inspired by the acclaimed Catholic spiritual writer Thomas Merton, centering prayer in its purity seeks nothing for the meditator. The meditator seeks simply and totally to give himself or herself to the Divine, to God (Fortney & Bonus, 2007; Pennington, 2006). Pennington (2006) gives an example of a centering prayer:

- Sitting relaxed and quiet with your eyes closed
- Being in faith and love to God
- Choosing a sacred word (such as *God, peace, love, nature*) as your intention to consent to God's presence and action within
- Being aware of your thoughts and gently returning to your sacred word
- Remaining in silence with your eyes closed for a couple of minutes at the end of your prayer period

Another example comes from *Morning Meditation* by James Webb (2007). He offers readers 12 guiding principles to help develop a one-on-one relationship with God and he believes that practicing morning meditation can help people reveal their part in co-creating their own destiny with God. Webb's 12 guiding principles include the following:

1. *Know what you want:* Focus on what you want, not on what you don't want.
2. *Choose to be happy:* Happiness is a thought in the now and independent of people, things, or circumstances.
3. *Play a game of make-believe:* Co-create your own destiny with the power of your thoughts.
4. *Use your powers for good:* Your enlightened presence can uplift the energy of your environment.
5. *Life is easy:* You can make your life complicated or choose to make it simple.
6. *You get to know only the next step:* Enjoy the precise moment of your journey.
7. *Choose your friends wisely:* Choose friends who uplift you and add positive value to your life.
8. *Work from within your core of creativity:* Contribute your gifts and talents to the rest of humanity, and you will find an unlimited supply of possibilities for yourself.

9. *Return to the basics:* Eat healthily, exercise daily, drink plenty of water, get enough sleep, and maintain a clean and organized home.
10. *Know that you are loved:* God loves you.
11. *There is only plan A:* You can have the life you choose to have.
12. *Have a theme song:* Singing uplifts the spirit; find your own theme song that energizes you.

Webb's morning meditations include some of the same practices as other forms of meditation, such as praying, reading, professing the Word, giving thanks, creating good thought, journaling, and listening to music.

Sufi Meditation

Sufism is a path of love and the ancient wisdom of the heart. According to Goleman (1988), "For the Sufi, the basic human weakness is being bound by the lower self" (p. 59). In the Sufi tradition, saints are those who have overcome their lower nature, and meditation is essential for novices who seek to escape their lower natures and purify their hearts (Goleman, 1988). The Sufi is on a journey back to God that takes place within the heart.

Sufis believe that meditation is essential to purify the heart, and they aim for a total and permanent purity. Vaughn-Lee (2006) states that Sufi meditation takes the meditator from the world of duality to the oneness within the heart; it is not limited by time, place, or form. In Sufi tradition, the mind is purified and disciplined through the continual practice of meditation. The first step is learning the art of listening—the art of being inwardly present, attentive, and empty. The next step is learning to be silent, because listening is born from silence, and in silence the meditator connects with the Beloved (Vaughn-Lee, 2006).

Sufi paths call for different meditation techniques. The two central practices of the Naqshbandi path are the silent *dhikr* (remembrance of God) and the silent meditation of the heart. Goleman (1988) notes that "the main meditation among Sufis is *zikr*, which means 'remembrance'" (p. 59). In this practice, the meditator believes that there is no god but God and the way to purity is by a constant remembrance of God. Remembrance of God involves repeating His name, thus purifying the seeker's mind and opening the heart to Him. As is common to most meditation systems, the goal of zikr is to overcome the mind's natural state of carelessness and inattention (Goleman, 1988).

MEDITATION TECHNIQUES

Although there are many ways to meditate and many forms of meditation, they all share the characteristic of intentionally training the attention and concentration. All meditative techniques involve conscious breathing and a focus on what is happening in each present moment until the mind becomes empty of thoughts, judgments, and past and future concerns (Reynolds, 2001).

In describing meditation, Dyer (2003) states that "the paramount reason for making meditation a part of our daily life is to join forces with our sacred energy and regain the power of our Source (God)" (p. 2). He discusses "the gap," which he defines as the place where miracles occur and the space between thoughts. Awaiting people in the gap is the experience of activating the higher dimensions of insight, intuition, and creativity and a conscious contact with God that creates a feeling of enchantment, bliss, relaxation, and peace.

Many people have difficulty getting into the gap due, in part, to the fact that silence is not cultivated in our society. It takes practice to quiet the mind. New meditators may find it helpful to remember the following guidelines (Dyer, 2003):

- There is no such thing as a bad meditation because it is valuable to spend any amount of time in silence.
- Meditation takes time, but your inner dialogue will shut down and you will slip into the gap.
- There is no right or wrong time to meditate.
- There is no correct length of time to meditate (approximately 30 minutes is usually optimal, but even a few minutes can be nurturing).
- There is no correct posture or place for meditating; it's whatever works for you.

Kaplan (1985) describes meditation as thinking in a controlled manner, deciding how you wish to direct the mind, and then doing it. While controlling the thoughts to stop thinking may sound simple, those who are new to the meditative experience find it amazingly difficult (Kaplan, 1985). Here are some additional suggestions for a successful meditation practice (Fortney & Bonus, 2007):

- Create a quiet and secluded sanctuary.
- Meditate on an empty stomach.
- Beginners should not meditate too long.
- Be consistent with regular meditation.
- Try meditating with others in a group.
- Choose a meditation form that resonates with your intuition, needs, and beliefs.

The following methods may help you enter into a meditative state:

- Breathing techniques
- Transcendental Meditation
- Mindfulness meditation
- Concentration meditation

- Moving and walking meditation
- Medical meditation
- Meditating using visualization
- Meditating with sound
- Creative and receptive meditation

Breathing Techniques

The breath is an almost universal object for meditation (Chilson, 2004). Christianity views breath as the presence of the Holy Spirit within each person. In Judaism the word for breath is *ruach* (the spirit of God). In Sanskrit the word for breath is *prana* (the intuitive wisdom beyond words or concepts). The Chinese word for breath is *qi*.

Using breathing techniques is one of the simplest meditation practices and an important component of most forms of meditation.

- One breathing technique involves counting each breath while breathing in and out. Each inhalation and exhalation together count as one breath. Usually the individual breathes in slowly through the nose (counting from 1 to 10) and breathes out slowly through the mouth (counting backward from 10 to 1).
- Meditation on the breath is a technique that cultivates both concentration and mindfulness. To start, become aware of your breath, each inhalation and exhalation. Feel the sensations in your nostrils or note the rise and fall of your stomach as you breathe. Do not try to control your breath, just be aware of it. If your mind wanders, gently bring it back to your breath. Let go of all other thoughts and distractions (Goleman, 1988).
- Another method is called spaced breathing, which involves taking as much time as possible between breaths. The individual breathes gently and slowly and counts to five for each inhalation, holds the breath for a count of five, and then exhales to a count of five (Reynolds, 2001; Taylor, 2002).

Transcendental Meditation (TM)

In 1957, His Holiness Maharishi Mahesh Yogi offered the world *Transcendental Meditation* (TM), a universal meditation technique based on a summation of the ancient Vedic wisdom of the Himalayas and the growth of scientific thinking in the Western world (Maharishi Mahesh Yogi, 2001). This technique originated over 1,200 years ago in India and had its origin in Advaita Vedanta, one of six traditional systems of ancient India. Shear (2006) describes

Transcendental Meditation as "an effortless mental technique that quickly and easily enables any ordinary person to experience the source of thought deep within his or her own mind" (p. 23).

For centuries, only a limited number of people had access to this technique. After the death of Swami Brahmananda Saraswati in the 20th century, his close disciple Maharishi Mahesh Yogi went to live in seclusion in the foothills of the Himalayas. When he returned a few years later, he began to teach the Transcendental Meditation technique. He considers duality as the fundamental cause of suffering, and his technique for transcending duality begins with the repetition of a mantra (a Sanskrit word or sound) selected specifically for each person (Goleman, 1988).

According to Shear (2006), the immediate goal of Transcendental Meditation is to "bring forth the latent potential each of our minds has to experience bliss, freedom, higher states of consciousness, and fulfillment in daily life. The broader goal is to provide the precondition for world peace" (p. 24). In this discipline, bliss is believed to arrive with the stillness of the mind. The goal of the mantra, according to the Maharishi, is transcendental consciousness, when the mind loses all contact with the outside and is content in this state (Goleman, 1988).

Over a 10-year span, the progression of the meditators' experiences inspired the Maharishi to identify seven distinct states of consciousness (Maharishi Mahesh Yogi, 2001):

- Waking
- Dreaming
- Sleeping
- Transcendental consciousness (The mind transcends even the finest aspect of thought, makes contact with Being, and becomes completely silent and at rest, yet fully awake inside.)
- Cosmic consciousness (The deep silence of transcendental consciousness is never lost, whether one is waking, sleeping, or dreaming.)
- God consciousness (Unbounded, unlimited love overflows in all directions for everything.)
- Unity consciousness (The individual experiences perfection of life, a life lived on the level of the ultimate Unity of all life, a life of all possibilities.)

Transcendental Meditation techniques allow the mind to progressively experience higher levels of thought until it experiences the source of thought (pure consciousness) (Freeman, 2004). Meditators usually practice 20 minutes in the morning and 20 minutes in the evening (Leddy, 2006).

Hundreds of research studies have demonstrated the following health benefits of a consistent Transcendental Meditation practice (Maharishi Mahesh Yogi, 2001; Riley, Ehling, & Sancier, 2004; Shear, 2006):

- Decreased need for medical treatment
- Decreased healthcare costs
- Reduced hospital admissions
- Increased blood flow to the brain
- More stable autonomic nervous system
- Positive psychological mood
- Enhancement of creativity and happiness
- Decreased anxiety
- Reduced hypertension
- Reduced stress-related issues
- Improved asthmatic conditions

Mindfulness Meditation

Traditionally rooted in Eastern meditation disciplines, *mindfulness meditation* is universal in practice and uses breath awareness as a starting point (Fortney & Bonus, 2007; Riley et al., 2004).

Jon Kabat-Zinn developed mindfulness meditation by drawing from the traditions of Zen and other Buddhist meditation practices (Kabat-Zinn, 1994; Leddy, 2006; Sierpina, 2001). In Buddhism, meditation is called the path of mindfulness, the path of right understanding, and the path of the wheel of truth (dharma). Kabat-Zinn (1994) describes mindfulness meditation as a way rather than a technique: "It is a Way of being, a Way of living, a Way of listening, a Way of walking along the path of life and being in harmony with things as they are" (p. 88). Kabat-Zinn adds, "Mindfulness has to do above all with attention and awareness, which are universal qualities" (p. xvii).

The practice of mindfulness meditation includes eight key factors: nonjudgment, being in the present moment, patience, beginner's mind, trust, nonstriving, acceptance, and letting go (Kabat-Zinn, 1994; Leddy, 2006). In mindfulness meditation, the meditator directs awareness to whatever presents itself, which could be an external object or sound or an internal sensation, emotion, or thought. The meditator notices the passing object or internal sensation but does not attach to it; he or she is aware of whatever may come. The result is a sense of resting in the present moment (Bright, 2002). The meditator observes without emotional reaction, judgment, or analysis. The goal is to observe the observer; that is, to get outside yourself and observe your own thought processes (Seaward, 2006).

Research has been conducted in small studies on mindfulness meditation for the treatment of anxiety and chronic pain. However, large-scale studies are needed to provide empirical evidence (Plews-Ogan, Owens, Goodman, Wolfe, & Schorling, 2005; van der Watt, Laugharne, & Janca, 2008).

Concentration Meditation

Concentration meditation is the process of bringing the mind to a single focus (Borysenko, 2001). This type of meditation is common to most religions and spiritual practices. The meditator focuses on an external object (such as a candle flame, picture, or music) or on something internal (such as the meditator's own breath, pulse, or heartbeat). Visualization is often called concentration meditation (Bright, 2002). The simplest form of concentration meditation is to sit quietly and focus one's attention on the breath (Trivieri & Anderson, 2002). As the meditator focuses on slowing down inhaling and exhaling, breathing becomes slower and deeper, and the mind becomes calm.

Seaward (2006) lists five actions that help the meditator focus on a single thought in concentration meditation:

- *Mental repetition:* A thought is produced over and over, most commonly by the use of a one-syllable mantra (e.g., "om," "one," "peace," "love") or a short positive phrase (e.g., "I feel good," "I am calm").
- *Visual concentration:* The meditator visually focuses on or stares at an object or image. Common visual objects include a candle flame, flower, seashell, or mandala (an intricately designed circular object).
- *Repeated sounds:* A sound is repeated continually to help focus the mind's attention (e.g., beating drum, chimes, Tibetan bells, Gregorian chants). Natural sounds include those of a waterfall, ocean waves, or rolling thunder.
- *Physical repetition:* Meditators use repetitive motion, such as some form of rhythmic exercise (e.g., running, walking, swimming). Pranayama or diaphragmatic breathing is also used.
- *Tactile repletion:* The meditator holds a small object (e.g., a stone, a shell, or beads).

Moving and Walking Meditation

In addition to performing meditation while sitting or lying down, a person can meditate while moving or walking.

Moving Meditation

Moving meditation includes yoga, Qigong, Therapeutic Touch, Sufi dancing, and Native American and shamanic ritual dance. Moving meditation helps the body get rid of high levels of stress chemicals, leaving it more relaxed (Achterberg, Dossey, & Kolkmeier, 1994).

Walking Meditation

Walking meditation is especially beneficial during times of crisis and trauma; it helps practitioners center themselves in the most challenging circumstances.

To perform walking meditation, practitioners can start by focusing on the footfall as a whole, or they can start with the left foot and begin walking slowly while synchronizing the breathing in and out with each step. Walking meditation may be practiced at any pace (Anselmo, 2005; Kabat-Zinn, 1994).

Walking the labyrinth is another form of meditation. It combines the actions of the body, mind, and spirit with the imagery of the circle and the spiral to create a purposeful path. An ancient activity, walking the labyrinth is reemerging in churches, schools, parks, and medical centers, where staff, clients, and families walk the labyrinth to reduce stress, relax, and deal with loss and grief. The meditative response to walking the labyrinth is both formal and ritualistic. It includes three phases:

1. *Releasing* occurs during the walk as the practitioner empties the mind and repeats a word, chant, or prayer.
2. *Receiving* occurs when the walker is in the center of the labyrinth (sitting or standing while inviting an opening to healing, connection, renewal).
3. *Returning* involves retracing one's steps in the opposite direction.

Walkers may experience a change of energy in mind, body, and spirit. The average labyrinth walk is about 20 minutes, and the intention is to evoke physiological, affective, and spiritual outcomes (Sandor & Froman, 2006).

Medical Meditation

Medical meditation, created by Dharma Singh Khalsa, MD, in 1979, is one of the newest and leading-edge advances in the field of integrative medicine. Using advanced meditative techniques in a modern clinical setting, medical meditation combines elements of meditation with Kundalini yoga to produce a practice that focuses on treating medical conditions (Khalsa & Stauth, 2001). By combining medical meditations with appropriate medical treatment, Khalsa created treatments for diabetes, hypertension, migraines, symptoms of premenstrual syndrome, and psoriasis.

The healing energy that medical meditation generates is a complete mind-body-spirit connection. It uses specific breathing patterns, movements, mantras, and mental focus to channel energy to specific glands, organs, and energy zones.

Meditating Using Visualization

Visualization techniques, another form of meditation, can include picturing a sacred place, focusing on an external object, or visualizing sacred symbols (Reynolds, 2001; Taylor, 2002).

- *Picturing a sacred place:* The place may be real or imaginary, such as a stream with water flowing over the boulders, a mountain landscape, an ocean scene, or the image of a forest. Contemplating this scene transports the individual to a meditative state.
- *Focusing on an external object:* This practice may involve keeping the eyes open and focusing on a single object (such as a candle flame) for a specific period of time.
- *Visualizing sacred symbols:* The meditator visualizes certain symbols and shapes regarded as sacred in his or her culture. For example, Hindus and Buddhists use a mandala, a graphic representation depicting the universe. Sacred symbols can help individuals connect with their deep subconscious awareness and create a meditative state.

Meditating with Sound

Meditation with sound is meditation using mantras, chanting, singing bowls, drums, or CDs to incorporate sound vibrations in the promotion of a meditative state of mind (Reynolds, 2001).

- *Mantras* involve synchronizing the breathing with the silent repetition of a sound, word, or phrase (such as sacred Sanskrit syllables and words like "om").
- *Chanting* involves repeating certain words or sounds aloud.
- *Singing bowls*, usually made of a unique alloy or quartz crystal, are rubbed or struck with a wooden stick to create soothing sounds that invoke a meditative state.
- *Drums* are beaten in rhythm with the breath or heartbeat to create a deep meditative state.

- *CDs* of music, nature sounds, or meditation instructions can help create a relaxed meditative state.

Creative and Receptive Meditation

Harbula (2005) divides the various meditation processes into two basic forms: creative and receptive meditation:

> Creative meditation can consist of any type of guided imagery or mental focus that creates an altered state of consciousness that is conducive to inner discovery or growth. Receptive meditation is the act of transcending the thought process completely, stilling the rational mind, and experiencing a quality of consciousness more subtle than thought. (p. 168)

Through receptive meditation, many have had mystical experiences or experienced cosmic consciousness (an awareness of the universal mind and one's unity with it). Most meditators practice a combination of creative and receptive meditation. For example, watching the breath or chanting can be considered a creative meditation designed to lead the meditator into a state of receptive meditation (Harbula, 2005).

HEALTH BENEFITS OF MEDITATION

The regular, consistent practice of meditation may improve a variety of medical conditions ranging from hypertension to chronic pain (Riley et al., 2004). Micozzi (2006) notes that "many studies have found that various practices of meditation appear to produce physical and psychological changes" (p. 293). The following physiological and psychological changes occur with regular meditation practice (Carlson, Speca, Patel, & Goodey, 2004; Eliopoulos, 2004; Freeman, 2004; Lane, Seskevich, & Pieper, 2007; Seaward, 2006; Trivieri & Anderson, 2002).

Physiological Benefits

- Decreased oxygen consumption
- Decreased blood lactate levels
- Decreased cortisol (a major stress hormone)
- Increased skin resistance
- Decreased heart and respiration rate
- Decreased blood pressure
- Decreased muscle tension
- Increased alpha waves

- Decreased pain
- Improved respiratory conditions

Psychological Benefits

- Improved mental health
- Reduced perception of stress
- Reduced anxiety and depression
- Increased degree of self-actualization
- Increased locus of control
- Improved sleep
- Increased sense of well-being
- Increased sense of peace
- Increased awareness and spiritual calm

KEY CONCEPTS

1. Meditation practices are used by diverse cultures all over the world, are rooted in the traditions of the great religions, and have been practiced for thousands of years to alleviate suffering and promote healing.
2. The goal of all meditation paths—whatever the method, ideology, or tradition—is to transform the meditator's consciousness.
3. When practiced in a disciplined manner, meditation provides many physiological and psychological benefits, such as a reduced perception of stress, improved immune and cardiovascular function, increased sense of peace, reduced anxiety, decreased blood pressure, and decreased pain.

QUESTIONS FOR REFLECTION

1. What are the differences between the types of meditation?
2. What are the physiological and psychological effects of meditation on the mind and body?
3. What types of meditation techniques have you practiced?

REFERENCES

Achterberg, J., Dossey, B., & Kolkmeier, L. (1994). *Rituals of healing: Using imagery for health and wellness.* New York: Bantam Books.

Anselmo, J. (2005). Relaxation: The first step to restore, renew, and self-heal. In B. M. Dossey, L. Keegan, & C. E. Guzzetta, *Holistic nursing: A handbook for practice* (4th ed., pp. 523–564). Sudbury, MA: Jones and Bartlett.

Borysenko, J. (2001). *Inner peace for busy people.* Carlsbad, CA: Hay House.

Borysenko, J., & Dveirin, G. (2007). *Your soul's compass.* Carlsbad, CA: Hay House.

Bright, M.A. (2002). *Holistic health and healing.* Philadelphia: F. A. Davis.

Carlson, L., Speca, M., Patel, K., & Goodey, E. (2004). Mindfulness-based stress reduction in relation to quality of life, mood, symptoms of stress and levels of cortisol dehydroeplandrosterone sulfate (DHEAS) and melatonin in breast and prostate cancer outpatients. *Psychoneuroendocrinology, 29*(4), 448–474.

Carson, J., Keefe, F., Lynch, T., Carson, K., Goli, V., Fras, A., et al. (2005). Loving-kindness meditation for chronic low back pain. *Journal of Holistic Nursing, 23*(3), 287–309.

Chilson, R. W. (2004). *Meditation: Exploring a great spiritual practice.* Notre Dame, IN: Sorin Books.

Cleary, T. (2000). *Taoist meditation: Methods for cultivating a healthy mind and body.* Boston: Shambhala.

Dalai Lama. (2003). *Stages of meditation.* Ithaca, NY: Snow Lion.

Dyer, W. (2003). *Getting in the gap: Making conscious contact with God through meditation.* Carlsbad, CA: Hay House.

Eliopoulos, C. (2004). *Invitation to holistic health: A guide to living a balanced life.* Sudbury, MA: Jones and Bartlett.

Fortney, L., & Bonus, K. (2007). Recommending meditation. In D. Rakel, *Integrative medicine* (pp. 1051–1071). Philadelphia: Saunders Elsevier.

Freeman, L. (2004). *Mosby's complementary and alternative medicine: A research-based approach* (2nd ed.). St. Louis, MO: Mosby.

Goleman, D. (1988). *The meditative mind.* New York: G. P. Putman's Sons.

Harbula, P. (2005). *The magic of the soul: Applying spiritual power to daily living.* Thousand Oaks, CA: Peak.

Jou, T. H. (2000). *The Tao of meditation: Way to enlightenment.* Scottsdale, AZ: Tai Chi Foundation.

Kabat-Zinn, J. (1994). *Wherever you go, there you are: Mindfulness meditation in everyday life.* New York: Hyperion.

Kaplan, A. (1985). *Jewish meditation: A practical guide.* New York: Schocken Books.

Khalsa, D., & Stauth, C. (2001). *Meditation as medicine: Activate the power of your natural healing force.* New York: Fireside.

Lane, J., Seskevich, J., & Pieper, C. (2007). Brief meditation training can improve perceived stress and negative mood. *Alternative Therapies in Health and Medicine, 13*(1), 38–44.

Leddy, S. K. (2006). *Integrative health promotion: Conceptual bases for nursing practice* (2nd ed.). Sudbury, MA: Jones and Bartlett.

Maharishi Mahesh Yogi. (2001). *Science of being and art of living: Transcendental Meditation.* New York: Plume.

Micozzi, M. S. (2006). *Fundamentals of complementary and integrative medicine* (3rd ed.). St. Louis, MO: Saunders Elsevier.

Odier, D. (2003). *Meditation techniques of the Buddhist and Taoist masters.* Rochester, VT: Inner Traditions.

Pennington, B. (2006). Centering prayer: An ancient Christian way of meditation. In J. Shear (Ed.), *The experience of meditation* (pp. 245–257). St. Paul, MN: Paragon House.

Plews-Ogan, M., Owens, J., Goodman, M., Wolfe, P., & Schorling, J. (2005). A pilot study evaluating mindfulness-based stress reduction and massage for the management of chronic pain. *Journal of General Internal Medicine, 20*(12), 1136–1138.

Reynolds, C. (2001). *Spiritual fitness.* London: Thorsons.

Riley, D., Ehling, D., & Sancier, K. (2004). Movement and body-centered therapies. In B. Kligler & R. Lee, *Integrative medicine: Principles for practice* (pp. 241–254). New York: McGraw-Hill.

Roshi, S. (2006). Zazen meditation in Japanese Rinzai Zen. In J. Shear (Ed.), *The experience of meditation* (pp. 1–21). St. Paul, MN: Paragon House.

Sandor, M., & Froman, R. (2006). Exploring the effects of walking the labyrinth. *Journal of Holistic Nursing, 24*(2), 103–110.

Seaward, B. L. (2006). *Managing stress: Principles and strategies for health and well-being* (5th ed.). Sudbury, MA: Jones and Bartlett.

Shear, J. (Ed.). (2006). *The experience of meditation.* St. Paul, MN: Paragon House.

Sierpina, V. (2001). *Integrative health care: Complementary and alternative therapies for the whole person.* Philadelphia: F. A. Davis.

Taylor, E. J. (2002). *Spiritual care: Nursing theory, research, and practice.* Upper Saddle River, NJ: Prentice Hall.

Trivieri, L., Jr., & Anderson, J. W. (Eds.). (2002). *Alternative medicine: The definitive guide* (2nd ed.). Berkeley, CA: Celestial Arts.

van der Watt, G., Laugharne, J., & Janca, A. (2008). Complementary and alternative medicine in the treatment of anxiety and depression. *Current Opinion in Psychiatry, 21*(1), 37–42.

Vaughn-Lee, L. (2006). The Sufi meditation of the heart. In J. Shear (Ed.), *The experience of meditation* (pp. 223–244). St. Paul, MN: Paragon House.

Webb, J. (2007). *Morning meditation: Develop an intimacy with God and discover your destiny.* Longwood, FL: Xulon Press.

CHAPTER 5

Place and Space: Healing Environments

Nature is but another name for health.
—Henry David Thoreau

LEARNING OBJECTIVES

1. Define *healing environment.*
2. Describe the historical evolution of healing environments.
3. Identify the outcomes of a healing environment.
4. Describe the roles of color, nature, and lighting in creating a healing environment.
5. Describe the roles of air quality, temperature, and smells in a healing environment.
6. Describe the roles of music, noise, buildings, and furnishings in a healing environment.
7. Define *wayfinding* and describe its importance in a healthy environment.
8. Describe specific considerations when designing a healing environment for children.
9. Describe the roles of communication and education in a healthy environment.
10. Explain the role of the healthcare provider in creating a healing environment.

INTRODUCTION

Schweitzer, Gilpin, and Frampton (2004) assert that people have probably been seeking a "safe shelter in which to heal" since the beginning of time. "When little could be done to treat the physical causes of illness or injury," they add, "a safe, supportive environment where natural or supernatural forces could aid the recuperative process to help the patient heal was vital" (p. S71). Today, we specifically design and build spaces that induce healing and restorative effects.

Florence Nightingale, the founder of modern nursing, said that nature alone cures and that all we need to do is put our clients in the best condition for nature to act on them. Nightingale was one of the first healthcare professionals to realize the impact of the environment on the client's ability to heal. She was also among the first to explore and document the healthcare professional's role in employing nature and the environment in such a way that clients could begin their healing journey. Nightingale understood the connection between body and mind, and she understood the environment's role in healing them. She knew that clients would recover more quickly if they were cared for in environments with natural light, cleanliness, and basic sanitation. She even created drawings and notes that changed hospital design (Stichler, 2001).

Healthcare providers have the power to create the kind of healing environment that allows clients to access their inner healer—that phenomenon of healing that transcends social, cultural, economic, time, and space barriers and promotes healing. Healthy environments and sacred spaces are powerful ways to support the inner healer and to utilize the environment to maximize its healing effects.

WHAT IS A HEALING ENVIRONMENT?

The word *healing* is derived from the Anglo-Saxon word *hael*, which means "to make whole" or "to become whole" (Daniels, Nosek, & Nicoll, 2007). Healing is not the same as curing (which means to rid of disease). Healing is meant to enhance all aspects of well-being, restore integrity to the person, and facilitate the creation of meaning in the individual's life (Geller & Warren, 2004). The healing process uses the individual's own inner healing abilities, and a healing environment allows clients to mobilize resources from their body, mind, and spirit to help them respond and adapt to their illness.

Many people need no analysis to identify a healing environment; they simply know when they are in one. They feel welcome, balanced, and at one with themselves and the world. They feel relaxed, stimulated, reassured, and invited to expand. They feel at home. Stichler (2001) notes, "Healing environments help to stimulate a positive awareness of one's self and enhance one's connections with nature, culture, and people. A healing environment allows for privacy and does not harm the patient with toxic materials, lighting, noise, or temperatures" (p. 3). Stichler goes on to state that healing environments:

- Provide meaningful and varying stimuli
- Encourage relaxation with the use of therapeutic sounds, calming colors, comfortable furniture, and a sense of harmony in the environment
- Are flexible and adaptable

- Can accommodate overnight guests or family members who support the client emotionally
- Are designed from the perspective of the client and family rather than for the staff

In its broadest sense, the term *environment* can mean everything within and external to an individual. This chapter focuses on the elements of a healing environment and specifically on the impact of healthy and unhealthy environments on clients and the providers who care for them.

How Healing Environments Impact Health

The concept that the environment could impact health and wellness was first publicly introduced in San Diego, California, in 1989 during the Symposium for Health Care Design. Before then, the terms *client friendly, homelike,* and *family centered* were used to describe healing environments, but these terms were not accurate and did not fully convey the integration of the whole person—the body, mind, and spirit—in a healthcare environment (Huelat, 2003). Huelat explains the difficulty in defining a healing environment:

> The most basic definition of a healing environment is also our oldest and most common conception of one: a place where doctors practice medicine—a hospital . . . Confusing a health-care facility for a healing environment is made easier by the fact that we tend to think "healing" and "curing" are synonymous; they are not. (pp. 2–3)

Healing extends far beyond the walls of healthcare facilities. According to Smith, Roehll, and Bonnell (2007), "a healing environment is intended to elicit a positive or healthy outcome upon the user" (p. 38). A healing environment supports people and promotes health and well-being. It is a vital part of maintaining a healthy lifestyle and is just as important as eating properly, exercising regularly, caring properly for ourselves, and having meaningful relationships and support systems. Healing environments promote a sense of relaxation and peace, and they are meant to open senses that have been restricted. Huelat (2003) notes, "Ultimately, the meaning of a healing environment resides in a unique and personal experience" (p. vii).

According to Frankel, Sung, and Hsu (2005), optimal healing environments are situations in which mutual respect and positive relationships exist between individuals and in which the qualities and resources of those relationships are used to enhance health. Optimal healing environments can include both general and specific physical, medical, psychological, social, and spiritual components (Kligler, 2004).

Human beings thrive in warm, loving environments and wither in cold, sterile ones. According to Neumann and Mensik (1993), "Healing institutions integrate sensitive and compassionate care, a nurturing environment, and healing modalities as well as curing into their patients' overall experience" (p. 2).

Sacred Spaces

Healing environments are often sacred spaces. Wright and Sayre-Adams (2000) define a sacred space as "a place where wonder can be revealed, where the divine can be revealed or experienced, and where we can get in touch with that which is larger than ourselves" (pp. 11–12). Throughout the ages, sacred spaces have taken many forms, such as Stonehenge, the Great Pyramids, the Holy Land, Native American burial grounds, and Tibetan temples. Each such place provides its visitors with a venue for introspection where renewal can occur. Truly sacred, healing spaces celebrate life and love and fill the senses.

The Healing Environment of Nature

A growing amount of research links mental, physical, and spiritual health directly to an association with nature. Nature may even be a powerful form of therapy for attention-deficit disorders and other maladies (Louv, 2005). Yet Western society often supports a disconnected existence in which the average civilized person spends the majority of time indoors, apart from any tangible sensory contact with the natural world. For example, in Western societies, many work environments do not allow windows to be opened to fresh air, and many houses are built on tiny lots with no open space or room for local wildlife. Healthcare environments are often painted in cold tones and filled with unfamiliar, stressful noises and smells.

In Western medicine, the connection between healing and nature was gradually superseded by increasingly technical approaches, such as surgery, machines, X-rays, and CAT scans. The idea that healing could come from access to nature was all but lost. In addition, with the world's population increasing rapidly to over 9 billion people, the human race has transformed the physical matter that makes up the earth by burning, cutting, digging, and otherwise changing it. The resulting disconnection from the natural world can leave people feeling estranged, unfulfilled, and stressed, and they sometimes seek artificial substitutes for natural experiences.

Human beings are intimately connected to planet Earth. In primitive societies, this connectedness was linked to a high survival rate. Humans are ecologically a product and likeness of nature, and we share the planet with every other living organism. An evolutionary framework called *biophilia* proposes that humans have an inborn response to animals and to natural settings in which they evolve. Our ability to thrive and be fulfilled depends on our relationship with nature (Jones & Haight, 2002). Human beings are part of nature, and as such, we are influenced by energy cycles within our physical bodies as well as by the vibrational or universal body that relates to the external world's electromagnetic field. As part of a living universe that has vibrational fields, human beings are sensitive to that environment. The environment of objects, conditions, and situations that surround us and the vibrational energy of the environment can have both a positive and negative effect on the body, mind, and spirit of an individual (Eliopoulos, 2004).

Healing environments are healthy environments. They provide a connection with nature and natural elements that contributes to our health and well-being. Healing environments allow us to preserve a greater sense of control, provide access to social support and positive distractions, and provide the ability to cope more effectively with stress. They are a crucial element of healing and health.

A Shift in Focus and Back Again

The relationship between the mind-body, nature, and healing has been demonstrated for many centuries by many cultures. According to Burkhardt and Nagai-Jacobson (2002), Marcus and Barnes (1999), Neumann and Mensik (1993), Nightingale (2007), Stichler (2001), and Schweitzer, Gilpin, and Frampton (2004):

- Over 2,000 years ago, the ancient Greeks worshiped the god of healing by building healing temples, such as the one at Epidaurus, among cypress groves near the ocean. These temples faced the ocean and took advantage of the sea breezes and the sun. Visitors to the temples used libraries, gardens, baths, theaters, gymnasiums, and special sleep rooms to heal. They took part in activities specially designed to restore their natural body rhythms, thus achieving harmony between body and mind. The ancient Greeks also created healing spas, where individuals could restore themselves using rest, relaxation, soaking in spas or herbal baths, massage therapy, and specific dietary interventions.
- During the Middle Ages in Europe, monasteries included elaborate gardens to provide pleasant, soothing distractions for the ill.
- The ancient Egyptians decorated their healing places with murals because they believed the murals helped people maintain their interest in life.
- Early Christians designed their hospitals after cathedrals so the people recuperating there would feel confident, spiritual, serene, and strong.

- In the Judaic, Christian, and Islamic religions, paradise is symbolized by a garden.
- European and American hospitals in the 1800s commonly contained gardens and plants as prominent features.
- Various European and Asian groups have embraced holistic healing through the use of light therapy, music, nutrition, and herbs.
- Native Americans believe in the sacredness of special places and espouse deep connections with wildlife and the natural world.
- Florence Nightingale believed that a healthy house had five essential characteristics: pure air, pure water, efficient drainage, cleanliness, and light. She believed that no home could be healthy without these and that the home would be unhealthy in proportion to their deficiency.

Despite the historic precedents, for much of the 19th and 20th centuries in the United States very few individuals paid attention to the relationship between healing and environment. Instead, Americans focused on specific environmental concerns. Physicians were taught the principle of "first do no harm," but they were not taught the elements of design that promote or impede healing. Hospitals were designed to deliver state-of-the-art treatment in the most efficient way, but traditionally little attention was paid to the psychological well-being of their clients (Schweitzer et al., 2004).

Environmental concerns in the United States have evolved since their early beginnings in the late 1800s, when individuals reacted to the devastation of what seemed to be an inexhaustible wilderness. In that early phase, concerns were focused on ecological issues and on humankind's negative effects on the natural world, and the national park system arose from this awareness (Keegan, 2005). However, gardens became less prevalent in hospitals during the early 1900s as major advances in medical science caused hospital administrators and architects to concentrate on creating buildings that reduced infection risk, effectively housed technology, and were functionally efficient.

Then came the 1960s and 1970s, when Rachel Carson exposed the dangers of the toxic insecticide DDT and attention was directed to the proliferation of hazardous materials such as polychlorinated biphenyls (PCBs), lead, mercury, and other heavy metals. The focus shifted to concerns about environmental risks to human health, including the risks associated with manufactured environments (such as homes, workplaces, and schools), and to issues such as air and water quality and noise levels. The 1980s brought concerns about a hole in the ozone layer and global warming, and awareness shifted to an emphasis on a *sustainable future*, defined as meeting "the needs of the present without compromising the needs of future generations" (Keegan, 2005, p. 276).

In the early 1990s, sick building syndrome was first identified. In a sick building, more people than normal have various symptoms or feel ill, and the etiology is not attributable to live agents, bacteria, or molds. The term *building-related illness* (BRI) was coined; it is used when symptoms of diagnosable illness (such as asthma) are identified and can be attributed directly to airborne building contaminants. Risk factors for sick building syndrome include the following (Girman, Vigna, & Lee, 2004):

- Low room humidity
- Low or excessive amounts of outdoor air
- Smoking in work areas
- Visible mold growth
- High room temperature
- Dusty atmosphere
- Low-frequency fluorescent lamps creating subliminal flicker
- Low-frequency noise
- Dusty atmosphere or gaseous emissions
- Large areas of soft furnishings, carpets, and fabrics
- No local control of heating or cooling
- Large areas of open shelving and exposed paper
- More than half the occupants using display screen equipment for more than 5 hours
- Buildings that are more than 15 years old

In addition to awareness about indoor air quality, pest management, hazards of construction products, water quality, and noise levels, global concern has arisen about the amount of resources allotted to each inhabitant of the planet. Keegan (2005) cites two specific areas of concern and action that represent the evolving field of environmentalism and human health:

- *Environmental ethics:* Concern about valuing the environment as it relates to humankind, other creatures, and the land
- *Restorative justice:* A practice that involves conscious and deliberate steps toward repairing damages

Awareness of the need for functionally efficient, aesthetically pleasing, hygienic environments has continued to grow in the healthcare community. One reason is the increasing importance placed on mind-body integration and science. With the knowledge that stress and psychosocial factors can significantly affect client outcomes, the importance of creating new healthcare facilities with attention to pleasant, soothing distractions and social support increases. For example, as mounting scientific evidence demonstrates that viewing gardens can measurably reduce stress and improve client outcomes, there has been a resurgence in providing gardens in healthcare facilities around the world.

Today, healthcare organizations and healthcare professionals are committed to providing healthy, healing environments for their clients. By increasing their awareness of environmental issues and holistic healthcare practices, healthcare professionals contribute to this effort. For example, Dr. William Thomas proposed the Eden Alternative, which creates habitats for those who live and work in long-term care facilities. Thomas feels that it is important to look to nature to provide nursing home residents with a human habitat, instead of the sterile environment in which many find themselves. Eden Alternative facilities and those that have adopted the Eden Alternative philosophy offer a healthy, enhanced environment by empowering organizational structure and incorporating indoor plants, gardening, resident animals, and children's activities into the daily lives of residents and staff (Barba, Tesh, & Courts, 2002).

Increasingly sicker clients challenge healthcare organizations to provide a higher level of care and to be more outcome oriented and cost conscious in their delivery of care. At the same time, a paradigm shift in healthcare delivery is also taking place. The traditional medical model of trying to cure disease is being replaced by the more holistic approach of healing the whole client. The creation of healing environments is a natural outgrowth of the centuries-old concept of mind-body healing, the environmental movement in the United States, recent studies in environmental psychology, and holistic practices (Neumann & Mensik, 1993). As hospitals and healthcare facilities transform their high-tech environments into comfortable, user-friendly spaces, clients and their families will be supported and empowered in their healing journey (Neumann & Mensik, 1993).

The Power of Design

Leibrock (2000) asserts that client outcomes are suffering from overbuilt U.S. healthcare institutions and staff-intensive client care protocols. Leibrock calls for "health-care models that improve patent outcomes, lower liability, and reduce costs" and adds that "empowering design details can reduce costs as patients take responsibilities for their health care and decrease their reliance on staff. . . . Without these details, healthcare facilities are places where patients are overexposed to strangers and separated from family, where independence is lost to providers or to disabling design" (pp. xv–xvi).

Studies suggest that all hospital clients (and visitors) have the following design-related needs (Miller & Swensson, 2002):

- *Physical comfort,* which includes appropriate room temperature, pleasant lighting, comfortable furniture, and freedom from unpleasant odors and harsh, annoying noise
- *Social contact,* which includes personal privacy (limiting what others see and hear of you) and controlling what you see and hear of others
- *Symbolic meaning,* which includes the array of nonverbal messages embodied in design (For example, a cramped, uncomfortable waiting room suggests that hospital administrators don't respect their clients very much.)
- *Wayfinding:* which includes the ability to find the way easily through the maze of equipment and hallways and to avoid inadvertently wandering into a restricted, embarrassing, or even frightening space

Every type of healthcare organization has found that healing environments result in cost containment, improved client outcomes, and reduced liability. These bottom-line issues have resulted in (Stichler, 2001):

- Reduced nursing time (and staffing costs)
- Reduced client lengths of stay
- Reduced staff turnover and increased staff retention (as well as lowered recruitment costs)
- Improved quality and clinical outcomes
- Improved staff morale and satisfaction
- Positive impacts on the healthcare experience for clients and families
- Improved client satisfaction
- Increased market share
- Increased charitable contributions
- Increased number of staff and volunteer applications

Studies in environmental psychology have shown that effectively designed healthcare settings can nurture, comfort, relax, strengthen, and add to a sense of well-being (Neumann & Mensik, 1993). These elements of design are no longer luxuries but essential elements of a healthy environment.

Health care has a long history of being intertwined with spirituality. Schweitzer et al. (2004) note that "from the temples of Asklepios, to the monastic hospitals of the Middle Ages, to the spiritual calling of Nightingale nurses, health and spirituality have been closely linked" (p. S72). Often overlooked, this element of care is an essential aspect of healing environments. For many clients, illness is not only a physical and emotional crisis, but a spiritual one as well. Clients may face their own mortality, life-changing diagnoses, or a feeling that they have been betrayed by God. With the exception of a chapel, few spaces in hospitals provide a place for reflection.

One way in which hospitals are meeting the needs of clients in a healing environment is through the Planetree model of care. Based on the beliefs that clients and consumers should have broad access to health and medical information, that they should be active participants in their health care, and that their families and friends should be actively involved in care, Planetree hospitals often have massage therapy, open medical records, gardens, and soft lighting as well as art on the walls and music in the air (Mycek, 2007). Mycek also notes that, "Planetree is about privacy, comfort, patient dignity, and empowerment" (p. 24).

Healthcare institutions have the power and ability to design healing environments and maintain fiscal viability while providing their clients with a powerful and effective tool to help with their recovery and healing journey (Neumann & Mensik, 1993). Creating a healing environment does not cost any more than creating an institutional environment, and its long-term benefits may actually help save money. For example, time and motion studies on nurses revealed that they spent many hours on documentation and seeking information rather than working in client rooms. With redesigned units that eliminated long corridors and great distances to nursing stations, nurses were able to spend less time walking and more time educating and working with clients and families. Designs that encourage positive interactions among staff members and between nurses and physicians, such as gardens and lounges, or that support the family relationships of staff members (such as day care and sick-child day care facilities) are all parts of a healing environment (Schweitzer et al., 2004).

CREATING A HEALING ENVIRONMENT

Healing environments do not simply exist. They can, however, be created in any setting (Stichler, 2001). The creation of a healing environment requires attention to specific design elements, to cultural- and age-specific interventions, and to the role of the healthcare provider. The physical environment, while an important part of healing, is intertwined with many other aspects of an optimal healing environment. A well-designed environment has a powerful impact on health by influencing the behaviors, actions, and interactions of clients, their families, and the staff who take care of them (Schweitzer et al., 2004).

The creation of a healing environment can occur in any space and includes consideration of the following:

- Color
- Nature
- Lighting

- Air quality and temperature
- Smells
- Music
- Noise
- Buildings and furnishings
- Wayfinding

Color

Color, one of the most powerful elements in our environment, affects us in many ways. Color is often the first thing we see when we walk into a room, and changing an area's color can affect its personality.

The response of the body and mind to color is influenced by cortical activation, the autonomic nervous system, and hormone activation. Color has been shown to affect heart rate, brainwave activity, respiration, and muscular tension as well as to evoke memories and associations, encourage introversion or extroversion, and induce anger or peacefulness (Venolia, 1988). In fact, color therapy is based on these effects.

As early as Neanderthal times, color was used for its sacred powers and to invoke aid and protection. In fact, according to Eliopoulos (2004), the history of color therapy dates from 1550 BC, when Egyptian priests used papyrus manuscripts to demonstrate how they used color in their healing temples. Ancient Greeks and Egyptians used colors in healing, and colored cloth was used to treat disease in the Middle Ages (Venolia, 1988). Nightingale used colored flowers for therapy, and the ancient Egyptians designed chambers with light prisms to heal the sick. In 1878, Edwin Babbit wrote a book on color therapy, or chromotherapy, which was met with both praise and skepticism. In the early 1900s, Dinshah Ghadiali developed *spectro-chrome tonation*, a system of attuned color waves that was finally accepted by the American Medical Association after 40 years of use.

Color therapy deals with disease by treating the body's etheric field. According to Leddy (2006), color therapy is based on the concept that disease, a chemical imbalance, and an inappropriate energy vibration are equivalent. Today we know that all the cells in the body vibrate. Vibrating colors generate fields of energy. Each color has its own wavelength, or vibration, and specific vibrations can raise, lower, or neutralize energy levels. Some combinations of vibrations are harmonizing, some are neutralizing, and some distort each other. Every organ has a specific energy level at which it functions best. Nature often provides inspiration but how color affects and influences us is still open to controversy.

Light and color are interrelated, and neither can exist without the other because each enhances the other's life and energy. The visible spectrum of light contains seven colors: red, orange, yellow, green, blue, indigo, and violet. These seven visible colors are often associated with specific emotions and conditions (Eliopoulos, 2004; Leddy, 2006; Venolia, 1988):

- *Red:* A primary color located at the infrared end of the visible light spectrum, red is associated with high energy, passion, excitement, and the nature symbol of earth. It activates all five senses and vibrates 436 trillion times per second.
- *Orange:* Associated with emotional expression, courage, optimism, warmth, and the nature symbol of sunset, orange raises the pulse rate but not the blood pressure. It stimulates the thyroid and bone growth as well as the energy in the lungs and stomach. It activates all five senses and vibrates 473 trillion times per second.
- *Yellow:* The third color from the infrared end of the spectrum, yellow is a stimulant for the muscles, lymph glands, and digestive organs. It is considered the color of the mind and can raise low-energy emotional states of depression, apathy, and discouragement. It is associated with optimism, intellect, enlightenment, happiness, and mental clarity. The nature symbol of the sun, yellow vibrates 510 trillion times per second.
- *Green:* This is the master color, found in the middle of the spectrum. Green is the stabilizing color for all dysfunctions and relieves tension. Associated with healing, peace, balance, nurturing, unconditional love, and the nature symbol of growth, green vibrates 584 trillion times per second.
- *Blue:* Associated with relaxation, serenity, wisdom, spirituality, loyalty, calming, and the nature symbol of sky and ocean, blue increases the elimination of toxins and stimulates intuitive powers. It is a vitality builder, it is the color of the spirit, and it activates the pineal gland. Blue vibrates 658 trillion times per second.
- *Indigo:* Associated with meditation, intuition, spirituality, and the nature symbol of sunset, indigo is a cooling color that activates the parathyroid and calms the thyroid. It has an anesthetic effect, reduces swelling, and is generally calming. Indigo vibrates 695 trillion times per second.
- *Violet:* With the shortest wavelength of the visible colors, violet calms the metabolic process, relaxes muscles, and has antibiotic characteristics. It aids in meditation and sleep and may act as a pain reliever. Associated with spirituality, universal power and healing, stress reduction, and the nature symbol of the violet flower, violet vibrates 731 trillion times per second.

The following guidelines about the use of color in healthcare environments *are only guidelines*. The needs of specific populations, as well as personal preferences, geographic location, practices, and age must be taken into consideration when using color to create healing spaces (Leddy, 2006; Leibrock, 2000; Neumann & Mensik, 1993).

- Warm colors (such as peach, soft yellows, or coral) can stimulate the appetite and encourage alertness, joy, optimism, creativity, and socialization; these colors are useful in such areas as dining rooms or meeting spaces.
- Light colors often make a room appear more spacious (Long, 2001).
- Blues, greens, and other cool colors are useful in areas designed to be restful, contemplative, and quiet (such as waiting rooms or meditation areas).
- Primary colors (red, yellow, and blue) and strong patterns are pleasing at first but can be overstimulating and may contribute to fatigue. Red, for some, may be associated with blood, emergencies, or trauma (Long, 2001).
- Individuals with color blindness have difficulty distinguishing between green and red.
- Green symbolizes growth, renewal, hope, healing, and peace, and it has been used to reduce tension and nervousness.
- Yellow, green, and purple tones are not flattering to the skin and reflect jaundiced skin tones.
- Texture makes tones appear darker.
- Intense colors should be used only for accents (such as door frames, levers, switches, or grab bars).
- The brain requires constant stimulation. Monotonous color schemes contribute to sensory deprivation, disorganization of brain function, deterioration of intelligence, and an inability to concentrate. They slow the healing process and are perceived as institutional.
- Color affects an individual's perception of time, size, weight, and volume. Rooms where pleasant activities take place (such as dining or recreation) benefit by having warm color schemes, because the activity seems to last longer. In rooms where monotonous tasks are performed, a cool color scheme can make time pass more quickly.

Other important factors to consider when selecting color for the healthcare environment include:

- An understanding of the healing properties of color
- The creation of a balanced color palette
- The use of artwork

- The use of a variety of materials, finishes, and lighting
- Access to outside views

Nature

Natural elements, time spent in connection with nature, views of nature, and natural lighting can have a powerful effect on the healing process. For example, clients in rooms with views of nature heal faster and leave the hospital earlier than those whose rooms have no view or a poor view (Neumann & Mensik, 1993). Staring at the same four walls can be as detrimental to a client's recovery as a chaotic hospital environment.

Nature has a distracting influence on clients and caregivers, provides relief, and taps into our most basic senses of life and living. Cancer clients, for example, respond positively to living, growing things in the environment because they are strong metaphors for life (Leibrock, 2000). In Japan, one healing intervention is called Shinrin-yoka, which means "walking in the forests to promote health." This form of relaxation is used by many older adults to reduce chronic stress, hostility, and depression (McCaffrey, 2007).

A healing environment should include natural elements such as indoor landscaping, water features, plants, flowers, or aquariums, as well as the incorporation of animal-assisted therapy (Leibrock, 2000). At a minimum, elements of nature should be accessible physically and/or sensually; examples include large windows that open onto gardens, skylights, and artwork that depicts natural elements. Another way to include natural elements is to use color values that reflect the natural progress and tonal relationships found in nature (Stewart, 2006). For example, ceilings should be a light color (reflecting the sky), wall colors should be a medium color (reflecting the forest and the plains), and flooring should be darker earth tones (reflecting the earth). If we jump into a pool or lake, we tend to swim toward the lighter color because we instinctively know that the light is up. When our instincts are reinforced, we feel confident and in control.

Gardens have been used by healthcare institutions to reduce stress, pain, anxiety, and depression and to improve the overall quality of life for chronic and terminal clients. Simply looking at nature or environments dominated by greenery, flowers, or water is significantly more effective in promoting recovery or restoration from stress than looking at scenes of rooms, buildings, or towns. Within only 3–5 minutes, a positive effect may occur in the form of psychological, emotional, and physiological changes, such as:

- Increased positive feelings and calmness
- Reduced negativity, fear, anger, or sadness

- Reduced stressful thoughts
- Positive changes in blood pressure, heart rates, heart activity, muscle tension, and brain electrical activity

Gardens and nature in hospitals also significantly heighten satisfaction with the healthcare provider and the overall quality of care. Elements that are likely to worsen a garden's effects include:

- Starkly built content
- Cigarette smoke
- Intrusive, incongruent urban or machine noise (traffic sounds, for example)
- Crowds
- Perceived insecurity or risk
- Prominent litter
- Abstract, ambiguous sculpture or other built features that can be interpreted in multiple ways (these can cause highly negative reactions)

Features that increase a garden's positive effects include (Venolia, 1988):

- Beauty
- Verdant foliage and fragrance
- Stone, wood, paths, and sacred geometry
- Water (not tumultuous)
- Congruent or harmonious nature sources (birds, breezes, water)
- An atmosphere that allows for privacy, encourages times of relaxation, stimulates positive self-awareness, and provides meaningful and varying stimuli

Gardens provide a sanctuary, a place to pause and reflect, to regain our equilibrium, and to appreciate our place in the world. A good garden space allows for some privacy, a focal point for contemplation, a consideration of scale, and some frame around the space (such as a screen, fence, hedge, or wall). If these elements are addressed, gardens become personal, spirit-nurturing oases (Messervy, 2006).

Lighting

Nearly all living things need light to exist. The body's natural rhythms are guided by the cycles of light and dark, and most creation myths involve darkness and light. The term *circadian* is Latin for "around the day" and refers to rhythms repeated every 24 hours. Circadian rhythms—which Trivieri and Anderson (2002) define as "regularly recurring, biological changes in our mental and physical behaviors over the course of the day" (p. 303)—are controlled by the body's biological clock and are associated with sleep-wake patterns as well as with fluctuations in alertness and drowsiness. They are also related to physiological processes such as blood pressure, body temperature, hormone levels, sexual development, nervous system functioning, and the immune system (Trivieri & Anderson, 2002; Venolia, 1988).

Neumann and Mensik (1993) note the importance of light on the body's rhythms:

> All living creatures are influenced by the rhythms of seasonal change and by their own intrinsic rhythms. Much of how humans perceive this change is based on daily light cycles, the rising and setting of the sun, the yearly changes in length of day, and even the rhythms of the tides. Chronobiology, the cyclical view of time and rhythms and their effect on the body, is important in the design of patient rooms. (p. 4)

The therapeutic value of light has been recognized for thousands of years. For example, the Assyrians, Babylonians, and Egyptians all practiced sunbathing (Venolia, 1988). Nightingale (2007) believed that second only to the need for fresh air was the client's need for light in order to heal and that what hurts clients most is a dark room. She stated, "The sun is not only a painter but a sculptor . . . light has quite real and tangible effects upon the human body . . . The cheerfulness of a room, the usefulness of light in treating disease is all-important" (p. 59).

Lighting is an important design feature for health and safety. Most artificial lighting, both incandescent and fluorescent, lacks the complete balanced spectrum of sunlight and interferes with the body's optimal absorption of nutrition. Called *malillumination,* this condition can contribute to fatigue, depression, hostility, alcoholism, drug abuse, Alzheimer's disease, cancer, hair loss, and tooth decay, and it has been linked to loss of muscle tone and strength. In some studies, melanoma has been linked to exposure to fluorescent light, not to exposure to natural sunlight (Trivieri & Anderson, 2002).

Lighting has healing properties, and light therapy has been used to treat many diseases such as certain viruses, seasonal affective disorder, depression, and insomnia. Natural sunlight and certain forms of light therapy can help the body reestablish its natural rhythm and are becoming an integral treatment for many health conditions. In addition, light's ability to activate certain biochemical substances in the body has formed the basis of treatment for skin disorders such as psoriasis and for certain forms of cancer (Trivieri & Anderson, 2002). Ultraviolet light can enhance healing, increase protein metabolism, lessen fatigue, reduce depression, improve sleep, stimulate white blood cell production, increase the release of endorphins, lower blood pressure, elevate mood, and promote emotional well-being. It can also help orient confused clients to time, day, weather, and space (Schweitzer et al., 2004; Stichler, 2001; Trivieri & Anderson, 2002).

As individuals age and experience visual changes, it becomes increasingly important for them to have continuous, subtle sensory stimulation. Their eyes may adjust to light more slowly or may be unable to distinguish changes in light levels. Sensitivity to glare increases, and lenses may undergo a yellow tinting that affects their color perception. Depth perception may be altered, and peripheral vision may decrease (Leibrock, 2000). Older individuals who are ill or stressed often experience disorientation, which effective lighting can lessen.

Healthy lighting has characteristics similar to those of natural light: it changes subtly in light spectrum, intensity, and distribution throughout the day. If healthy lighting is combined with sensory stimulation in the form of smell, sound, and touch, and if it is synchronized with the biological clock, the individual benefits because the sensory perceptions are meaningful.

Lighting in client care areas is important for appropriate assessments of client conditions. New healthcare design codes and regulations require that every client room has a window to the outside. Guidelines for incorporating healthy lighting features into a healing environment include the following (Leibrock, 2000):

- Keep lighting levels consistent and adjustable from space to space.
- Utilize night lights in bedrooms and corridors and install lights near bed perimeters or on nightstands for easy access.
- Because many accidents occur in the bathroom, be certain that lighting is appropriate (without glare) and sufficient. (Steam-filled showers, for example, may decrease visibility, but vapor-proof light fixtures in shower stall ceilings and exhaust fans can reduce steam and improve visibility.)
- Prevent contrast glare by using shields or frosted globes on lights.
- Allow as much natural light into the area as possible with windows, skylights, and atriums; use full-spectrum fluorescent lighting if natural lighting is not possible.
- Keep blinds and drapes open if possible.
- Use sufficient lighting in areas requiring concentration or decision making and in areas of potential danger.
- Buy only incandescent lamps.
- Install dimmers on light switches to reduce glare and to allow clients, family, and staff to control the direction and amount of light.
- Eliminate glare on computer screens by using a nonglare fixture.
- Use appropriate lighting for the client population. (For example, studies have shown that clients with Alzheimer's disease become agitated under fluorescent lighting.)

- Avoid the use of cool fluorescent lights around individuals with cataracts because fluorescents emphasize the blue-green tones that are most difficult to see.
- Use lighting with spectrums as close as possible to those of daylight. (This can reduce depression, fatigue, hyperactivity, and some incidence of disease, as well as increase calcium absorption and reaction time to light. Circadian rhythm can be disrupted by inadequate exposure to natural light.)
- Conceal fixtures whenever possible. (Light is more effective as a healing tool when the light is seen but its source is not.)

Air Quality and Temperature

Florence Nightingale (2007) said, "The very first canon of nursing . . . the first essential to the patient, without which all the rest you can do for him is as nothing . . . is this: *To Keep the Air He Breathes as Pure as the External Air, Without Chilling Him*" (p. 12). Nightingale knew that fresh air of the appropriate temperature was essential to a person's ability to heal and remain well. She went on to say, "To attempt to keep a ward warm at the expense of making the sick repeatedly breathe their own hot, humid, putrescent atmosphere is a certain way to delay recovery or to destroy life" (p. 14).

Every day, we take approximately 24,000 breaths of air. This is equal to 2 gallons of air per minute or 3,000 gallons of air per day. Because breathing is essential to life, we need to be sure that the quality of every breath we take is optimal (Girman et al., 2004). The Clean Air Act of 1970 authorized the Environmental Protection Agency (EPA) to set standards for six different outdoor air contaminants: ground level ozone, particulate matter, carbon monoxide, nitrogen oxide, sulfur dioxide, and lead. These standards are referred to as the National Ambient Air Quality Standards. The Pollutant Standard Index also measures air pollution, including indoor air pollutants (environmental tobacco smoke, mold spores, and mercury) (Girman et al., 2004).

Indoor air pollution can pose many health risks and produce significant health effects, including the following (Girman et al., 2004; Schweitzer et al., 2004):

- Heart disease
- Lung cancer
- Stroke
- Rhinoconjunctivitis in children
- Eye, nose, and throat irritation
- Asthma development

- Headaches
- Damage to kidneys, liver, and the central nervous system
- Asthma-related mortality

Asthma, for example, is one of the most common health problems resulting from indoor pollution. The indoor levels of pollutants may be two to five times higher (and sometimes up to 100 times higher) than outdoor levels. Since most people spend up to 95% of their time indoors, the effects of exposure can be dramatic. During the past 20–30 years, our exposure to indoor air pollutants has increased because of many factors, including:

- Reduced ventilation to save money
- Reduced maintenance on current systems to save money
- The use of synthetic building materials and furnishings
- The use of personal care products
- The use of pesticides and household cleaning supplies
- Construction and renovation to seal buildings tightly

Healing environments provide good air quality to those who inhabit them. Guidelines for improving air quality include the following (Girman et al., 2004; Keegan, 2005; Leibrock, 2000; Neumann & Mensik, 1993; Nightingale, 2007; Schweitzer et al., 2004):

- Open windows to improve ventilation.
- Clean air ducts regularly.
- Test regularly for gas leaks.
- Maintain equipment and perform repairs in a timely manner.
- Use plants liberally and, whenever possible, provide clients with access to outdoor areas (such as solariums, outdoor gardens, and roof gardens).
- Use air filters, ionizers, or ozone purifiers.
- Clean carpets and upholstery regularly.
- Accelerate the off-gassing of new materials (fabrics, carpets, upholstery, etc.) by leaving the house, room, or facility; turning up the heat; closing the windows; "cooking" the environment for 24 hours; and then opening the windows to ventilate it.
- Promptly remove any asbestos.
- Use aromatherapy.
- Prohibit smoking. (Passive smoking, or the exposure to tobacco smoke produced by others, places nonsmokers at the same risk for illnesses as those who smoke. Cigarette smoking is associated with an increase in significantly higher all-cause mortality rates. Healing environments should be smoke free.)

Pleasant temperatures are also important in a healthcare environment. Temperature and humidity can dramatically affect comfort levels and the ability to sleep well, and clients should be able to control both. Without humidity, dry air (less than 20–30% relative humidity) can increase susceptibility to colds and flu. Excess humidity (above 70% relative humidity) can promote the spread of viral infections by providing microorganisms with the warm, moist environment they need for survival. Blankets, blanket warmers, and fans can be provided in areas where body temperatures may fluctuate or in rooms that are normally kept cool (such as operating rooms, recovery rooms, intensive care units, or emergency rooms).

Smells

The sense of smell is inexorably linked with environments. Information received through the sense of smell triggers both physiological and psychological effects. More than any other sense, smell is also linked with memory and emotions at both the conscious and subconscious levels. For example, the Proust phenomenon is named after a French author who described how the smell of tea-soaked cake lifted him from a sad state of mind to happy memories of his childhood. Other odors alert us to danger (the smell of fire), stimulate our appetite (the smell of freshly baked cookies), and can even arouse our desire for the opposite sex (the smell of perfumes or pheromones). Mothers bond with their newborn infants by nuzzling them, and babies identify their mothers through the distinctive smell of their breast milk.

Hospitals and healthcare clinics are well known for their often unpleasant odors or chemical smells. Florence Nightingale (2007) wrote that the smell from sick or diseased individuals "is highly noxious and dangerous" (p. 17). Since smell is acutely retained in memory (even more than sounds or visual images), strong smelling cleaning agents should not be used near clients. Pleasant odors, flower arrangements, and plants can reduce stress, absorb odors, and help clean the air; they are important components of any healing environment (Neumann & Mensik, 1993). Pleasing aromas can reduce blood pressure, slow respiration, and lower pain perception levels. They have even been shown to reduce client-related anxiety during magnetic resonance imaging. Negative smells stimulate anxiety, fear, and stress (Schweitzer et al., 2004).

Cleanliness and a state of order affect the perception of both clients and visitors, who often assume, rightly or wrongly, that a clean and orderly healthcare environment equates to excellent care. Keeping a facility clean and in good repair is a challenge, yet an environment that cannot remain clean cannot be considered a healing environment (Huelat, 2003).

Music

Music is a powerful healing tool that has been linked to medicine throughout history. In Greek mythology, Apollo was the god of music, and his son, Asclepius, was the god of healing and medicine. Music has accompanied armies as they marched to battle, and it has been played during rites of initiation, at funeral ceremonies, and on harvest and feast days. Today, music is incorporated into surgical suites, physician's offices, and many healthcare facilities as a holistic, stress-reducing measure (Eliopoulos, 2004; Keegan, 2005).

The music used in a healing environment must be chosen carefully to account for individual preferences and responses and cultural variations. Not all music is healing. The loud volume of rock music contributes to hearing loss. Classical music is generally less harmful to the body but it is not always healing. Music without words is most effective in healing environments. However, the best way to select healing music is to become aware of your subtle physical and emotional responses when you listen to a piece.

The use of music in healing environments is explored further in chapter 9.

Noise

Venolia (1988) observes that our advancing civilization has gotten noisier over time: "As far as we know, human hearing evolved in a relatively quiet setting . . . very loud noises were the exception. The sounds that were heard all carried meaning to the hearer, and the ability to detect subtle sounds was important for both survival and pleasure . . . Even as civilization advanced, the sonic environment remained fairly unpolluted until recently" (p. 84). Now, in a typical day, human beings rarely experience quiet. Our homes, towns, cities, and work environments rarely allow us to escape noise, the sound level is often harmful, and the background noise rarely contains useful information.

Some define noise as complex sound waves while others define it as unwanted or undesirable sound without agreeable musical quality (Buelow, 2001; Stichler, 2001; Venolia, 1988). Is music noise? Is a symphony noise? What about the noise created by a car's tires as it travels on the freeway? The effects of noise are difficult to measure, and its definition can be subjective. Psychologically, the impact of a sound is not entirely a function of its loudness. According to Venolia (1988), noise is more easily tolerated if it is under one's control, if it has some relation to the listener, or if it is perceived as contributing to a positive outcome. For example, your own lawnmower is less annoying than your neighbor's, and a fan noise is more meaningful if it is cooling the room. Noise is also relatively more tolerable if it is considered unavoidable (such as rain) but it is much more annoying if it is isolated, steady, or repetitive (such as drops from a leaky faucet). Annoyance is also cumulative. If you listen to noise all day long, you are more likely to be irritated by a single loud noise during the ensuing quiet evening.

Noise pollution is equally difficult to define. According to Cabrera and Lee (2000), noise pollution is an impurity of unpleasant sounds, and it is transient. There are differing opinions about how much noise pollution is too much. Although individual noises can be measured in terms of decibel levels, the cumulative effect of noise exposure is difficult to determine. Whatever the definition, environmental noise can affect the psychological and physiological well-being of an individual. It is considered a pollutant, one of the most pervasive in the United States, and a hazard to human health and hearing.

Most individuals are not aware of the hazardous effects of noise, yet even everyday sounds like street traffic or conversation can be stressful and cause unpleasant effects. One study examined the effects on children of living in environments with low-level noise, like train and car traffic, and found that those children released more stress hormone (cortisol) while sleeping than those who lived in more tranquil environments. Noise also affects cardiovascular health (Weil, 2006) and causes the release of adrenocorticosteroids, epinephrine, and norepinephrine. It can negatively impact a developing fetus and can also cause the following (Buelow, 2001; Cabrera & Lee, 2000; Keegan, 2005; Leibrock, 2000; Reiling et al., 2004; Venolia, 1988):

- Increased blood pressure
- Altered heartbeats
- Decreased immunity and immune system recovery
- Increased cerebral blood flow
- Increased blood cortisol and cholesterol levels
- Disturbed digestion and upset stomach or ulcers
- Fatigue and poor work performance
- Increased respiratory rate
- Increased pain perception
- Increase need for medication
- Intensified effects of drugs, alcohol, aging, and carbon monoxide

Noise is one of the most insidious environmental stressors in the hospital environment and a primary cause of sleep deprivation and disturbance among clients. It contributes to confusion, falls, increased lengths of stay, and increased use of medication and restraints. Sudden noises, like trays falling or doors slamming, can cause a startle reflex in clients with accompanying increased blood pressure, increased heart rate, vasoconstriction, and muscle flexion (Mazer, 2005; Robinson, Weitzel, & Henderson, 2005; Schweitzer et al., 2004). Prolonged exposure to noise increases stress, reduces safety, and affects sleep, resulting in decreased memory function; increased agitation and mental confusion; and delayed tissue healing, bone synthesis, and red blood cell formation (Robinson et al., 2005).

Rest and sleep are integral components of a healing environment, yet most healthcare environments provide little opportunity for them. Noise levels are high, privacy is minimal, and many strangers come through the room each day, often without much awareness of the noise they make during their care. In a typical hospital environment, the average healthcare worker and client hear beepers, alarms, machines, bed rails, ice machines, televisions, pneumatic tubes, carts, telephones, and voices from staff and even roommates. These sounds are considered normal by healthcare workers; however, depending on their age, hearing ability, medication level, culture, and fears, most clients do not consider these sounds normal or restful—and they are making their opinions known. Client satisfaction scores reveal that clients complain about noise twice as often as they complain about anything else in the hospital, including food.

Sleep is crucial if the body's tissues are to heal. Deep sleep releases growth hormone, an essential element of cell division and protein synthesis. Approximately 70% of the body's daily secretion of growth hormone occurs during sleep. Growth hormone also supports bone synthesis and red blood cell formation (Robinson et al., 2005). If wounds or body tissues are to heal, they require this hormone. Therefore, healing environments support sleep and keep noise to minimal levels.

Noise in the healthcare environment also affects healthcare providers. The Joint Commission cites noise as a potential risk for nursing errors, impacting the nurse's ability to hear doctor's orders, clearly understand clients, and remain focused. Noise also contributes to stress reactions such as exhaustion, burnout, depression, and irritability at home. Noisy environments contribute to staff members becoming less interpersonally engaged, less caring, and less reflective. Cognition is impeded, perseverance in addressing complex tasks is lost, and staffers tend to seek simple solutions (Fick & Vance, 2006; Mazer, 2005; Reiling et al., 2004; Schweitzer et al., 2004).

Noise levels are measured in decibels; the higher the decibel level, the louder the noise. Sounds louder than 80–85 decibels are considered hazardous (Daniels et al., 2007; Trivieri & Anderson, 2002). Consider the average decibel levels for everyday sounds shown in table 5-1 (Cabrera & Lee, 2000; Cmiel, Gasser, & Neveau, 2004; Daniels et al., 2007; Robinson et al., 2005). The noise generated by staff during the average shift change has been measured at 113 decibels—as loud as that of a jackhammer (Robinson et al., 2005).

Noise-induced hearing loss (NIHL) is a gradual, painless, permanent disorder affecting all age groups, including the aging adult. NIHL reduces efficiency in performing daily tasks, contributes to fatigue and irritability, and

Table 5-1 Average Decibel (dB) Levels for Everyday Sounds

Type of Noise	Rating	Decibel Level
Whispering, quiet library	Faint	10–20 dB
Normal conversation, quiet woodland	Faint	30 dB
Moderate rainfall	Moderate	50 dB
Loud conversation	Moderate	60 dB
Vacuum cleaner, busy traffic	Very loud	70 dB
Alarm clock	Very loud	80 dB
Lawn mower, motorcycle, hair dryer	Very loud	90 dB
Airplane taking off, snowmobile, portable X-ray machine	Extremely loud	100 dB
Rock music	Extremely loud	110 dB
Amplified rock music, chainsaw	Painful	120 dB
Jackhammer	Painful	110–130 dB
Firearms, jet engine	Painful	140 dB
Rock music peak	Painful	150 dB

contributes to communication difficulties. NIHL is appearing much earlier than it did 30 years ago, and it affects many parts of the body other than the ears (Leibrock, 2000).

Prevention and education are key factors in reducing NIHL. One intervention, called the Sh-h-h-h Project (Robinson et al., 2005), is designed to reduce noise and promote rest and sleep. Interventions include closed doors, relaxing music, warm blankets, back rubs, warm drinks, aromatherapy, and sleep baskets that contain earplugs.

The Environmental Protection Agency (EPA) recommends that continuous background noise in healthcare environments not exceed 35 decibels during the day and 40 decibels at night (Mazer, 2005). The following suggestions are additional ways to reduce NIHL and to create a healthy environment for clients (Eliopoulos, 2004; Fick & Vance, 2006; Leibrock, 2000; Mazer, 2005; Neumann & Mensik, 1993; Robinson et al., 2005; Stichler, 2001; Weil, 2006; Yee, 2006):

- Install carpeting, which can reduce ambient noise by up to 70%, prevent the generation of surface noise, and reduce the levels of impact noise (such as that generated by footsteps on the floor).
- Cover a wall with draperies, which can absorb nearly half the ambient noise in a space.
- Limit client exposure to noise by keeping radios, televisions, paging systems, telephones, loudspeakers, slamming doors, and even footsteps in the hallway as quiet as possible. Even conversations from the nurses' sta-

tion or staff lounge can be disruptive to an ailing individual and should be evaluated. Speak in lowered tones.

- Use padding under noisy machines (such as keyboards, blenders, or large equipment that vibrates).
- Reduce or eliminate the use of overhead paging systems and replace them with vibrating pagers or vibrating cell phones.
- Design work and healing spaces to reduce noise. For example, long, rectangular rooms increase sound reflection while irregularly shaped recessed areas along walls and ceilings diffuse sound waves. Use alcoves for storage carts, clean linen, and other supplies, since they reduce the noise caused by opening and closing doors. Utilize anterooms as part of client isolation rooms. Utilize sound-absorbing ceiling tiles. Incorporate a separate relaxation lounge for caregivers, and decentralize nursing stations.
- Close doors to clients' rooms when possible.
- Be a responsible consumer and look for noise ratings when purchasing products.
- Have hearing tested annually.
- Use sound-masking devices such as wind chimes, water, or music.
- Wear hearing protectors when exposed to loud noises.
- Educate others about noise, and take action before noise levels become disturbing. Staff working in a noisy environment tend to speak more loudly, thereby increasing the noise level and creating a vicious cycle of noise.
- If you cannot escape noise, block out unwanted or unpleasant noise by using noise-canceling headphones or a machine that creates white noise (which contains all frequencies and masks other sounds). CDs with nature sounds can also be helpful. Music or sounds played this way should never be so loud that you cannot hear others talking around you.

Buildings and Furnishings

The design elements and construction aspects of 21st-century healthcare facilities are undergoing a revolution. More institutions are looking for ways to integrate aesthetics with their organizational mission to create a healing environment for clients and staff (Litch, 2007). Feng shui—one of the earliest, well-documented, and continuous philosophies of environmental psychology—can positively impact building types and designs. Stewart (2006) notes that feng shui:

> . . . embraces the belief that we are one with nature and that all energy is interconnected. It teaches that the energy of our natural and built environments affects our individual human energy . . . we are happier and more productive when our environment recreates the balance of elements found in nature. (p. 30)

A building's design affects not only human beings, but also its surroundings. A healthy building minimizes its impact on its occupants, the surrounding community, and the earth. Some healthcare institutions promote healthy people by minimizing the disruption associated with construction practices. Knowing that physical and visual connections to the natural environment provide social, psychological, and physical benefits for clients, staff, and visitors, these institutions protect and enhance the site's existing natural areas as a therapeutic resource. The Clarion West Medical Center in Indiana, for example, designed and built a hospital that integrated a healing environment with the materials and colors of nature (Litch, 2007).

What people see when they enter a client room also affects their attitude. For example, a light-filled room with large windows will probably have a more positive effect than a dark room in which the toilet is one of the first things seen. People feel more comfortable walking on a gently curving exterior path than navigating one that has unnatural 90-degree turns (Stewart, 2006).

Other research supports design elements that impact client safety—an important aspect of a healing environment (Schweitzer et al., 2004):

- Private rooms in the intensive care unit decrease infection rates, improve staff communication, improve client satisfaction scores, decrease medication errors, and provide for family inclusion in care.
- Wider client bathroom doors that accommodate a staff person ambulating with the client decrease client falls.
- Rooms that allow staff to provide care to clients with a variety of needs minimize the need to transfer clients between units, thereby reducing medication errors.
- Designs that encourage physical activity reduce depression.

Buildings and furnishings need to be clean and uncluttered. Choosing furniture that can be effectively cleaned and maintained is important. Clutter is a major stress factor that can irritate the nervous system and disturb both the visual and vibrational energy fields (Eliopoulos, 2004; Huelat, 2003).

Furniture, accessories, art, and flowers help create a homelike atmosphere in the healthcare setting and can influence a client's outlook, contribute to comfort and a sense of safety, and increase orientation to an often unfamiliar environment. Nightingale states (2007) that beautiful objects and a variety of objects, which she called "fancies of the patient," are the most valuable indications of what is necessary for the client's recovery. She states that people are affected by form, color, and light and that these things are an actual means of recovery.

The following homelike elements can contribute to a healing environment (Leibrock, 2000; Neumann & Mensik, 1993; Nightingale, 2007; Schweitzer et al., 2004; Stichler, 2001):

- Clocks, calendars, family photos, and get well cards: These items can reduce or prevent disorientation.
- Beloved objects that are cherished, regardless of their value: These items can hold an honored place in a sacred space. Clients or staff may find that a special shell from the beach, flowers or plants, candles, photographs, or other objects make important additions to a space and can evoke wonderful memories that enhance a space.
- Chairs and recliners that offer neck and lumbar support, have sturdy construction, and are easy to get into and out of: For some spaces, sensuous, luxurious fabrics; soft pillows; and comfortable chairs are just what a client needs.
- Upholstery that is comfortable, visually appealing, and easy to maintain
- Art that contributes to the ambience of an environment and strengthens the link between the local community, staff, clients, and visitors: Select and position art to fit the needs of the viewer. Art that focuses on natural scenes is the most restful. Avoid ambiguous or uncertain art, emotionally negative or provocative subjects, forms that are optically unstable, close-up animals staring directly at the viewer, and outdoor scenes with overcast or foreboding weather. Minimize bold patterns since medicated or confused clients can view them as threatening. Choose art that produces a restful, calm feeling, and place it consciously. Figurative art should have emotionally positive facial expressions. Group scenes should depict friendly, caring, or nurturing relationships.
- Assisted living apartments that offer the option of having personal collections
- Relationships with children and pets
- Homelike architectural details (such as bay windows, balconies, and porches)
- Bathroom safety and efficiency features (such as heated toilet seats, automatic flush levers, safety grab bars, and an internal odor exhaust system)
- Safety features to prevent falls (such as proper lighting and non-slip floor mats)
- Mobility features and appropriate space requirements for the disabled
- Universal kitchen design elements (such as roller-equipped drawers, adjustable counter heights, and easily reachable storage)
- Refrigerators, couches, tables, and reading lamps that resemble homelike surroundings

Special equipment used in client care areas is also part of the furnishings of a healing environment and must be selected to reduce the need to expend excess energy, encourage independence, and be safe and effective. In psychiatric hospitals, for example, where clients are potentially violent, furnishings that cannot be turned into weapons may be specifically chosen. Specialized knowledge about furnishing selection is also needed to address the needs of certain populations such as bariatric clients, children, and the elderly.

Privacy is an important element of effective client care and of a healing environment. Making sure clients are appropriately covered when they are ambulating, bathing, and toileting is essential. In addition, controlling visitors to provide privacy and client dignity supports the client's need to heal (Stichler, 2001).

Wayfinding

Wayfinding means knowing where you are, knowing your destination, following the best route, recognizing your destination, and finding your way back out. Good wayfinding creates a clear sense of order and place in an environment that is often frightening, confusing, and complex. If the main entry doors to a facility are easily visible and welcoming, people often feel more comfortable, confident, and less lost as they find their way to their appointment or hospital stay. Hunting for the entrance only increases their anxiety (Stewart, 2006).

Wayfinding is an important component of a healing healthcare environment, since disorientation can result in increased fatigue; headaches; anxiety, increased feelings of stress, frustration, and helplessness; or, in extreme situations, death. Consider the ailing elderly client with a walker who likes being punctual and is already late as she searches the maze-like hallways of the hospital for the laboratory, or the ambulance driver who is transporting a seriously ill person and cannot quickly find the emergency room entrance to the local hospital. The use of universal, appropriate navigational tools, signage, artwork, visual clues, and symbols prevent wayfinding confusion for the healthcare professional and the client (Leibrock, 2000; Long, 2001; Schweitzer et al., 2004). An environmental design solution should work for the most vulnerable client.

Wayfinding can be improved by following a few simple guidelines (Huelat, 2003; Leibrock, 2000; Stewart, 2006):

- Develop a facilities master and site plan.
- The form of a building provides the strongest wayfinding cues. Limit the number of corridors and use items in personal collections (such as artifacts, sculptures, photographs, or paintings) to provide important orientation cues.
- Unique client room entrances can help everyone distinguish a specific room from others on a long corridor. Unique floor tiles, room carpet that is a different color from the hallway carpet, or private client mailboxes at the room entrance are just some ways to differentiate.

- Atriums and galleries (instead of long corridors) are effective wayfinding tools because of their often distinctive designs.
- A paving pattern that includes bands running perpendicularly to the flow of traffic slows the traffic down and may require more signage than a pattern that runs parallel to and reinforces the main traffic flow.
- Consistent lighting, floor stripes, and the use of colors, color coding, and patterns can differentiate the sections of a healthcare environment.
- Outdoor play areas or gardens can serve as strong reference points to help with orientation to a building.
- Signs should have only one symbol. They should provide information, direction, identification of an area, or regulatory information. Signage should be easily identifiable, and international symbols should be used whenever possible.
- Graphics should include the facility's name or logo, which should also be on signs, printed materials, and badges worn by staff members. Lettering should be easy to read. This consistency helps to convey the facility's message.
- Directional artwork and continuous finishes can lead people to specific destinations. For example, getting off an elevator and seeing a large photograph of a baby tells people that they are near the nursery.
- Since clients are often prone, it is more important to differentiate between walls and ceilings (by using different colored paint or different textures and surfaces) than it is to differentiate between walls and the floor.
- A view of the sky and the ground helps maintain circadian rhythms in clients and prevents hallucinations and disorientation.
- Clocks and calendars can improve time orientation. Writing the date and time on a white board is also effective. It is not helpful to mark off the days on a calendar, however, because this can contribute to a client's sense of loss of another day.
- Signs that use tactile and audible cues as well as visual ones are important to individuals with differences in vision, reading, and learning abilities.

CHILDREN AND HEALING ENVIRONMENTS

When creating healing environments, one client population deserves special attention: children. Children are not just little adults, and they have special environmental needs. For example, children who are exposed (safely) to ultraviolet (UV) light tend to have fewer colds, grow faster, and experience better physical and mental development than those who are not exposed to UV light.

Children differ from adults in many of their physiological and psychological responses to environmental elements and toxins.

- Children are more sensitive than adults to gradients in temperature and to toxic elements in the environment (Venolia, 1988).
- Children breathe more rapidly than adults, making them more susceptible to airborne environmental toxins.
- Children drink more fluids per body weight than adults, increasing their susceptibility to contaminants such as pesticides found in drinking water, milk, and juices.
- Children play on the floor, grass, and playground, increasing their exposure to lead-based paint dust, cleaning product residues, fertilizers, herbicides, and pesticides in the ground.
- Children also differ in their responses to colors, design elements, and the unfamiliar sights and sounds often found in healthcare environments.

Children's developmental levels play an important role in their interpretation of the environment. When creating healing environments, healthcare providers must consider children's unique needs and special vulnerabilities, along with the needs of their parents. For example, having parents in the room calls for regular beds; storage shelves; soft, homelike lighting; outlets for computers; and appropriately sized chairs.

Healing environments for children need to include a philosophy of family-centered care. Families are the social support network for children and are critical to their healing. Special spaces for families and visitors, visiting policies, and spaces for activities and distractions (such as fountains, aquaria, art, gardens, and reading materials) are essential (Long, 2001).

One hospital, the William Beaumont Hospital in Royal Oak, Michigan, completed a 4,000-square-foot garden in their William and Marie Carls Children's Medical Center. The fifth-floor pediatric garden "extends the concept of healing gardens to incorporate the power of multi-sensory stimulation, play, diversion and laughter" (Metz, 2006, p. 22). A central garden is surrounded by four smaller gardens, each designed to accommodate a specific population. For example, the teen section includes a Cyber Café Garden, and the Quiet Garden, adjacent to the neonatal intensive care unit, includes a special space for infant care. This project includes music, liquid crystal display (LCD) monitors, special-effects lighting, technology, bright colors, and movable seating and benches. The design was based on input from children, parents, family caregivers, physicians, nurses, and hospital staff, and it has been enthusiastically received by clients, staff, and families (Metz, 2006).

COMMUNICATION AND EDUCATION

Neumann and Mensik (1993) note that "access to information is crucial to a healing environment. The information itself and the sense of control that communicating can bring will positively affect the healing process" (pp. 4–5). Consider the following suggestions to provide effective communication and appropriate education to clients:

- Communication must be private as well as audible. Provide for quiet spaces conducive to personal and professional conversations and consultations.
- Accommodation must be made for individuals with hearing impairments. Flashing lights on telephones, closed-captioned televisions, text telephones, strobe lights for smoke alarms, or substituting shaking pillows or beds for alarm clocks are just some suggestions that contribute to a healing environment for the hearing impaired.
- Nurses and other staff should present a culturally appropriate welcoming presence to clients and visitors while ensuring confidentiality. Smiles, pleasant and approachable demeanors, and a willingness to go the extra mile all contribute to the client's sense that the healthcare provider cares and is truly committed to his or her healing.
- Call buttons and other controls should be within reach and lit for nighttime use.
- Phones should be close at hand.
- Educational material should be culturally appropriate and written for a variety of learning levels.

Prevention and wellness depend on educated clients making responsible choices. When individuals take responsibility for their health, pressure on the staff is lowered, and hospital stays and staff turnover can be reduced. Printed information, classes, and support groups are just some of the many ways in which education can be delivered to clients (Leibrock, 2000).

Staff education is also critical. Unless an organization's culture supports a change to the environment, the change may not be successful. Staff, including nurses, may find the changes difficult to understand and incorporate into their practice, but they must view the benefits as outweighing the challenges. While the concept of healing environments is not yet mainstream, it is a growing movement.

THE HEALTHCARE PROVIDER AS A HEALING ENVIRONMENT

The healthcare provider can be one of the most powerful tools for healing in the client's environment. Quinn (2005) asserts that the "energy fields of the two interact and form a new pattern of inter-penetration, spirit within spirit" (p. 50).

Nurses, in particular, can have a tremendous impact on the client. Quinn (2005) also states, "Simply by virtue of the role, a nurse has all the ritual power of the shaman of other cultures. The nurse is guardian of the patient's journey through illness and healing; the keeper and bestower of information, medicines, and treatments; the mediator of the system, and the comings and goings of others in the system" (p. 49).

Healing is a process of being or becoming whole, and it requires the emergence of a process of connection or right relationship between the healthcare provider and the client. This right relationship encourages true healing and the dynamic process of emergence into something new, rather than a simple return to prior states of being (Quinn, 2005). Respect, compassion, empathy, effective communication, appropriate clinical skills, and positive intent are essential elements in this process.

The concept of optimal healing environments (OHEs) includes many elements, but two key elements are the relationship between healer and client and the relationship between healers and their inner selves (Bolles & Maley, 2004). Every healing effort and every healing intention starts within the healthcare professional who has an accepting, mindful, and warmhearted relationship with his or her self. This principle recognizes the symmetry between an individual's relationship with the outer world and the relationship with his or her inner world.

As healers, people are the most important aspect of any healing environment because they provide care, understanding, and counsel (Huelat, 2003). Viewed in this light, healthcare providers are not simply separate selves doing something to the client; they are often an integral part of the client's healing journey. This quality of being with the client requires attention to the healthcare provider's own healing environment, both internally and externally (Keegan, 2005).

A healing presence supports a healing environment. A healing presence is an interpersonal, intrapersonal, and transpersonal transcendent phenomenon that leads to a beneficial, therapeutic, and/or positive spiritual change within another person and within the healer (McDonough-Means, Kreitzer, & Bell, 2004).

Healers who support a healing environment also support meaningful client and family relationships. For example, for the last several decades, fathers have been permitted into delivery rooms. Less restrictive visiting hours, especially in critical care, emergency, and recovery areas, unite family members with their extremely ill loved ones at a time when they are needed the most. Good design creates sufficient space for family access. Separating clients with walls rather than curtains allows for privacy and enhances interactions among family members (Schweitzer et al., 2004). Clients and their families may be undergoing a tremendously difficult ordeal. Yet, if care is delivered in a way that incorporates all the elements of a healing environment (including positive, supportive staff), the experience can be a healing one. Healing environments, with all of their elements, are a crucial part of this dynamic process.

THE FUTURE OF HEALING ENVIRONMENTS

Just as the world around us affects our behavior, we affect our surroundings with our thoughts, emotions, and actions. Urbanization may be one of the most important environmental influences on behavior in the 21st century. As a species, we must adapt to unprecedented technological and social changes, and we must continually redefine what a good, or healing, environment is in our community, in a forest, in an office, in our schools, and in our homes. With increasingly complex existences, we need places that support rather than fragment our lives, places that balance the technology and urbanization with the natural, personal, and healthful.

KEY CONCEPTS

1. A healing environment is intended to elicit a positive or healthy outcome for the user; it is one in which people are supported and nurtured and health and well-being are promoted. Elements of a healing environment include color, nature, lighting, air quality and temperature, smells, music, noise, buildings and furnishings, and wayfinding. Healing environments for children need to embody a philosophy of family-centered care.
2. Healthcare providers are not separate selves, doing something to the client. They are often an integral part of the client's healing journey, and the quality of being with clients requires attention to their own healing environments, both internally and externally.
3. A healing presence supports a healing environment. A healing presence is an interpersonal, intrapersonal, and transpersonal transcendent phenomenon that leads to a beneficial, therapeutic, and/or positive spiritual change within another person and within the healer.

QUESTIONS FOR REFLECTION

1. What is a healing environment?
2. What roles do the elements of color, lighting, and noise play in the development of a healing environment?
3. How can a healthcare provider contribute to a healing environment?

REFERENCES

Barba, B. E., Tesh, A. S., & Courts, N. F. (2002, March). Promoting thriving in nursing homes: The Eden alternative. *Journal of Gerontological Nursing, 28*(3), 7–13.

Bolles, S., & Maley, M. (2004). Designing relational models of collaborative integrative medicine that support healing processes. Toward optimal healing environments in health care: Second American Samueli Symposium, January 22–24, 2004. *Journal of Alternative and Complementary Medicine, 10*(Suppl. 1), S61–S69.

Buelow, M. (2001). Noise level measurements in four Phoenix emergency departments. *Journal of Emergency Medicine, 27*(1), 26.

Burkhardt, M. A., & Nagai-Jacobson, M. G. (2002). *Spirituality: Living our connectedness.* Albany, NY: Delmar Thomson Learning.

Cabrera, I. N., & Lee, M. H. M. (2000, April). Reducing noise pollution in the hospital setting by establishing a department of sound: A survey of recent research on the effects of noise and music in health care. *Preventive Medicine, 30*(4), 339–345.

Cmiel, C. A., Gasser, D. M., & Neveau, A. J. (2004). Noise control: A nursing team's approach to sleep promotion. *American Journal of Nursing, 104*(2), 40–48.

Daniels, R., Nosek, L. J., & Nicoll, L. H. (2007). *Contemporary medical-surgical nursing.* Clifton Park, NY: Thomson Delmar Learning.

Eliopoulos, C. (2004). *Invitation to holistic health: A guide to living a balanced life.* Sudbury, MA: Jones and Bartlett.

Fick, D. D., & Vance, G. L. (2006, August). Quiet zone. *Health Facilities Management, 19*(8), 21–24.

Frankel, R. M., Sung, S. H., & Hsu, J. T. (2005). Patients, doctors, and videotape: A prescription for creating optimal healing environments? Developing healing relationships: Third American Samueli Symposium. *Journal of Alternative and Complementary Medicine, 11*(Suppl. 1), S31–S39.

Geller, G., & Warren, L. R. (2004). Toward an optimal healing environment in pediatric rehabilitation. Toward optimal healing environments in health care: Second American Samueli Symposium, January 22–24, 2004. *Journal of Alternative and Complementary Medicine, 10*(Suppl. 1), S179–S192.

Girman, A., Vigna, L., & Lee, R. (2004). Selected issues in environmental medicine. In B. Kligler & R. Lee, *Integrative medicine: Principles for practice* (pp. 339–367). New York: McGraw-Hill.

Huelat, B. J. (2003). *Healing environments: Design for the body, mind, and spirit.* Alexandria, VA: Medezyn.

Jones, M. M., & Haight, B. K. (2002, March). Environmental transformations: An integrative review. *Journal of Gerontological Nursing, 28*(3), 23–27.

Keegan, L. (2005). Environment. In B. M. Dossey, L. Keegan, & C. E. Guzzetta, *Holistic nursing: A handbook for practice* (4th ed., pp. 275–303). Sudbury, MA: Jones and Bartlett.

Kligler, B. (2004). The role of the optimal healing environment in the care of patients with diabetes mellitus type II. Toward optimal healing environments in health care: Second American Samueli Symposium, January 22–24, 2004. *Journal of Alternative and Complementary Medicine, 10*(Suppl. 1), S223–S229.

Leddy, S. K. (2006). *Integrative health promotion: Conceptual bases for nursing practice* (2nd ed.). Sudbury, MA: Jones and Bartlett.

Leibrock, C. A. (2000). *Design details for health.* New York: John Wiley and Sons.

Litch, B. K. (2007, July/August). The marriage of form and function: Creating a healing environment. *Healthcare Executive, 22*(4), 20–27.

Long, R. (2001). Healing by design: Eight key considerations for building therapeutic environments. *Health Facilities Management, 14*(11), 20–22.

Louv, R. (2005). *Last child in the woods.* Chapel Hill, NC: Algonquin.

Marcus, C. C., & Barnes, M. (1999). Introduction: Historical and cultural perspective on healing gardens. In C. C. Marcus & M. Barnes (Eds.), *Healing gardens: Therapeutic benefits and design recommendations* (pp. 1–26). New York: John Wiley and Sons.

Mazer, S. (2005). Stop the noise: Reduce errors by creating a quieter hospital environment. *Patient Safety and Quality Healthcare, 2*(2), 36–39.

McCaffrey, R. (2007). The effect of healing gardens and art therapy on older adults with mild to moderate depression. *Holistic Nursing Practice, 21*(2), 79–84.

McDonough-Means, S. I., Kreitzer, J. J., & Bell, I. R. (2004). Fostering a healing presence and investigating its mediators. Toward optimal healing environments in health care: Second American Samueli Symposium, January 22–24, 2004. *Journal of Alternative and Complementary Medicine, 10*(Suppl. 1), S25–S41.

Messervy, J. M. (2006, April/May). Soul garden. *Body + Soul,* 56–60.

Metz, R. K. (2006, July/August). Garden for all seasons. *Medical Construction and Design, 2*(4), 18–22.

Miller, R. L., & Swensson, E. S. (2002). *Hospital and healthcare facility design* (2nd ed.). New York: W. W. Norton.

Mycek, S. (2007, March). Under the spreading Planetree. *Trustee, 60*(3), 22–25.

Neumann, T., & Mensik, K. (1993, Spring). The healing power of design. *Innovator,* pp. 2–5. (Available from the Center for Nursing Innovation and Corporate Communications, St. Luke's Episcopal Hospital, Houston, TX)

Nightingale, F. (2007). *Notes on nursing: What it is, and what it is not. With an introduction by Anita S. Kessler, RN, MSN, M.Ed.* Radford, VA: Wilder.

Quinn, J. F. (2005). Transpersonal human caring and healing. In B. M. Dossey, L. Keegan, & C. E. Guzzetta, *Holistic nursing: A handbook for practice* (4th ed., pp. 275–303). Sudbury, MA: Jones and Bartlett.

Reiling, J. G., Knutzen, B. L., Wallen, T. K., McCullough S., Miller, R., & Chernos, S. (2004). Enhancing the traditional hospital design process: A focus on patient safety. *Joint Commission Journal on Quality and Safety, 30*(3), 115–124.

Robinson, S. B., Weitzel, T., & Henderson, L. (2005, November/December). The sh-h-h-h-project: Nonpharmacological interventions. *Holistic Nursing Practice, 19*(6), 263–266.

Schweitzer, M., Gilpin, L., & Frampton, S. (2004). Healing spaces: Elements of environmental design that make an impact on health. *Journal of Alternative and Complementary Medicine, 10*(Suppl. 1), S71–S83.

Smith, J., Roehll, G., & Bonnell, L. M. (2007). Design with nature. *Healthcare Design, 7*(1), 36–41.

Stewart, B. L. (2006). The benefits of feng shui. *Medical Construction and Design, 2*(4), 30–33.

Stichler, J. F. (2001). Creating healing environments in critical care units. *Critical Care Nursing Quarterly, 24*(3), 1–20.

Trivieri, L., Jr., & Anderson, J. W. (Eds.). (2002). *Alternative medicine: The definitive guide* (2nd ed.). Berkeley, CA: Celestial Arts.

Venolia, C. (1988). *Healing environments: Your guide to indoor well-being.* Berkeley, CA: Celestial Arts.

Weil, A. (2006, April). My advice for quieting noise pollution. *Self healing: Creating optimum health for your body and soul,* 1.

Wright, S. G., & Sayre-Adams, J. (2000). *Sacred space: Right relationship and spirituality in healthcare.* Edinburgh: Churchill Livingstone.

Yee, R. (2006). *Healthcare spaces no. 3.* New York: Visual Reference.

CHAPTER 6

Traditional Chinese Medicine: An Ancient Approach to Healing

The way that can be told is not the eternal Way.
—Lao Tsu

LEARNING OBJECTIVES

1. Describe the differences between viewpoints in Western medicine and traditional Chinese medicine (TCM).
2. Compare and contrast the concepts of yin and yang.
3. List the five elements of five elements theory and explain their characteristics.
4. State the characteristics of the basic substances of qi, jing, blood, body fluids, and shen.
5. Describe the role of the basic substances in the body.
6. Identify the organs of the zang-fu system and describe their functions.
7. Explain the meridian or channel system and its role in TCM.
8. List the internal and external causes of disharmony according to TCM.
9. Describe the four types of examinations used in TCM.
10. Explain the most common treatment methods used in TCM, including acupuncture, moxibustion, cupping, acupressure, herbalism, Qigong, Tai Chi Chuan, and lifestyle modifications.

INTRODUCTION

Traditional Chinese medicine (TCM) originated thousands of years ago. Dating back over 3,000 years to 1000 BC in the Shang Dynasty, it has a long, rich history of development and it has been examined, tested, manipulated, and modified throughout its long use. Employed by a quarter of the world's population, it is the "oldest literate, professional, continuously practiced medicine in the world" (Bright, 2002, p. 261). Consider the following evidence and observations about TCM (Cassidy, 2002; Micozzi, 2006; Williams, 1996):

- Archeological digs reveal acupuncture needles, and unearthed bones show inscriptions of medical conditions.
- Huang Di's book, *The Yellow Emperor's Inner Classic (Huang Di Nei Jing)*, dates to the third century BC but contains much older material, including listings and discussion on the principles of yin and yang, the five phases, and the effects of the seasons on the human body as well as the therapeutic value of acupuncture, moxibustion, and more than 100 extracts from herbal, mineral, and animal sources.
- Many of the postures of Qigong (a TCM practice similar to yoga) were developed from observations of animal behavior. The movements of wild geese, for example, form the basis of dayan Qigong, which relates these movements to acupuncture points and the energy body.
- Many shamanic practices, especially those of ancient Asia, are believed to be at the foundation of TCM.

Many healthcare practitioners are familiar with the Western scientific view of medicine and unfamiliar with TCM, even though it has been practiced for several thousand years (Micozzi, 2006). While TCM may seem exotic and unusual, it is based on a profound philosophy and a rich tradition of empirical study (Williams, 1996). Today this medicine is so popular and easily available that some call it mainstream (Cassidy, 2002).

Because we tend to make sense of the world from our individual viewpoints, we may often make intellectual errors when dealing with medical systems that have been developed in other cultures. To avoid errors, healthcare providers and other caregivers must understand the medical systems embedded in their own and other cultures.

DIFFERENCES BETWEEN TCM AND WESTERN MEDICINE

Although TCM and Western medicine are being integrated in Asia, Europe, and the United States, there are fundamental differences between the two systems.

- Western medicine typically cures disease by external forces, whereas TCM attempts to reinforce and stimulate the body's internal strength to cure disease.
- The Western scientific view of medicine is based on the philosophy of reductionism, which seeks to understand all life by isolating it into its smaller parts. The Chinese view of medicine is based on the Taoist belief that everything in the universe is mutually interactive and interdependent. Williams (1996) notes that "nothing is excluded; nothing is analyzed or interpreted without reference to the whole . . . As human beings we exist as an integral part of an energetic—energy-filled—universe" (p. 13).

- While the Western view of medicine has resulted in many amazing advances in the treatment of diseases, it often lacks the insight resulting from a view that incorporates all aspects of the human being (Williams, 1996). TCM, on the other hand, takes a holistic view of the human being, approaching the person as a whole, comprised of body, mind, and spirit. It proposes that the forces of nature must be kept in balance and harmony according to natural laws and the larger universe. In TCM, the emphasis is on health rather than on disease (Dossey, Keegan, & Guzzetta, 2005; Williams, 1996).

Many believe that Western medicine is useful for treating acute illnesses while TCM is more appropriate for treating chronic illnesses. However, more and more healthcare practitioners in the West are incorporating the use of TCM in their treatment of clients, and more and more clients are seeking the services of TCM practitioners in their search for relief from various medical conditions (Williams, 1996).

BASIC CONCEPTS OF TCM

TCM is based on the relationship between symptoms, diseases, and patterns. Symptoms tell the TCM practitioner that something in the body-mind is diseased or out of balance; the goal is to bring the entire organism back into balance. Patterns allow the practitioner to see the whole person and provide treatments that are safe and effective (Flaws & Sionneau, 2001).

Comprised of integrated ideas, theories, assumptions, and modalities such as acupuncture, acupressure, herbal medicine, and Qigong, TCM has produced a highly sophisticated, heterogeneous set of practices designed to cure illness and maintain health and well-being (Cassidy, 2002; Williams, 1996). Because TCM involves complex and subtle philosophies and principles that differ from those of Western medicine, it is important to understand its underlying framework in order to comprehend TCM (Williams, 1996; Yanchi & Lianrong, 1998). The following sections explain its key underpinnings.

Energetic Concept of Qi

Qi (pronounced *chee*) is a fundamental concept in TCM. Qi is the basic substance that makes up the human body and an essential material that circulates constantly with strong energy. Qi maintains life activities (Yanchi & Lianrong, 1998). An illness is caused by a disturbance of the qi within the body (Micozzi, 2006).

From the Western point of view, energy is measurable and synonymous with vigorous action. However, qi means more than that in TCM. Consider the following (Bright, 2002; Cassidy, 2002; Williams, 1996; Yanchi & Lianrong, 1998):

- Everything in the universe has qi, but qi is not considered a particle or substance. Qi varies with its distribution, origin, and function.
- Qi begins with original or primary qi (yuan qi), also called prenatal or before-heaven qi. This qi is inherited from our parents at conception and nourished by food after birth. If original or primary qi is congenitally deficient or depleted because of chronic illness, pathological changes can occur in the body.
- Pectoral qi is composed mainly of clear qi and is inhaled by the lung.
- Essential qi is transformed by the stomach and spleen from the essence of food and drink.
- Two sources of postnatal qi are food or substance (gu qi) and inhaled air or clean qi (kong qi). These two mix to form gathering or aggregative qi (zong qi), which nourishes the heart and lungs and thus promotes respiration and blood circulation.
- Nutritive qi (ying qi) evolves from gathering qi. It originates from the essential elements of food transformed by the spleen and stomach. It is secreted by the body fluids, circulates inside the blood vessels, and nourishes all tissues in the body, including the extremities and the five zang and six fu organs.
- Defensive qi (wei qi), which circulates outside the body, warms and nourishes tissues and organs, adjusts the opening and closing of body pores, and protects the body from factors that can cause disharmony, such as exogenous pathogenic factors.

Qi has five main functions (Williams, 1996):

- It is a source of all body activity and movement.
- It warms the body and maintains normal body temperature.
- It protects the body from harmful external environmental factors.
- It transforms food and air into other vital substances (such as qi itself, blood, and body fluids).
- It helps hold organs, vessels, and body tissues in their correct place so they function properly.

There are four types of qi disharmony (Williams, 1996):

- *Deficient qi* results in a body's inability to effectively carry out necessary functions. For example, an aging person may have a qi deficiency that results in a chronic cold.

- *Sinking qi* results when a deficiency is so tremendous that the organ no longer functions. An organ prolapse is an example of sinking qi.
- *Stagnant qi* results when the qi flow to an organ is impaired, sluggish, or blocked. For example, an injury to the arm may result in swelling and pain.
- *Rebellious qi* occurs when qi flows in the wrong direction. For example, a rebellious stomach qi results in hiccups, nausea, or vomiting.

Yin and Yang Theory

Part of the Chinese worldview since ancient times, yin and yang are fundamental to TCM (Bright, 2002). These concepts are derived from observing the physical world and from the Taoist philosophy that nature and wholeness are comprised of the union of mutually dependent opposite pairs (Fontaine, 2000). Yin and yang theory classifies the healthcare practitioner's examination findings and guides the client's treatment because the goal is to foster a balance and harmony between yin and yang (Cassidy, 2002).

The natures of yin and yang are relative. They always exist together as variable proportions of each other, just as the concept of hot has no meaning without cold and day has no meaning without night. In addition, the concepts of yin and yang support the emphasis of TCM on process rather than structure. Thus, yin and yang describe a dynamic interaction between all aspects of nature and the universe. Yin and yang are always waxing and waning, and they express the idea of opposing but complementary phenomena that exist in a state of dynamic equilibrium (Cassidy, 2002; Micozzi, 2006; Trivieri & Anderson, 2002; Williams, 1996).

- Yin translates as "shady side of the mountain" and represents substance more than energy. It is associated with cold, earth, moon, night, autumn, winter, female, rest, downwardness, and passivity (Bright, 2002; Fontaine, 2000; Freeman, 2004; Micozzi, 2006; Williams, 1996).
- Yang translates as "sunny side of the mountain" and represents warmth, light, heaven, sun, summer, male, fast, excitement, upwardness, and vigor (Bright, 2002; Fontaine, 2000; Freeman, 2004; Williams, 1996).

In theory, all yin and yang can be subdivided into aspects that are themselves yin and yang. For example, the front of the body is considered yin in relation to the back (which is yang), but the upper front of the body (the chest) is considered to be yang in relation to the lower front (the abdomen).

An important concept is the dynamic interaction between yin and yang. Change is at the root of all of nature. As an example, Williams (1996) notes that "the seed (yin) grows into the plant (yang), which itself dies back into the earth (yin). This takes place within the changes of the seasons—winter (yin) transforms through the spring into summer (yang), which in turn transforms through the fall into the winter again" (p. 26). Disharmony and illness result when this dynamic change (transformation) is prevented from occurring. Conversely, a healthy body is characterized by a dynamic balance between yin and yang aspects (Williams, 1996).

Five Elements Theory

The metaphor about yin, yang, and the seasons can also be articulated in TCM's system of the five elements. The five elements are (Cassidy, 2002; Sierpina, 2001; Williams, 1996; Yanchi, 1995):

- *Wood*, representing germination, growth, extension, softness, flexibility, rootedness
- *Fire*, representing dryness, heat, ascension, movement
- *Earth*, representing growth, nourishment, change, fertility
- *Metal*, representing cutting, strength, firmness, hardness, conduction
- *Water*, representing wetness, moisture, coolness, descending, flowing, yielding

Each element corresponds to an element in the natural world, in yin and yang, and in the human body (Williams, 1996). For example, fire corresponds to heat and to the heart. The interrelationships between the elements are a model for demonstrating how the processes in the body support each other. The five elements are used to interpret the relationship between the physiology and pathology of the human body and the natural environment. For example, an angry person who tends to shout has a greenish complexion and tends to respond to stimulation of the meridian points of the liver and gallbladder (Cassidy, 2002).

When the five elements are used to describe how the body processes support each other, they are described through the sheng and ke cycles (Williams, 1996):

- The *sheng cycle* (often referred to as the mother and son cycle) is one of mutual production or promotion (Williams, 1996). In this cycle, every element is created by another element (the mother). It, in turn, creates another element (the child, or son). This creative cycle has no beginning or end (Cassidy, 2002).
- The *ke cycle* is one of mutual control. In the relationship between the elements in the natural world, each element is part of a process of dynamic equilibrium (Williams, 1996). Each element controls and is controlled by

another element. This cycle also has no beginning and no end. To strengthen the energy of a weak element, meridians of the element can be tonified (strengthened), the meridian of the element's mother can be tonified, or the meridians of the element's controller can be weakened (Cassidy, 2002).

Basic Substances Theory

Western medicine views the body as a system of physical structures (bones, muscles, skin, and specific organs) and views health and disease in terms of a cause-and-effect model. The Chinese approach to the human body is quite different. In TCM, the body's processes rather than its structures are considered crucial in understanding health and disease.

While the energy and five elements theories are one way to assess the balance or imbalance of qi in the body, another method is to view the body as an energy system in which various substances interact to create a whole physical structure. This theory is called the *basic substances theory*, and it encompasses the substances qi, jing (essence), xue (blood), jin ye (body fluids), and shen (spirit).

- *Qi:* Already discussed in some detail, qi, in the basic substances theory, is responsible for movement, protection, transportation, and warmth (Cassidy, 2002).
- *Jing (essence):* Essence is the foundation of all aspects of organic life. People are born with essence, which is similar to the Western concept of genes, DNA, and heredity. Essence is the cells' basic material, it supports life, and it is restored by food and rest (Fontaine, 2000). If essence is plentiful, a strong life force is present, and the organism is radiant and healthy. Jing is associated with the slow, developmental changes that accompany an organism's growth from fetus to old age and death. Jing governs an individual's growth, reproduction, and development throughout life; it determines the strength of our constitution or our ability to withstand infection or illness (Bright, 2002; Williams, 1996).
- *Xue (blood):* In TCM, blood is not just the physical substance normally recognized in Western medicine. Blood nourishes, moistens, and lubricates the body, and it contributes to the development of the mind (shen) to produce clear, stable thought processes and a positive state of mind. Food and drink are transformed into blood by means of the action of the spleen and the marrow (Bright, 2002; Cassidy, 2002; Williams, 1996).
- *Jin ye (body fluids):* Body fluids include all normal liquid in the body (such as saliva, gastric fluid, intestinal fluid, joint cavity fluid, tears, nasal

discharge, sweat, and urine). Body fluids originate from the ingestion of food and liquids, and they moisten and nourish the body (Bright, 2002; Cassidy, 2002).

- *Shen (spirit):* Shen, the mind or spirit of the individual, is considered the gift of heaven. Since TCM distinguishes among several aspects of the spirit, shen probably best represents the mind and aspects of human consciousness, thoughts, beliefs, and emotional well-being. Shen is the inner glow, or radiance, that others perceive (Bright, 2002; Fontaine, 2000).

Jing, qi, and shen are collectively called the three treasures in TCM because they are believed to be the essential elements of any individual. Individuals who are physically fit, mentally sharp, and alert are said to have their three treasures in harmony (Fontaine, 2000; Williams, 1996).

The Zang-fu System

The zang-fu system is comprised of the:

- Zang (or yin) solid organs
- Fu (or yang) hollow organs
- Extra fu organs (the extra fu)

Each zang organ is linked to or has a corresponding fu organ.

In TCM, an organ system is part of a dynamic energy process in the body (Williams, 1996). The zang and fu organs represent not only specific anatomical organs but also the physiology and pathology of body systems (Yanchi, 1995).

The Zang (Yin) Organs

The five zang (or yin) organs are the lungs, heart, spleen, liver, and kidneys. The pericardium is also considered a yin organ. These organs lie deep in the body and function mainly to manufacture, store, and regulate the fundamental substances of qi, blood, and body fluids (Williams, 1996; Yanchi, 1995). The following is a brief description of the functions of the zang organs (Bright, 2002; Cassidy, 2002; Williams, 1996; Yanchi, 1995).

- The lungs (called the receiver of pure qi from heaven) dominate qi and control respiration, regulate the body's rhythm, control the dispersion of body fluids (such as sweat), and send body fluids down to the kidneys. They also regulate the passage of water through the body, control the quality of the skin and the hair, and open to the nose.
- The heart (called the supreme controller) dominates the blood and controls the blood vessels. The heart also contributes to healthy circulation

and shen (spirit), governs the mind, opens into the tongue (the mirror of the heart), and is manifested in the face.

- The spleen (called the controller of transportation) governs the transportation and transformation of food leading to the production of qi and blood. The spleen ensures that muscles and limbs have good tone and shape. It opens into the mouth, ensures a good sense of taste, ensures clarity of thought and ideas, and is manifested on the lips.
- The liver (called the controller of planning) regulates the amount of blood in circulation. The liver controls the smooth flow of qi, helps regulate the evenness of temperament, and controls the ability of the tendons and ligaments to expand and contract. The spleen opens to the eyes and is manifested in the quality of the nails.
- The kidneys (called the controller of water) store the essence. They dominate reproduction, growth, and development; regulate fluid balance in the body; and dominate the anus and urethra. The kidneys open into the ears and are manifested in the quality of hearing and hair.

The Fu (Yang) Organs

The six fu (or yang) organs are the small intestine, large intestine, gallbladder, bladder, stomach, and the san jiao ("triple warmer" or "triple heater"), which has no anatomical counterpart in Western medicine. These organs are close to the body's surface and receive, separate, distribute, and excrete body substances. They digest food, absorb nutrients, and transport and excrete waste (Yanchi, 1995). They are important in the dynamic process of movement and change.

The following is a brief description of the functions of the fu organs (Bright, 2002; Cassidy, 2002; Williams, 1996; Yanchi, 1995):

- The small intestine (called the transformer of matter and separator of the pure from the impure) digests food and separates pure from impure food.
- The large intestine (called the drainer of the dregs) receives waste, absorbs the pure food, and transports and excretes waste.
- The gallbladder (called the decision maker and judge) stores bile and assists the liver in maintaining free-flowing qi.
- The bladder (called the controller of the storage of water) stores urine and controls excretion.
- The stomach (called the controller of rotting and ripening) receives and stores food and sends qi downward for processing.
- The san jiao (also called the triple heater or the official of balance and harmony) coordinates the transformation and transportation of qi and body fluids and regulates body temperature.

The Extra Fu Organs

The extra fu organs are the brain, uterus, marrow, bone, blood vessels, and gallbladder (the gallbladder is considered both a fu and extra fu organ). They are not as important in terms of process as the other two groups (Williams, 1996).

The Meridian (Channel) System

Meridians are pathways in which qi and blood circulate. The meridian system consists of 12 main channels (or vessels), 8 extra channels, 15 collaterals, 12 divergent channels, and the musculo-tendinous and cutaneous regions of the 12 regular channels. Physiologically, these channels and collaterals are thought of as a series of connecting passages through which qi and blood circulate throughout the body (Cassidy, 2002; Williams, 1996; Yanchi, 1995; Yanchi & Lianrong, 1998).

Since TCM operates at a very subtle energy level, the meridians are not the same as arteries, veins, and capillaries, and they do not correspond to any anatomic map in Western medicine. Instead, the meridian system is an energy distribution network that is, itself, also energetic (Moyers, 1993; Williams, 1996). A common analogy is that qi is like a river flowing toward its ultimate source, the ocean. During its course, it is shallow, deep, quick flowing, and slow flowing but always following its natural path.

Meridians represent areas of high qi concentration where the energy is dynamic. Any block to that energy flow results in an imbalance that manifests itself in illness or disease. Along the channels or meridians, access points, or energy vortices, allow qi to be removed or drawn into the body. These vortices are the acupuncture points that can be used to directly cause changes in the human body's energy system with resulting physical effects.

The channel system performs three functions in the body (Williams, 1996; Yanchi, 1995):

- Communication among related parts of the body
- Regulation of the activities of the zang-fu organs
- Distribution of qi

The 12 regular channels of the meridian system correspond to the five yin organs, the six yang organs, and the pericardium. Each channel communicates with its corresponding organ (Williams, 1996).

Three yin organs and three yang organs relate to each arm and leg. According to Williams (1996):

- Qi flows from the chest along the three arm yin channels to the hands, where they connect with the three paired arm yang channels.
- From there they flow upward to the head, where they connect with the three corresponding leg yang channels and flow down the body to the feet.
- There they connect with the corresponding leg yin channels and flow up again to the chest to complete the cycle.

At times qi and blood flow is at its maximum in each given channel, and the practitioner uses this information when diagnosing illness and developing treatment strategies.

CAUSES OF DISHARMONY

The concept of *disharmony*, which has evolved over the centuries, refers to a state or condition of being out of balance or not in harmony. By following various established diagnostic procedures, TCM practitioners can construct a detailed assessment of the status of all the internal organs without the aid of laboratory tests or other modern technology. They then use various methods to treat the disharmony and restore balance to the body. Disharmony can result from internal, external, or miscellaneous causes (Williams, 1996).

Internal (Endogenous) Causes

The seven internal causes of disharmony, also known as the seven emotions, cause illnesses that result from intense, prolonged, or suppressed feelings. Basically psychological in nature, they represent the inner life of an individual. They include the following emotions (Cassidy, 2002; Micozzi, 2006; Williams, 1996; Yanchi, 1995):

- *Sadness (or melancholy):* Associated with depression, fatigue, amenorrhea, shortness of breath, asthma, allergies, colds, and flu, sadness takes its toll primarily on the lung.
- *Grief:* Associated with upper respiratory diseases (such as emphysema, allergies, asthma), colds, and flu, extreme grief injures the lung.
- *Pensiveness:* Associated with digestive disorders, edema, low appetite, and fatigue, pensiveness injures the spleen.
- *Fear:* Associated with lower back pain, kidney damage, palpitations, insomnia, anxiety, and joint pain, fear injures the kidney.
- *Fright:* Associated with breathlessness, anxiety, insomnia, lower back pain, joint pain, and kidney damage, fright affects the heart.

- *Anger:* Associated with headaches, mental confusion, dizziness, and hypertension, anger affects the liver.
- *Joy:* Associated with heart damage, hysteria, muddled thought, and insomnia, overjoy produces adverse effects primarily on the heart.

While all of these emotions can be appropriate reactions to life situations, when the reactions become fixed, habitual, exaggerated, or inappropriate in any way, they may disrupt qi, affect balance, and lead to illness (Cassidy, 2002).

External (Exogenous) Causes

The six external causes of disease or disharmony, also called the six evils, relate to climatic conditions. While healthy, balanced individuals adapt to these conditions, they can overcome qi in weakened, imbalanced clients, penetrating the individual and resulting in illness (Cassidy, 2002; Yanchi, 1995).

The external causes of disharmony include the following (Cassidy, 2002; Micozzi, 2006; Williams, 1996; Yanchi, 1995):

- *Wind* is associated with chills, fever, colds, flu, nasal congestion, headaches, allergies, arthritic and rheumatic conditions, dizziness, and vertigo.
- *Cold* is associated with colds, cough, upper respiratory allergies, poor circulation, anemia, muscular pain and spasm, and poor digestion.
- *Heat* is associated with hypertension, hyperthyroid, ulcers, colitis, profuse sweating, convulsions, inflamed arthritic joints, flu, and skin rashes.
- *Dampness* is associated with obesity, cyst or tumor formation, and an increased production of phlegm.
- *Dryness* is associated with disorders of the lungs, sinuses, large intestine, skin, digestion, and reproductive organs.
- *Summer heat* is associated with dizziness, convulsions, general malaise, heat stroke, nausea, extreme thirst, and exhaustion.

Miscellaneous Causes

The miscellaneous causes of disharmony and disease include the following (Cassidy, 2002; Micozzi, 2006; Williams, 1996):

- Genetic and congenital factors
- Lifestyle factors (such as stress)
- Excessive or stressful work
- Excessive or inappropriate exercise
- Trauma

- Dietary irregularities
- Excessive sexual activity
- Unforeseen events (such as plagues, poisoning, animal bites and stings, parasites, epidemics, accidents, injuries, pollution, and food contamination)

DIAGNOSTIC TECHNIQUES

TCM practitioners utilize four types of examinations to assess their clients: inspection (looking), auscultation and olfaction (listening and smelling), inquiry (questioning), and palpation (touching). Once they gather information from the four examinations, the practitioners organize it to understand the energies and disharmonies observed. The most common organizational patterns used by TCM practitioners are the eight-principle patterns (applied to the zang-fu system), the five-element patterns, and the channel patterns. The four examinations and the eight-principle approach (the most commonly used pattern in both East and West) are described in the following sections (Williams, 1996; Yanchi, 1995).

The Four Examinations

The order in which the TCM practitioner conducts the four types of examination is not arbitrary. It follows the hierarchy of the senses: the eyes for looking, the ears and nose for listening and smelling, the mouth for questioning, and the hands for feeling. Each of the four types is described in the following sections (Bright, 2002; Cassidy, 2002; Fontaine, 2000; Micozzi, 2006; Nielsen & Hammerschlag, 2004; Williams, 1996; Yanchi, 1995).

Inspection (Looking)

The first step in assessment is observing the individual. Inspection involves assessing the physical and spiritual aspects of a client. Physical appearance can provide many important clues about the person's health. Weight, level of activity, posture, gait, pallor, hair condition, facial condition, and the condition of the tongue are all significant. For example, dry skin may indicate a blood deficiency, and swollen skin can indicate qi stagnation or a deficiency of kidney yang. Observation of spirit, clarity of thought, coordination, and vigor provide insight into the individual's strength or loss of spirit.

The tongue is considered to be the visual gateway to the body's interior. In TCM, the entire body is mapped out on the tongue; that is, various organ systems correspond to various parts of the tongue and can be assessed by looking at the tongue. For example, the tip of the tongue corresponds to the heart, and the center back portion of the tongue corresponds to the kidneys and bladder. The tongue is inspected for color, shape, markings, and coatings (fur or moss) to provide the practitioner with information about the individual's state of balance.

Auscultation and Olfaction (Listening and Smelling)

These two aspects of the examination are grouped together because the Chinese word for this examination doesn't distinguish between them. They involve listening to the quality of the client's voice, the speed of conversation, and the rate and intensity of breathing, and noticing the presence of any odors from the ears, nose, genitals, urine, stool, or parts of the body. The odor of the breath is considered an indicator of balance or imbalance. The stronger the odor, the more serious the imbalance.

Inquiry (Questioning)

Of the four examinations, inquiry is the one most similar to (and therefore familiar to) Western practitioners. It is also the part of the exam that takes the most time. When assessing an individual's health, the practitioner can gain important information by asking about health and lifestyle. Questions should be asked about the condition of a client's social, emotional, and spiritual health, as well as his or her physical health, including the following:

- Sensing: Seeing, hearing, tasting, touching, thinking, feeling
- Digestion: What, when, and how food is eaten and to what degree of satisfaction
- Bowels and excreta: Regularity, shape, color, smell, and sensation
- Fluid intake, thirst levels, perspiration, tears
- Urination: Frequency, color, sensation, and stream
- Sleep patterns and energy levels
- Pain: Location, frequency, severity, and responsiveness
- Body temperature
- Lifestyle features: Vitality, activity, work, and pleasure
- Emotional features
- Menses: Regularity, length, color
- Sexual desire and activity

Palpation (Touching)

In the last aspect of the examination, the practitioner conducts the actual laying on of hands and works with the client to examine the entire body, especially the pulses. Body temperature, body moisture, and painful areas along meridian lines are assessed. Cold skin, for example, might suggest a cold disharmony, while moist skin can suggest a lung disharmony. Pain along a meridian may suggest a local channel problem.

Pulse diagnosis provides important information about a person's overall condition and is probably the most well known part of the four examinations. The pulse is considered an expression of the qi moving the blood. Since qi and blood represent yin and yang, any imbalance in yin or yang and any abnormality in qi or blood are manifested as an altered pulse.

This exam has many regional and situational variations. Twenty-eight (or 29, depending on the source) pulse qualities on the six pulse positions (three on each wrist) can be assessed, including the rate, volume, depth, width (between the fingers), strength, and rhythm. A thready, thin pulse could suggest a blood deficiency. A slippery pulse (one that slips along under the fingers like a thin fluid) could indicate an internal damp spleen disharmony. Other pulse descriptions include gliding, string-like, soggy, or large. These pulses can be recorded accurately with modern technology: the six-channel oscilloscope.

Once information is gathered from the four examinations, the TCM practitioner must organize the information to understand the energies and disharmonies observed.

The Eight Principles

This method of understanding disharmonies uses four interdependent pairs of characteristics (Williams, 1996):

- Yin and yang
- Interior and exterior
- Cold and hot
- Deficiency and excess

The combination of these pairs is always dynamic and can change over time; thus the use of this method requires flexibility so energy changes can be tracked.

The most common problems result from an excess or deficiency of either heat or cold. Treatment focuses on reducing the excess or restoring the deficiency. If too much heat is present, the excess is expelled or cooled. If too much cold is present, the excess is either expelled or warmed (Williams, 1996).

TREATMENT METHODS

Ideally, disharmonies should be prevented. However, when they do occur, they can be treated with several methods:

- Acupuncture
- Moxibustion
- Cupping
- Acupressure
- Herbalism
- Qigong
- Tai Chi Chuan
- Lifestyle modifications

Acupuncture

TCM practitioners have used acupuncture to influence qi for several thousand years. Until President Richard M. Nixon's visit to China in 1972, the practice of acupuncture to treat pathophysiological conditions in the United States was rare. However, acupuncture continues to grow in the United States due to research regarding its efficacy, consumer demand, recognition by the National Institutes of Health and The Joint Commission, and the training and licensing of acupuncturists (Nielsen & Hammerschlag, 2004).

The general theory of acupuncture purports that disease is caused by disruptions and imbalances in the flow of qi through the body. Acupuncture attempts to unblock congested energy pathways, thus allowing a freely flowing energy current (Seaward, 2006). The therapeutic goal of acupuncture is to improve and regulate qi by strategically placing needles along the meridians that conduct energy between body surfaces and deep internal organs (Leddy, 2006; Micozzi, 2006).

Acupuncture is based on a significant amount of scientific evidence derived from the systematic observation of the effects of needles placed on specific *ashi* points on the body. Initially, the needles were made from sharpened stones, animal bones, or bamboo, and they were used to remove blocked meridians and regulate qi flow. The aim is to tone, disperse, sedate, warm, cool, guide, or drain qi (Cassidy, 2002). Specific ashi points have been identified and their actions recorded, but the practice continues to be refined and developed even today (Williams, 1996).

In acupuncture, the practitioner's skill and intent are crucial. Before the session, the experienced practitioner conducts a diagnostic interview and makes a complete assessment (Williams, 1996). The practitioner's intent must be positive, and his or her concentration must be focused while performing the procedure.

The needle must be correctly located and manipulated to elicit the desired therapeutic effect. It can be rotated, flicked, or stroked; the technique chosen depends on the practitioner's personal preference and experience. Practitioners use various methods to select points for treating a client. When the qi is accessed, both client and practitioner may be able to detect the sensation. While the sensation is difficult to describe, some individuals who have undergone Chinese styles of acupuncture have said it feels like a small pinch followed by a sensation of itching, tingling, numbness, ache, traveling warmth, or heaviness (Cassidy, 2002; Micozzi, 2006; Williams, 1996). The client can use his or her recall of the sensation to advise the practitioner as to when the needle has reached the correct point. The practitioner can use the needle to reinforce a deficiency of qi, reduce an excess of qi, or smooth out qi that is not overly excessive or deficient (Williams, 1996). The practitioner may also use pressure, friction, suction, heat, or electromagnetic energy to stimulate specific anatomic points (Fontaine, 2000).

Acupuncture is effective in treating postoperative pain (including dental procedures) as well as the nausea and vomiting that result from chemotherapy. It is also useful as an adjunct treatment or acceptable alternative for the following conditions (Benor, 2004; Fontaine, 2000; Lu, 2005; Sierpina, 2001):

- Acute and chronic pain
- Motion disabilities, stroke rehabilitation, myofascial pain, osteoarthritis, low-back pain, carpal tunnel syndrome, and tennis elbow
- Respiratory and cardiovascular conditions, including asthma, chronic obstructive pulmonary disease (COPD), palpitations, and hypertension
- Eye, ear, nose, and throat disorders (conjunctivitis, tinnitus, Meinier's disease, rhinitis, sore throat)
- Gastrointestinal disorders (gastritis, ulcers, colitis, constipation, irritable bowel syndrome)
- Urogenital conditions (premenstrual syndrome, endometriosis, menopausal symptoms, prostatitis, incontinence, erectile problems)
- Skin disorders (eczema, shingles, urticaria)
- Addictive disorders and withdrawal syndromes

Acupuncture is contraindicated in those clients with hemophilia, pregnancy, severe psychotic conditions, and acute cardiovascular disorders or in those who have recently taken drugs or alcohol (Fontaine, 2000; Williams, 1996).

Acupuncture practitioners use rigorous standards of sterilization for their equipment. In fact, many practitioners use disposable needles packed in foil packs with guide tubes. The needles may be made from stainless steel and can range in thickness and in length, depending on the style of acupuncture used (Cassidy, 2002; Williams, 1996).

Anyone considering the use of acupuncture should check the registry of their state or country's professional licensing body to ensure that the practitioner is registered and in good standing and to determine whether any complaints have been filed. The training, accreditation, and registration of TCM practitioners vary from country to country and, in the United States, from state to state. Fully registered practitioners have, however, undertaken specific training in the practice of TCM and have met curricula standards for Western anatomy, physiology, and pathology. These practitioners perform acupuncture and massage, prescribe Chinese herbs, teach Qigong, provide dietary and lifestyle advice, adhere to a rigorous standard of ethical conduct, and carry comprehensive professional indemnity insurance.

Moxibustion

Moxibustion is a collective name for any procedure in which heat is applied to the body surface. Classically, the procedure involves using a dried herb, or moxa (usually mugwort, or *Artemisia vulgaris*), which is burned either directly on the skin or indirectly above the skin over specific acupuncture points. The word *moxibustion* is derived from the Japanese term *moe kusa* ("burning herb") (Cassidy, 2002).

The herb is harvested at a specific time (usually during the early summer months) and the leaves are dried, allowed to age, crushed, and then sifted (Williams, 1996). Moxibustion is used extensively to treat yang deficiency and excess cold and to nourish qi and blood. The three variations of moxibustion are:

- Direct (nonscarring)
- Indirect
- Scarring

Direct (Nonscarring) Moxibustion

The most refined moxa is used for direct application to the skin and consists of the soft underside of the herb leaf. The moxa is formed into small cones, lit, and placed on the skin. The cone is allowed to burn down until the client's skin turns red and the client feels the heat. The ash is then removed and a new cone is lit. This process is repeated for the duration of the treatment (Williams, 1996). This method is particularly useful to treat asthma and hypertension (Cassidy, 2002).

Indirect Moxibustion

Indirect moxibustion includes all methods that do not burn moxa directly on the skin (Cassidy, 2002). This method typically uses a lower grade of moxa either above the skin or on another medium between the moxa and the skin.

The choice of media depends on the practitioner's experience and the condition being treated, and it can include the following (Cassidy, 2002; Micozzi, 2006; Williams, 1996):

- Salt
- Garlic
- Ginger
- Bean cake
- Clay

In indirect moxibustion, moxa sticks or rolls (which can be the length of large cigars) are lit and rotated about an inch above the skin or moved in a circular or pecking motion for anywhere from several to 15 minutes. The client can be taught to use moxa rolls safely at home as an adjunct to office therapy (Cassidy, 2002; Micozzi, 2006; Williams, 1996).

Moxa sticks can also be burned on the handle of a stainless steel needle, which is then inserted into an acupuncture point. This warms the skin and draws the heat into the channel. A moxa box can also be used: moxa is placed into a box and heated, and the box is placed over a specific body part (Williams, 1996).

Scarring Moxibustion

In this procedure, moxa is applied directly to the skin, ignited, and allowed to burn all the way down. This process can be repeated several times (Cassidy, 2002).

While this method results in scarring of the skin, it is not part of the regular practice of moxibustion in the West. Although ancient wisdom dictates that blister formation and scarring are essential if healing is to be achieved, modern Western practitioners find that equally effective treatments can be achieved without scarring (Williams, 1996).

Cupping

Cupping is an ancient procedure used by folk medicine healers as well as by modern practitioners. It is particularly useful for treating headache, dizziness, cough, rheumatic pain, indigestion, abdominal pain, and stomachache (Lu, 2005). Cupping is commonly used to supplement acupuncture (Cassidy, 2002; Micozzi, 2006).

A vacuum is created by burning a cotton ball in a cup, which is made of strong, rounded glass, earthenware, or bamboo, and then quickly discarding the cotton ball and placing the cup firmly over the acupuncture point (for 5–10 minutes) so the cup attaches to the skin surface. The vacuum causes the cup to adhere to the skin, which is drawn up into the cup, encouraging the flow of qi and blood in the area. The strength of the vacuum depends on the amount of oxygen in the cup and on the practitioner's skill in quickly placing the cup on the client's skin (Cassidy, 2002; Lu, 2005; Williams, 1996). Moving the cup around the skin areas while the vacuum remains intact can reinforce the effects, obtaining more generalized qi and blood movement (Lu, 2005; Williams, 1996).

Cupping is avoided in the following conditions (Cassidy, 2002):

- In clients with high fevers
- In clients with blood dyscrasias
- In clients with a history of convulsions
- Over the abdomen and lower back of pregnant clients
- Over the large blood vessels
- Over any skin with signs of edema, sores, ulcers, or allergic reactions

Acupressure

Acupressure is based on the same general principles as acupuncture, but the qi is manipulated through massage instead of with needles. Varying forms of pressure are used, depending on whether the goal is to tonify, reduce, or calm the qi. Many massage techniques are used in TCM. For example, cavity-press techniques apply pressure to an acupuncture point for specific systemic changes. Other forms of acupressure massage include the following (Williams, 1996):

- *Tui na:* The use of pressure, manipulation, and other techniques to treat disharmonies
- *Shiatsu:* The use of pressure to more than 600 acupuncture points by the finger, thumb, or palm of the hand
- *Zero balancing:* The use of a specific sequence of well-defined protocols to encourage energetic harmony in the body

Acupressure is effective in treating the following conditions (Fontaine, 2000; Williams, 1996):

- Common colds
- Insomnia
- Leg cramps
- Painful menses
- Minor headaches
- Mild nausea and/or vomiting and diarrhea

- Joint and muscle aches and pains, arthritis, and stiff neck
- Asthma
- Nasal bleeding

According to Williams (1996), the techniques of acupressure are usually safe but the following precautions are important to note:

- Never massage or use acupressure on someone with an acute infection or severe cardiovascular or liver disease.
- Do not use acupressure or massage on areas with lesions, sores, lumps, or tumors or on areas that have been burned to any degree.
- Avoid massage on individuals who exhibit psychotic illness or evidence of severe mental illness.
- Take extreme care when using massage or acupressure on pregnant or menstruating clients.
- Take care when using massage or acupressure on frail or elderly clients.

Herbalism in TCM

Evidence of the use of herbal preparations dates to 2000 BC, to a shamanic culture that used plant, animal, and mineral substances to heal individuals. During this time, Emperor Chi'en Nung (also spelled Shen Nong and called the Divine Farmer) described over 300 medicinal plants in his book *Pen Tsao*. During the next several hundred years, the use of these substances was further refined, and by AD 659 a comprehensive *materia medica* was developed. This document listed the various substances as well as their actions and properties (Williams, 1996).

Herbal medicine is an integral part of TCM, which uses more than 1,000 different herbs (Cassidy, 2002). Not all plants are herbs, and not all herbs are plants. Herbal remedies can be made from (often controversially) animal parts and mineral parts, as well as many parts of plants (including the roots, stems/stalks, bark, leaves, fruit, and seeds). For example, herbs can be made from any of the following (Williams, 1996):

- Watermelon skin
- Gardenias
- Lily bulbs
- Lotus seeds
- Rose hips
- Mother of pearl
- Hornets' nests
- Fossilized animal bone

- Praying mantis egg cases
- Geckos
- Cuttlefish bones
- Abalone shells
- Indigo
- Oyster shells
- Talcum
- Amber
- Frankincense
- Pumice

Herbs can be used in the following forms (Cassidy, 2002; Fontaine, 2000; Williams, 1996):

- In their raw, dried form (which is then cooked in a soup, drained, and ingested)
- In powdered form (often taken as a capsule)
- As a tincture (suspended in 25–60% alcohol)
- As a patented preparation (in pill, spray, cream, or poultice form)

Botanical products are a $1.5 billion industry in the United States. While an estimated 60–70% of Americans take botanical products, only about one-third of these individuals inform their practitioners about their use (Kuhn, 2002).

Since herbs can be bought over the counter and self-prescribed, most people in the United States believe herbs are natural and harmless—something to be grown in the garden. This Western view of herbs can be quite misleading. Approximately 33% of medications used in the United States were developed from plants, including digitalis, morphine, atropine, and several chemotherapeutic agents. Herbs can affect multiple body functions, and the potential for misuse is high (Cassidy, 2002).

Even though precautions or contraindications are associated with the use of many herbs and some are toxic if misused, herbal medicine is safe when used properly. Because herbs are sold as food supplements, companies are not required to prove their efficacy, determine their side effects, or determine the possible interactions that may occur with other products. Healthcare practitioners must be educated about the effects of herbs and the possible interactions between herbs and other medications that their clients may be taking (Cassidy, 2002; Kuhn, 2002).

Properties of Herbs

Herbs perform highly specific actions, and certain herbs can perform different functions at the same time. For example, herbs can be used as antiviral, antibacterial, antifungal, and anticancer treatments and they can be used to treat pain, aid digestion, lower cholesterol, treat colds and flu, increase resistance to disease, enhance the immune function, improve circulation, regulate menstruation, and increase energy (Fontaine, 2000).

Herbal practitioners must take into account multiple factors as they develop a specific formula for an individual, since the formula will be uniquely designed to possess different qualities and properties and to target specific disharmonies. Williams (1996) notes that "the Chinese herbal formula is a complex cocktail of energetic qualities, functions, directions, and foci, and it takes skill to pick ingredients and dosage at the correct level . . . to address the symptoms of a patient's disharmony" (p. 165).

Chinese herbs can be classified according to several characteristics (Williams, 1996):

- Four energies (qi) of herbs
- Five tastes of herbs
- Four movements of herbs

Four Energies (Qi) of Herbs

The four energies of herbs (cold, cool, warm, and hot) relate to their energetic qualities, actions, and perceived temperatures. For example, cool or cold herbs relieve conditions related to an excess of heat in the body. Some herbs are neither hot nor cold and are thus neutral herbs; fu ling (poria) is one example. Since the qualities of herbs are not absolute, they are best described in relation to their position on an energetic continuum. Thus an herb can be slightly cool, very cool, cold, and so on.

Five Tastes of Herbs

The five tastes of herbs relate to their action on the body's qi:

- Pungent or acrid herbs (such as hong hua, or safflower) disperse and promote the movement of qi and stimulate the blood.
- Sweet herbs (such as ren shen, or ginseng root) tone and strengthen qi and nourish the blood.
- Sour/astringent herbs (such as wu wei zi, or schisandra fruit) control the function of zang-fu and absorb certain body substances.
- Bitter herbs (such as huo po, or magnolia bark) reduce excess qi and dry excess moisture.
- Salty herbs (such as mang xiao, or Glauber's salt) are believed to soften lumps.

Four Movements of Herbs

Herbs are used to treat specific body parts or facilitate the movement of other active herbal ingredients, and thus they have four basic movements. Herbs that can ascend and float, and so move upward and outward, influence the extremities and upper body. Herbs that descend, or move downward and inward, influence the interior and lower body. The functions of herbs (and their resulting movements) are influenced by:

- How the herb is prepared (for example, fried or prepared with salt)
- How it is cooked (glass or earthenware pots are best, although stainless steel is acceptable)
- How it is processed

Herbs should never be cooked in the microwave because this method of preparation can impair their energetic qualities (Williams, 1996).

Qigong

Qigong (pronounced *chee-gong*) is translated as qi ("energy") and gong ("discipline") (Lu, 2005). Fontaine (2000) describes Qigong as "the art and science of using breath, movement, self-massage, and meditation to cleanse, strengthen, and circulate vital life energy and blood" (p. 59).

Qigong is similar to yoga in India and has been called acupuncture without needles. By practicing Qigong and working with the mind, body, and spirit, an individual can achieve perfect harmony, resulting in a long, healthy, energetic life (Cassidy, 2002). The Chinese believe that qi is everywhere all the time, floating, flowing, innervating, and energizing everything around us. A vital life force, qi is responsible for healthy functioning; it is essential to Chinese life and governs all parts of daily life (Williams, 1996). The Chinese believe that good qi is taken in through air and food, while bad qi is expelled. The practice of Qigong helps individuals take in good qi and expel bad qi. Early morning is the best time to take in good qi, and ideally intake should be done close to nature. Practitioners don't have to stand outside on a beach, in the forest, or in a garden; any natural space, however small, can promote qi and serve as the backdrop for taking in good qi (Williams, 1996).

Qigong can be broadly categorized as internal (meditation with visualization to guide the energy) or external (meditation along with movement). Some of the postures are static while other movements flow smoothly from one posture to another. Some are quite dynamic, some are inspired by animals (such as the wild goose or swimming dragon), some are inspired by natural phenomena (water, trees, clouds), and some include meditations based on the sun and the moon. When practiced regularly, Qigong movements create a sense of balance in the meridian system by opening blocks and clearing congestion. The body's energy system can therefore function at an optimal level of well-being (Lu, 2005; Seaward, 2006; Williams, 1996).

The regular practice of Qigong can improve physical and mental well-being and may enable a person to (Benor, 2004):

- Improve relaxation, muscle tone, and breathing
- Contribute to improvements in musculoskeletal pain, asthma, and cancer
- Reduce stress and tension
- Reduce blood pressure
- Improve mental attitude
- Improve the flow of qi in the body

Diseases and medical conditions that have benefited from Qigong include the following (Micozzi, 2006):

- Allergies
- Asthma
- Bone fractures
- Cancer
- Cardiovascular disorders
- Cervical spondylosis
- Deafness

Qigong is also discussed in chapter 3.

Tai Chi Chuan

Dating back thousands of years, Tai Chi Chuan ("supreme ultimate fist" or "supreme ultimate boxing art") is a type of exercise that promotes the unrestricted and peaceful flow of energy throughout the body, thus helping to maintain a state of good health (Seaward, 2006).

Tai Chi Chuan and its graceful, fluid movements are probably more familiar to most Westerners than the movements of Qigong. Although Tai Chi Chuan and Qigong share a common philosophy, Tai Chi Chuan is a dynamic form of Qigong and a powerful and effective martial art, intended to create perfect harmony between yin and yang energies, promote the smooth and abundant flow of qi throughout the body, and maintain optimal health (Williams, 1996).

Tai Chi Chuan is thought to have originated as a fighting art with the Taoist monk Chang San Feng in the 14th century. The most common styles are the long and short forms of Yang, Wu, Sun, Chen, and Wudang, and each style has its own postures, sequences, and moves. As with all aspects of TCM, it is important to find an experienced and knowledgeable instructor who can effectively teach the subtleties and complexities of this art (Williams, 1996).

Tai Chi Chuan is discussed further in chapter 12.

Lifestyle Modifications

Few people would argue with the idea that having a healthy lifestyle—eating properly, exercising regularly, practicing relaxation techniques for stress reduction, and having a positive support network—can help us maintain a vital, healthy mind, body, and spirit. A healthy lifestyle supports the healthy flow of qi and supports a balance between extremes. Imbalances such as too much exercise or extreme dieting, for example, can lead to imbalance and disharmony in the body.

Exercise and TCM

The presence or absence of physical exercise in our lives can greatly affect our health. Moderate exercise helps to circulate blood and qi throughout the body, while the lack of exercise can lead to the stagnation of qi, and excessive exercise can weaken the body. TCM promotes regular, gentle, flowing exercise and body movement, such as Qigong, Tai Chi Chuan, walking, gentle jogging, swimming, and cycling. It calls for avoiding activities (such as weightlifting) that push the body to the limits of its capabilities and that stress it, and dressing properly for the type of weather in which activities are undertaken (Lu, 2005; Williams, 1996). In TCM, walking is the simplest form of exercise, suitable for all seekers of longevity and a must for older adults.

Meditation and TCM

Meditation is an excellent activity for reducing stress and balancing the mind, body, and spirit. The word *meditate* is derived from the Latin word *mederi*, which means "to cure" (Bright, 2002). A fundamental concept in Taoist thinking or Qigong practice is that qi follows intent. If the mind is calm, the qi is calm. If the mind is scattered, the qi becomes weak and unsubstantial. Meditation involves a conscious awareness of the breath and of the mind's intent.

There are numerous forms of meditation and individuals must experiment with different forms to determine which is most effective for them (Williams, 1996). For example, in *concentration meditation*, the meditator focuses on something specific in the internal or external environments—a sound, a word, music, a picture, a candle flame, or an object. Concentration meditation can also involve visualizing something imaginary (such as a peaceful landscape). In *mindful meditation*, the meditator directs awareness to whatever presents itself. The object of awareness is noted but not focused upon (Bright, 2002).

Meditation takes practice, but anyone can learn it and use it to produce an energized and healthy mind and body (Williams, 1996).

Meditation is discussed in detail in chapter 4.

Diet and TCM

In TCM, diet therapy is an adjunct to acupuncture and herbal medicine. Food is believed to sustain the body's qi and to promote health and vitality. Dietary interventions, the simplest and most easily accessible types of treatments, can be individualized according to the individual's particular disharmony. For example, food selection and preparation are of particular significance. TCM emphasizes the importance of cooking food lightly. Digestion is believed to "cook" the food, so overcooking and cooking with excess fats or oils are viewed as unhealthy (Cassidy, 2002; Fontaine, 2000; Williams, 1996).

The thermal nature of foods is described in terms of how an individual feels after eating them and of their yin and yang energies. For example, watermelon is believed to cool a person, and lamb chops may warm the eater. Warm, pungent, and sweet-flavored foods are considered yang, whereas cool foods and those with bitter or salty flavors are yin. A healthy diet is varied and includes a minimum of seven fruits and vegetables a day to avoid a hot or cold imbalance (Cassidy, 2002; Fontaine, 2000).

TCM also emphasizes the importance of eating a diet rich in cooked grains and vegetables and containing only a small amount of meat and dairy products. The overconsumption of hot and spicy foods is considered unhealthy, as is overeating in general. Food should be eaten at regular intervals, should be chewed slowly and thoroughly, and should be completely digested before sleeping. Fresh organic produce, foods local to an individual's area, and seasonal fruits and vegetables are preferred (Williams, 1996).

The Future of TCM

Few TCM practitioners are adept at using all the treatment modalities available. Most are trained in one specialty. It is important to consult a fully qualified practitioner when seeking treatment.

The future of TCM looks promising. Western traditions can be integrated with TCM to create what some are calling integral TCM.

KEY CONCEPTS

1. An understanding of TCM results in a higher level of care provided to clients.
2. Healthcare professionals who gain an understanding of TCM find that they are better able to understand the therapies used by TCM practitioners, the basis for those therapies, which therapies are useful for certain conditions, and why Chinese medical practitioners prescribe as they do.
3. Healthcare practitioners may also find that, as they gain a deeper understanding of TCM techniques and increase their knowledge about the importance of living in harmony with nature (and human nature), eating, sleeping, working, and exercising in a healthy way, they are able to incorporate these aspects into their own lifestyle and reap the benefits as well.

QUESTIONS FOR REFLECTION

1. How do the four types of examination used in TCM compare to Western types of examination?
2. What common treatment methods in TCM have you experienced?
3. Describe how you envision the integration of TCM with Western traditions.

REFERENCES

Benor, D. J. (2004). *Consciousness, bioenergy, and healing.* Medford, NJ: Wholistic Healing.

Bright, M. A. (2002). *Holistic health and healing.* Philadelphia: F. A. Davis.

Cassidy, C. M. (2002). *Contemporary TCM and acupuncture.* New York: Churchill Livingstone.

Dossey, B. M., Keegan, L., & Guzzetta, C. E. (2005). *Holistic nursing: A handbook for practice* (4th ed.). Sudbury, MA: Jones and Bartlett.

Flaws, B., & Sionneau, P. (2001). *The treatment of modern Western medical diseases with TCM.* Boulder, CO: Blue Poppy Press.

Fontaine, K. L. (2000). *Healing practices: Alternative therapies for nursing*. Upper Saddle River, NJ: Prentice Hall.

Freeman, L. (2004). *Mosby's complementary and alternative medicine: A research-based approach* (2nd ed.). St. Louis, MO: Mosby.

Kuhn, M. A. (2002, April). Herbal remedies: Drug-herb interactions. *Critical care nurse, 22*(2), 22–32.

Leddy, S. K. (2006). *Integrative health promotion: Conceptual bases for nursing practice* (2nd ed.). Sudbury, MA: Jones and Bartlett.

Lu, H. C. (2005). *Traditional TCM: An authoritative and comprehensive guide.* Laguna Beach, CA: Basic Health.

Micozzi, M. S. (2006). *Fundamentals of complementary and integrative medicine* (3rd ed.). Philadelphia: Saunders Elsevier.

Moyers, B. (1993). *Healing and the mind.* New York: Doubleday.

Nielsen, A. & Hammerschlag, R. (2004). Acupuncture and East Asian medicine. In B. Kligler & R. Lee, *Integrative medicine: Principles for practice* (pp. 241–254). New York: McGraw-Hill.

Seaward, B. L. (2006). *Managing stress: Principles and strategies for health and well-being* (5th ed.). Sudbury, MA: Jones and Bartlett.

Sierpina, V. (2001). *Integrative health care: Complementary and alternative therapies for the whole person.* Philadelphia: F. A. Davis.

Trivieri, L., Jr., & Anderson, J. W. (Eds.). (2002). *Alternative medicine: The definitive guide* (2nd ed.). Berkeley, CA: Celestial Arts.

Williams, T. (1996). *The complete illustrated guide to TCM.* Rockport, MA: Element Books.

Yanchi, L. (1995). *The essential book of Traditional TCM: Vol. 1. Theory.* New York: Columbia University Press and People's Medical Publishing House.

Yanchi, L., & Lianrong, D. (1998). *Basic theories of Traditional TCM.* (Edited by Beijing University of Traditional TCM). Beijing: Academy Press [Xue Yuan].

CHAPTER 7

Ayurvedic Medicine: Ancient Foundations of Health Care

If anything is sacred, the human body is sacred.
—WALT WHITMAN

LEARNING OBJECTIVES

1. Define the term *Ayurveda* and describe the origins of Ayurvedic medicine.
2. Explain the five elements of Ayurveda.
3. Describe the tridoshas and their relationship to an individual's characteristics and health.
4. Describe the three gunas.
5. Identify the roles of the seven dhatus and the three malas.
6. Define the term *ojas*.
7. Describe the three causes of disease according to Ayurvedic medicine.
8. State the six stages of the disease process in Ayurvedic medicine.
9. Describe the diagnostic techniques used by the Ayurvedic practitioner.
10. Explain the treatment modalities used in Ayurvedic medicine and the importance of their timing when utilized.
11. Explain the educational standards related to Ayurvedic medicine practitioners in the United States today.

INTRODUCTION

Ayurveda (pronounced *aa-yoor-vay-da*) is not only a science but also a religion and a philosophy. Lad (1998) defines philosophy as the love of truth, science as the discovery of truth through experiment, and religion as experiencing truth and applying it to daily living. According to Lad (2004), the religion of Ayurveda denotes the beliefs and disciplines that support a state of being in which the individual is open to all aspects of life; the philosophy of Ayurveda deals with the love of truth and the sacredness of the life journey. Morrison

(1995) says that Ayurveda is "a science of life which focuses on the subtle energies in all things—not only in living and inorganic things, but also in our thoughts, emotions, and actions" (p. 8). She also states that Ayurveda stresses "that we are all born with an individual constitution that is unique: an integral part of our being, a fixed point which is our personal baseline for health" (p. 8).

Ayurveda is a whole medical system that seeks to integrate and balance the body, mind, and spirit. Rather than asking, "What disease does my client have?" Ayurvedic practitioners strive to know who their clients are from the perspective of how they are constituted. *Constitution* is a key word in Ayurvedic medicine and refers to our overall health profile, including our strengths and susceptibilities. Once assessed and identified, the client's constitution becomes the foundation for all clinical decisions. The person's metabolic body type is first identified, and then a specific treatment plan is designed to bring the person back into harmony with the environment. Ayurvedic treatment plans include dietary changes, exercises, yoga, meditation, massage, herbal tonics and sweat baths, medicated enemas, and medicated inhalations (Trivieri & Anderson, 2002).

There are two main types of Ayurveda: traditional and maharishi. The latter is based on translations from the classical texts of Maharishi Mahesh Yogi. Both types support the basic principles of Ayurveda, but the maharishi type:

- Stresses the role of supreme consciousness in maintaining health and promotes Transcendental Meditation (TM) as a method for experiencing the consciousness of the universe
- Believes in the importance of positive emotions
- Supports being in tune with the natural rhythms of the body

The traditional form of Ayurveda is the focus of this chapter.

WHAT IS AYURVEDA?

Ayurveda is a combination of science, religion, and philosophy that details the many physical, mental, emotional, and spiritual components necessary for holistic health (Lad, 2004; Warrier & Gunawant, 1997). It is the oldest complete medical system in the world (Pai, Shanbhag, & Archarya, 2004; Shealy, 1996), with recorded origins dating back 3,500–4,000 years to 1200–800 BC. It has been practiced in India and Sri Lanka for at least 5,000 years and has recently become popular in Western cultures (Lad, 2004). With roots in ancient Indian civilization and Hindu philosophy, Ayurveda has been extremely influential in the development of all other Asian medical systems (Shealy, 1996). Ayurveda is based on the Samkhy philosophy of creation. The word *Samkhya* is derived from two Sanskrit words: *sat*, meaning "truth," and *khya*, meaning "to know" (Lad, 2004).

The word *Ayurveda* is derived from the Sanskrit words *ayus*, meaning "life" or "all aspects of life from birth to death" (representing a combination of the body, the sense organs, the mind, and the soul), and *vid* or *veda*, meaning "knowledge" (representing ancient knowledge about the rhythm and structure of the universe as well as knowledge of the secrets of sickness and health) (Basuray, 2002; Fontaine, 2000; Lad, 2004; Qutab, 2002). Thus, Ayurveda literally means "knowledge of life." According to Pai et al. (2004), Ayurveda is "a science in which the knowledge of the body (sarira), senses (indriya), mind (sattva), and soul (atma) are defined into one meaningful system" (p. 219).

Lad (1998) adds that both male and female energies are present in all living organisms and inanimate objects:

> According to Ayurveda, the source of all existence is the universal Cosmic Consciousness that manifests as male and female energy. Purusha, often associated with male energy, is choiceless, passive, pure awareness. Prakruti, the female energy, is active, choiceful consciousness. Both . . . are eternal, timeless, and immeasurable. (p. 7)

The basic principle of Ayurveda is to prevent illness by maintaining a balance between the mind, body, and consciousness. This balance is achieved through proper nutrition (including herbal remedies), drinking, diet, and lifestyle. Health, then, is "not just the absence of disease but the state of enjoying uninterrupted physical, mental, and spiritual happiness" (Pai et al., 2004, p. 219).

Ayurveda's Origins

Ayurveda is derived from the Vedas (the four oldest documented scriptures written in Sanskrit), the classical religious texts of Hinduism, Buddhist curative practices, and Islamic medical science. It is believed to be the world's oldest existing literature, handed down from the Hindu gods to the enlightened sages of the day (rishis), who were seers of truth whose teachings were transmitted orally from teacher to disciple and then later put into Sanskrit poetry (Basuray, 2002; Lad, 2004; Pai et al., 2004). The rishis were concerned about the increasing ill health in the world and sought, through meditation, to understand the foundations of human health and physiology so they could help prevent suffering (Sharma & Clark, 1998). Their meditations resulted in the four Vedas:

- Rig Veda
- Sama Veda

- Yajur Veda
- Atharva Veda

The Vedas address the topics of health, spirituality, and ethical living as well as the sciences of archery, fine arts, architecture, astrology, and yoga (Pai et al., 2004). Atharva Veda and Rig Veda are considered the first two magico-religious scriptures (Zysk, 2006). Prior to the Vedas, diseases were believed to be the result of possession by various demon entities. Ayurveda is part of the fourth Veda, written about 800 BC (Warrier & Gunawant, 1997).

Three important classical texts emerged as a result of the Vedic knowledge (Pai et al., 2004): *Charaka Samhita*, *Sushruta Samhita*, and *Ashtanga Samgraha*. The first two bear the names of Charak and Sushruta, well-known physicians whose writings became the working guidelines for the practice of Ayurvedic medicine.

- *Charaka Samhita:* Although written in 700 BC—over 2,000 years before the invention of the modern microscope—this most famous of all Ayurvedic texts contains details about cells and 20 different microscopic organisms that were believed to cause disease. Written on the subject of general medicine, it defines disease according to etiology, clinical presentation, pathophysiology, and prognosis, and it prescribes treatments for the diseases, including herbal medications, diet, and behavioral lifestyle recommendations (Pai et al., 2004).
- *Sushruta Samhita:* The second classical Ayurvedic text describes surgical techniques, equipment, suturing procedures, and the importance of hygiene during and after a surgical procedure (Morrison, 1995; Warrier & Gunawant, 1997). Written about 600 BC, it is named after the author who is considered the father of plastic surgery. It describes operative techniques and procedures, types of surgical instruments, and nearly 760 botanical sources of medicines. It also describes the first science of massage therapy and vital body points, which were later adopted into Chinese acupuncture (Pai et al., 2004).
- *Ashtanga Samgraha:* The name of the third classical text means "collection of the eight branches or specialties" of Ayurvedic medicine and was written about AD 700. These branches mirror the fields of modern medicine practiced today and include (Lad, 2004; Pai et al., 2004; Qutab, 2002; Warrier & Gunawant, 1997): *Salyachikitsa* (surgery), *Kayachikitsa* (general, or internal, medicine), *Bhuta Vidya* (psychology), *Balaroga Chikitsa* (pediatrics, obstetrics, and gynecology), *Shalakya Chikitsa* (otorhinolaryngology and ophthalmology), *Rasayana Chikitsa* (geriatrics and rejuvenation), *Agandatantra* (toxicology), and *Vajikarana Chikitsa* (fertility and sexual health).

As a result of these writings, two schools of Ayurveda evolved over the following centuries: the school of physicians (Atreya) and the school of surgeons (Dhanvantari). Because of these schools, Ayurveda was transformed into a scientifically verifiable and classifiable medical system. Deeply rooted in the myths, legends, religion, and typical daily life of India, Ayurveda is considered one of the greatest gifts that the ancient Indian sages left to humanity (Qutab, 2002).

Ayurveda Today

Ayurveda is a traditional, comprehensive, holistic national system of medicine practiced in India and Sri Lanka. Its emphasis is on the mind, body, and spirit. Self-realization, or spiritual healing, is its ultimate goal (Qutab, 2002; Warrier & Gunawant, 1997). Ayurveda is a prescription for living and a loosely organized set of traditions that can be highly individualized among both clients and practitioners (Sharma & Clark, 1998).

Ayurvedic medicine posits a fundamental connection between the microcosm and the macrocosm. Human beings are considered a tiny representation of the universe, containing within themselves everything that makes up the world around them. The interconnectedness of humans and their surrounding world makes it impossible to understand one without the other (Fontaine, 2000; Lad, 2004; Zysk, 2006). In Ayurveda, human beings are believed to be born in a state of perfect harmony and balance, but they lose this perfection through improper diet or a lifestyle that does not suit their natural constitution or temperament. Ayurveda aims not only to cure diseases but also to enhance health, creative growth, and well-being. Practitioners believe in the importance of preventing illness and disharmony before they occur.

In Ayurvedic medicine, every aspect of a person's lifestyle is assessed, including diet, personal habits, work and home situations, sex life, spirituality, hobbies, and relationships. Treatment is individualized, and no one treatment works for the same ailment in every person. The skill of the practitioner lies in his or her ability to diagnose the cause of disharmony or imbalance, to identify the person's constituent type, to determine the correct balance of the individual's doshas (bioenergetic forces that determine his or her physical constitution), and then to decide on the appropriate treatment (Warrier & Gunawant, 1997).

THE PRINCIPLES OF AYURVEDA

In Ayurvedic medicine, everything is composed of five elements, or panchamahabhutas, that interact, giving rise to all that exists. In humans, these five elements combine to form the following (Pai et al., 2004; Warrier & Gunawant, 1997; Zysk, 2006):

- *Three doshas (tridoshas):* Bioenergetic forces that determine an individual's physical constitution (or prakrti)
- *Three gunas:* Qualities of the mind that determine mental and spiritual health
- *Seven dhatus (structural elements):* Tissues that sustain the body
- *Three malas:* Waste products

In addition, there are:

- *Ojas:* End products of perfect digestion
- *Agnis:* Metabolic transformations (enzymes)
- *Srotas:* Bodily communication channels or vessels

All of these energies must be balanced for the individual to live a healthy, balanced life. In Indian philosophy, the purpose of life is to achieve dharma (virtue), artha (wealth), kama (enjoyment), and moksha (salvation). As a science, Ayurveda sets forth clear principles and practices for achieving a useful, creative, healthy life (Warrier & Gunawant, 1997).

The Five Elements

According to Ayurvedic teaching, everything in the universe is composed of five elements, or panchamahabhutas. Individually called bhutas, these elements are central to the Ayurvedic theory of creation and they combine with the soul to create a living being. The five elements and their corresponding qualities are as follows (Fontaine, 2000; Lad, 2004; Morrison, 1995; Pai et al., 2004; Warrier & Gunawant, 1997):

- *Akasha (space or ether):* Clear and subtle, the first element corresponds to spaces or cavities in the body, such as the mouth, nostrils, thorax, abdomen, respiratory tract, and cells.
- *Vayu (air):* Cold, mobile, and rough, the second element corresponds to movement (especially of the muscles), pulsations (especially of the heart), expansion and contraction of the lungs and intestines, and cellular movement.
- *Agni (fire):* The third element is hot and light, and it corresponds to metabolism and enzyme functioning, intelligence, the functioning of the digestive system, and temperature regulation.
- *Jala (water):* The fourth element is liquid and soft, corresponding to plasma, blood, saliva, digestive juices, salivary glands, mucous membranes and cytoplasm, the fluid inside the cells, and anything that is liquid, moving, slow, soft, smooth, oily, slimy, or related to sweat or urine.

- *Prithvi (earth):* Dense, heavy, and hard, the fifth element corresponds to solid body structures such as bones, nails, teeth, muscles, cartilage, tendons, skin, and hair.

These elements are *not* the same as their counterpart physical elements that are more familiar in the Western view of life (Warrier & Gunawant, 1997). All five elements are present in all matter in the universe to varying degrees and are present in any one substance. Water provides the classic example. Ice, the solid state of water, represents the earth principle. Latent heat (fire) liquefies ice, manifesting the water principle. Heat eventually turns water into steam, manifesting the air principle, and steam disappears into space (Lad, 2004). As Morrison (1995) explains, the five elements are part of the "dynamic dance of creation: they are constantly changing and interacting. A change in one element affects the others" (p. 22). The five elements, their qualities, their related sense organs and faculties, and their properties and actions are listed in table 7-1 (Lad, 2004; Morrison, 1995; Warrier & Gunawant, 1997).

The combination of these elements gives rise to the formation of the three metabolic body types, or tridoshas (Trivieri & Anderson, 2002).

The Tridoshas

Ayurvedic medicine is based on the principle that, just as no two fingerprints are alike, every individual has a unique composition related to the energies in his or her body (Sharma & Clark, 1998). A healthy individual has a balanced composition that can adequately defend itself against disharmony or illness. A poorly balanced individual is susceptible to both physical and psychological illness. This concept is similar to the Western medicine view of homeostasis, which states that all vital mechanisms have only one objective: to preserve the constant conditions of their internal environment. However, while modern Western medicine focuses on destroying pathogens as a way to prevent disease, Ayurveda focuses on making the body's defenses as strong as possible to promote balance and avoid disease (Sharma & Clark, 1998).

Ayurvedic medicine proposes that three doshas (tridoshas) determine the unique composition (prakriti) of every individual and provide the foundation for promoting balance. An excess or shortage of a dosha can result in disease (Sharma & Clark, 1998; Zysk, 2006).

The tridoshas are known by their Sanskrit names:

- *Vata*, which governs air and space
- *Pitta*, which governs fire and water
- *Kapha*, which governs water and earth

Table 7-1 The Five Elements

Element	Quality	Sense Organs	Sensory Faculties	Properties	Actions
Space	Sound	Ears	Auditory	Smooth, soft, subtle, porous, no distinct taste	Produces softness, lightness, and porous qualities. The main action is speech, and the organs of action are the tongue, vocal cords, and mouth.
Air	Touch	Skin and hands	Tactile	Rough, light, dry, cold, soluble, slightly bitter tasting	Removes sliminess; produces lightness, dryness, and emaciation. The main action is holding, and the main organ of action is the hand.
Fire	Sight	Eyes	Visual	Heat producing, pungent, rough, pungent tasting	Produces burning sensation, helps digestion and maturation, increases temperature, improves eyesight. The main action is walking, and the main organ of action is the foot.
Water	Taste	Tongue	Gustatory	Cold, fluid, moist, slimy, sweet tasting with astringent, sour, and saline taste	Produces moisture, acts as emollient and purgative. The main action is procreation, and the main organs of action are the genitals.
Earth	Smell	Nose	Olfactory	Heavy, firm, immobile, compact, thick, strong, sweet tasting	Increases firmness, strength, and acts as purgative. The main action is excretion, and the main organ of action is the anus.

Each individual is controlled by all three doshas to some extent, but one (the parental dosha) is usually dominant; sometimes two are dominant. This dominance results in seven normal body constitutions (Fontaine, 2000; Lad, 2004; Warrier & Gunawant, 1997; Zysk, 2006):

- Vata
- Pitta
- Kapha
- Vata-pitta
- Pitta-kapha
- Vata-kapha
- Sama (a balanced, and extremely rare, dosha)

The tridoshas govern all the biological, psychological, and physiological functions of the body, mind, and consciousness (Lad, 2004; Trivieri & Anderson, 2002; Warrier & Gunawant, 1997; Zysk, 2006). In addition to determining an individual's constitution (which is genetic and cannot be changed), the doshas also determine the following (Lad, 2004; Trivieri & Anderson, 2002; Warrier & Gunawant, 1997):

- An individual's unique characteristics, such as hair color, body shape, food preferences, and the types of foods that the person should eat
- The creation, maintenance, and destruction of bodily tissue and the elimination of waste from the body
- Psychological phenomena such as fear, anger, and greed, as well as love, compassion, and understanding
- The types of illnesses to which an individual is most susceptible

Ayurvedic medicine strives to help individuals learn about their own constitutions and emphasizes its positive aspects so that an imbalance state (vikrti) does not occur (Warrier & Gunawant, 1997). An explanation of each dosha follows.

Vata

Vata is derived from the Sanskrit word *vaayu*, meaning "to move" or "wind" (Lad, 2004; Zysk, 2006). Vata is the most important of the tridoshas because it plays a important role in all homeostatic mechanisms. It is said to be the king dosha since it leads the other doshas, which are considered lame and cannot move on their own. Aggravated vata can agitate and dislocate the other doshas. Aggravated vata is therefore more likely to cause disease than other aggravated doshas are (Sharma & Clark, 1998).

Vata is associated with the air and space elements. The principle of kinetic energy and movement, it is responsible for the physical and mental movements of the body. Vata governs breathing, blinking of the eyelids, pulsations of the heart, and circulation throughout the body; it carries nourishment to the body, supports body structure and tissues, and separates nutrients from waste products in the body (Lad, 2004; Sharma & Clark, 1998; Warrier & Gunawant, 1997; Zysk, 2006).

Vata is considered the intelligence that channels perceptions through the proper sensory organs, converts them to psychological events, and then determines the proper responses of the organs. It promotes a healthy balance between thoughts and emotions, and it generates creativity, activity, and clear understanding. Vata is located below the naval, and its principal seat is the colon (Zysk, 1996). It governs such feelings and emotions as freshness, nervousness, fear, anxiety, pain, and tremors. The large intestine, pelvic cavity, bones, skin, ears, and thighs are the seats of vata (Lad, 2004; Trivieri & Anderson, 2002).

The characteristics and properties of vata include (Lad 2004; Trivieri & Anderson, 2002; Warrier & Gunawant, 1997; Zysk, 2006):

- Roughness
- Coolness
- Dryness
- Lightness
- Subtlety
- Mobility
- Enthusiasm
- Intuitiveness
- Activities (like walking and lifting)
- Elimination of body discharges

Changeability is a key characteristic of the vata metabolic type. Unpredictability and variability in size, shape, mood, and action are trademarks (Trivieri & Anderson, 2002). Vata people often exhibit the following characteristics and personality traits (Lad, 2004; Sharma & Clark, 1998; Trivieri & Anderson, 2002; Warrier & Gunawant, 1997):

- A thin, light build; an active, restless mind; rough, dry, dark skin; prominent features, joints, tendons, and veins; a small thin mouth with large, crooked, or protruding teeth; dull, dark eyes; and curly hair
- Rapid speech
- Avoidance of confrontation
- Aversion to cold weather
- Active and sensitive natures
- Irregular eating and sleeping habits (eat and sleep at all hours)

- Ability to learn quickly and forget quickly
- Self-expression through sport and creative pursuits
- Overindulgence in pleasurable activities
- The most sexual natures of the three prakrtis
- Little sleep requirement and sleep may often be interrupted
- Frequent feelings of fear, anxiety, and unpredictable temper
- Changeable beliefs
- Preference for sweet, sour, and salty foods
- Moderate thirst
- Frequent constipation and irregular digestive powers

Signs of a balanced vata include exhilaration, alertness, the proper coordination of body functions, normal digestion and elimination, normal respiration, controlled and precise mental activity, and sound sleep (Sharma & Clark, 1998).

Disturbances in vata can result in the following (Sharma & Clark, 1998; Warrier & Gunawant, 1997; Zysk, 2006):

- Dry or rough skin
- Insomnia
- Constipation and bloating
- Fatigue of a nonspecific origin
- Arthritis
- Persistent bodily discharges
- Shortness of breath, dry cough, or respiratory problems
- Anxiety, fatigue, mental agitation, confusion, or impaired memory
- Low body weight
- Intolerance of cold
- Tension headaches

Pitta

The word *pitta* is derived from a Sanskrit word meaning "to heat" or "to burn." Pitta is associated with the elements of fire and water. It is responsible for all of the body's metabolic activities (such as digestion and hormone functions), biochemical reactions (such as glycolysis, the tricarboxylic acid cycle, and the respiratory chain), and the production of heat. Located between the navel and the chest, its principal seat is the stomach (Lad, 2004; Sharma & Clark, 1998; Warrier & Gunawant, 1997; Zysk, 2006).

The characteristics and properties of pitta include (Lad, 2004; Trivieri & Anderson, 2002; Warrier & Gunawant, 1997; Zysk, 2006):

- Heat
- Sharpness or irritability

- Liquidity
- Slight oiliness
- Fleshy and unpleasant smell
- Intelligence
- Pride
- Hair that grays early
- An aggressive nature

The pitta person may have the following characteristics or personality traits (Fontaine, 2000; Lad, 2004; Sharma & Clark, 1998; Trivieri & Anderson, 2002; Warrier & Gunawant, 1997):

- Medium height and build
- Soft, fair skin
- Light brown or reddish hair
- Small yellowish teeth and medium-sized mouth
- Penetrating green, gray, or yellowish eyes
- A tendency to speak clearly but often sharply
- The enjoyment of light but uninterrupted sleep
- Intelligence, often with aggressiveness
- Often a reddish complexion with moles and freckles
- Thin, fair hair and early graying or balding
- Good, clear memory
- Sometimes fanatical in their beliefs
- The tendency to be jealous, aggressive, and easily irritated
- A love of eating and of eating a lot
- A preference for sweet, bitter, and sharp-tasting foods
- An unquenchable thirst
- Regular, soft, loose bowel movements
- Emotional intensity

A disturbance in pitta can result in (Warrier & Gunawant, 1997):

- Rashes
- Inflammatory skin disease
- Inflammatory bowel disease
- Impaired vision
- Peptic ulcers
- Heartburn
- Excessive body heat
- Confusion
- Irritability or anger
- Premature graying or baldness

Kapha

Kapha is the Sanskrit word for "phlegm" or "bodily water." It also means "to embrace" or "to hold together" because this dosha is responsible for the body's strength, cohesion, and construction. Kapha is stable in nature and is the source of the body's developmental and reproductive activity. It regulates vata and pitta and controls patience, sexual power, and strength. It is composed of the elements of water and earth (Lad, 2004; Zysk, 2006). Kapha is related, microscopically, to anatomical connections in the cell, such as the cell membrane, synapses, intracellular matrix, and membranes of the organelles (Sharma & Clark, 1998). Kapha lubricates the joints, provides moisture to the skin, helps heal wounds, supports memory retention, and maintains immunity (Lad, 2004). Kapha brings about sturdiness, plumpness, enthusiasm, wisdom, and virility, providing the body with strength, softness, contentment, peace, and satisfaction (Warrier & Gunawant, 1997).

The characteristics and properties of kapha include (Lad, 2004; Trivieri & Anderson, 2002; Zysk, 2006):

- Heaviness
- Coldness
- Stability
- Denseness
- Softness
- Smoothness

The kapha person may have the following characteristics or personality traits (Fontaine, 2000; Lad, 2004; Sharma & Clark, 1998; Trivieri & Anderson, 2002; Warrier & Gunawant, 1997):

- Large body frame and excess weight
- Thick, pale, cool, and oily skin
- Thick, wavy, and oily hair
- A large mouth with full lips
- Large and attractive eyes with thick, dark lashes
- A tendency to be slow to learn and slow to forget
- The need for a lot of sleep
- Aversion to damp weather
- A long memory
- Lethargy or even laziness
- Poor short-term recall
- The ability to be dogmatic in their beliefs
- The ability to be calm and caring but also greedy, jealous, envious, and possessive

- A slow and steady appetite
- A tendency to enjoy bitter, pungent, and sharp tastes
- Slow bowel movements
- The tendency to be very loving and emotionally secure
- Slowness to anger but, once angered, slowness to calm down
- A sense of honor and a tendency to keep their words

Disorders that result from a disturbance of kapha include (Sharma & Clark, 1998; Warrier & Gunawant, 1997):

- Oily skin
- Obesity
- Weariness and lethargy
- Excessive sleep
- Cysts and other growths
- Asthma
- Sinus congestion and nasal allergies
- Slow digestion

Disharmonies Caused by Abnormal Doshas

Lad (2004) writes that "health is order; disease is disorder" (p. 37). Within every body is a continuous interaction between order and disorder, and the internal environment constantly reacts with the external environment. Disorder (or disease) results when the internal and external environments are out of balance.

Individual behavior and emotional patterns are often caused by years of beliefs, family values, ideas passed from generation to generation, and cultural influences. These patterns can lead to an unbalanced, poor quality of life that can result in many common ailments and chronic conditions. The most powerful unbalanced state is that of an unbalanced vata, followed by an unbalanced pitta, and finally by an unbalanced kapha (Warrier & Gunawant, 1997). This section describes unbalanced behavioral patterns that can lead to diseases or conditions.

Unbalanced Vata

Behaviors that aggravate vata include (Warrier & Gunawant, 1997):

- Having too many late nights (resulting in excessive fatigue and anxiety)
- Getting too much exercise (dancing, aerobic activity, running, etc.)
- Eating too many leafy vegetables or uncooked foods or vegetables
- Having insufficient time alone or in meditation

- Making and taking too many long telephone conversations, especially on mobile phones
- Indulging in excessive sexual activity
- Having no routine
- Lacking touch, emotional support, or family support
- Engaging in too many emotionally charged relationships
- Watching too much television, videos, or movies

Diseases and conditions caused by an unbalanced vata include (Morrison, 1995; Warrier & Gunawant, 1997):

- Cracked nails or feet
- Problems with the feet
- Sciatica
- Gastrointestinal difficulties (diarrhea, constipation, stomach pain, rectal prolapse)
- Cardiac arrhythmias
- Chest pain
- Stiff joints
- Earaches
- Deafness
- Cataracts
- Toothaches
- Headaches
- Dry mouth
- Sleeplessness
- Mental instability
- Fear, anxiety, fatigue, or excess worry

Unbalanced Pitta

Behaviors that aggravate pitta include (Warrier & Gunawant, 1997):

- Getting too much sun exposure
- Wearing too much clothing in the summer
- Eating too many spicy foods
- Drinking alcohol excessively
- Drinking insufficient amounts of water
- Indulging in too many arguments
- Taking part in too few outdoor activities, particularly in green fields and near rivers
- Not developing a firm, loving, and secure relationship devoid of jealousy and competition

Conditions or diseases caused by an unbalanced pitta include the following (Morrison, 1995; Warrier & Gunawant, 1997):

- Irritability, being hypercritical, and anger
- High temperature
- Burning sensations (in the shoulder, skin, chest, or anywhere on the body)
- Cracking or itching skin
- Genital herpes
- Jaundice
- Foul odor of the mouth
- Excessive thirst
- Excess stomach acid
- Pharyngitis or stomatitis
- Conjunctivitis

Unbalanced Kapha

Behaviors that aggravates kapha include (Warrier & Gunawant, 1997):

- Getting insufficient exercise
- Engaging in an inactive or lethargic lifestyle
- Overindulging in sweet foods and drinks
- Sleeping too much (especially in later morning or afternoons)
- Overeating (especially rich food)
- Eating too many cold foods
- Getting wet in rain or snow
- Wearing damp clothes or not drying properly after a bath or swim
- Depending excessively on a loving relationship

Conditions or diseases caused by an unbalanced kapha include (Morrison, 1995; Warrier & Gunawant, 1997):

- Anorexia nervosa
- Drowsiness or excessive sleep
- Laziness
- Timidity
- Excess salivation
- Excess bodily secretions
- Obesity
- Nausea
- Bloating
- Urticaria
- Goiter

- Atherosclerosis
- A sweet taste in the mouth

The Three Gunas

Just as the physical body has three major doshas and a dosha prakrti (body constitution), the mind has seven gunas: sattva, rajas, tamas, sattva-rajas, sattva-tamas, rajas-tamas, and sattva-rajas-tamas (Qutab, 2002). The first three are the major gunas. These essential components of the mind are the foundation for all existence, and they have specific influences (Lad, 2004; Pai et al., 2004; Sharma & Clark, 1998; Warrier & Gunawant, 1997; Zysk, 2006):

- *Sattva:* Essence, love, clarity, compassion, balance, and positive influence
- *Rajas:* Energy, movement, or the incentive to be active
- *Tamas:* Inertia or the slowing of activity

Like doshas, the gunas have specific characteristics based on an individual's manasa prakrti (psychological constitution). These characteristics are basically determined genetically, and each individual is a mixture of all three properties. While their influence is universal, one of the gunas is usually predominant, and so the individual's manasa prakrti can be either sattvika, rajasika, or tamasika prakrti. Since sattva is pure and cannot be disturbed, disturbances are caused by imbalances of rajas and tamas (Sharma & Clark, 1998; Warrier & Gunawant, 1997).

Sattva and the Sattvika Individual

The characteristics of sattva include lightness, consciousness, pleasure, clarity, and freedom from disease (Warrier & Gunawant, 1997). Sattva activates the senses and is responsible for the perception of knowledge. Sattvika individuals are considered spiritual and noble, and their astrological sign may influence their personalities. These individuals can be (Qutab, 2002; Sharma & Clark, 1998; Warrier & Gunawant, 1997):

- Passionate
- Highly intellectual with a powerful memory
- Wealthy
- Skillful
- Grateful
- Free from anxiety
- Courageous
- Patient
- Articulate

- Polite
- Religious
- Farsighted with a love of dance, music, song, and fragrances (perfumes and flowers)
- Angry, greedy, ignorant, and jealous

Anything that increases sattva in the mind is considered valuable, while anything that reduces it (thereby increasing rajas or tamas) should be moderated (Sharma & Clark, 1998).

Rajas and the Rajasika Individual

The characteristics of rajas include motion, stimulation, and responsibility for all desires, wishes, and ambitions (Warrier & Gunawant, 1997).

An imbalance of rajas can result in psychiatric illnesses. Rajasika individuals are very intellectual, brave, action oriented, worldly, and passionate. They always strive for more and so can be ambitious, hot-tempered, self-indulgent, cruel, envious, ruthless, and gluttonous (in painful or pleasurable pursuits). They may have an excessive appetite for food and sleep. These individuals can have a frightening appearance, and they enjoy physical and verbal disguises. Like the other types, their astrological sign can influence their natures, and they can have an element of pitta in their physical constitution (Qutab, 2002; Warrier & Gunawant, 1997).

Tamas and the Tamasika Individual

The characteristics of tamas include heaviness, resistance, delusions, laziness, apathy, and sleep (Warrier & Gunawant, 1997).

These individuals can be described as practical, down-to-earth, or salt of the earth. Their dominant element is vata. They prefer an easy, relaxed lifestyle and dislike the routine of an office job or any constraining activity. They are not curious about anything, are not particularly intelligent, and avoid cleanliness. They can become dependent on pleasurable activities (including sex or drug use), and they avoid confrontation. The tamasika individual can be intolerant, unreliable, and envious (Qutab, 2002; Warrier & Gunawant, 1997).

The Seven Dhatus

Ayurvedic medicine states that seven vital dhatus, or tissues, sustain the body and that the doshas are located in and govern these specific tissues. More accurately, dhatus are the fundamental principles that support the various bodily tissues (Lad, 2004; Sharma & Clark, 1998; Zysk, 2006). The Sanskrit word *dhatu* means "constructing element," and these seven elements are responsible for the entire structure of the body. They maintain the function of the body's organs and systems, and they play a role in development.

Each dhatu is formed from the previous tissue in ascending order of complexity (Lad, 2004; Zysk, 2006):

- *Rasa*, meaning "sap" or "juice," is the principle upholding the first products of digestion, such as chyle, lymph, and plasma; it functions to nourish the tissues, organs, and systems of the body.
- *Rakta* is the principle upholding blood; it functions to invigorate the body by oxygenating the tissues.
- *Mamsa* is the principle upholding flesh or muscle; it functions to stabilize and strengthen the body.
- *Meda* is the principle upholding fat (adipose tissue); it functions to lubricate the body.
- *Asthi* is the principle upholding bone (cartilage); it functions to support the body.
- *Majja* is the principle upholding bone marrow and the nervous system; it functions to support communication among the body's cells and organs.
- *Shukra* is the principle upholding male and female sexual fluids; it functions in a reproductive and immune capacity.

Trivieri and Anderson (2002) offer another way to look at the dhatus:

- Vata is motion that activates the physical systems and the nerve force and allows the body to breathe and circulate blood. The seats of this dosha are the large intestine, pelvic cavity, bones, skin, ears, and thighs.
- Pitta is metabolism, food, air, and water processing and is responsible for the body's endocrine and enzymatic activity. The seats of this dosha are the small intestine, stomach, sweat glands, blood, skin, and eyes.
- Kapha offers nourishment and protection for the body and is the structure of bones, tendons, muscle, and fat that hold the body together. The seats of this dosha are the chest, lungs, and cerebral spinal fluid.

The Three Malas

The three waste products, or malas, that result from digested and processed food and drink are urine (mootra), feces (purisha), and sweat (sweda). A fourth category of waste products includes fatty excretions from the skin and intestines, ear wax, nasal mucus, saliva, tears, hair, and nails (Lad, 2004; Sharma & Clark, 1998; Zysk, 2006). According to Ayurvedic medicine, individuals should evacuate their bowels once a day and evacuate their bladder at least six times a day (Zysk, 2006). Ayurveda considers digestion to be the most important function in the human body, since it sustains the organism; it considers improper digestion to be the principal cause of all maladies (Zysk, 2006). According to Sharma and Clark (1998):

- Feces and urine are the waste products of anna (food).
- Sweat is associated with meda (fat).
- Mucus is said to be the waste product of rasa (chyle) and associated with kapha dosha.
- Khamalas is excreta from outer orifices and is said to be associated with mamsa (muscle).
- Hair is said to be the waste product of asthi (bone).
- Bile is said to be the waste product of rakta (blood) and associated with pitta dosha.

Excreting the malas cleanses the body, so individuals are cautioned against suppressing these natural body functions, which include sneezing, yawning, burping, urinating, defecating, and passing gases (Fontaine, 2000). In addition, the buildup of toxins and waste products in the body, referred to as ama, can block the body's communication channels (srotas) (Pai et al., 2004).

Ojas

The word *ojas* means "vitality" or "bodily strength" (Morrison, 1995). Ojas nourishes and strengthens the body and is considered its most important biochemical substance (Sharma & Clark, 1998). Considered to be the end product of perfect digestion and metabolism, ojas is actually more important than that. Sharma and Clark (1998) define it as "a 'lamp at the door' between consciousness and matter, connecting them and thus ensuring that the sequence of natural law is expressed properly in the body" (p. 30).

Ojas is described as a white, oily substance that is maximized by an individual's level of consciousness (the more enlightened one is, the more ojas is produced), by good digestion, and by a balanced diet. Foods such as milk, ghee (clarified butter), and rice increase ojas, while other foods (such as alcohol) decrease it. Food eaten in a warm, supportive, uplifting atmosphere also increases ojas. To be avoided are factors that decrease ojas, such as (Morrison, 1995; Sharma & Clark, 1998):

- Negative emotions of any kind
- Stress
- Excessive exercise
- Fasting

- Overexposure to sun and wind
- Overindulgence in sexual activity
- Alcoholic beverages
- Injury or trauma to the body
- Excessive loss of body fluids (such as blood)

Agnis and Srotas

Ayurvedic medicine also believes that 13 agnis (enzymes) assist in the digestive process and 13 types of srotas (vessels or channels of the body) enable all substances to circulate (Zysk, 2006).

Metabolic Transformation: Agni

Agni is considered to be the fire that burns within an individual's body and mind and stimulates all the biological processes of life. Because agni includes the digestion and absorption of food in the gastrointestinal tract and cellular transformations, it covers the whole sequence of chemical interactions and changes in the body and mind. The four levels of agni range from the gross digestion of food to the molecular metabolism and transformation of food. There are three types of agni (Zysk, 2006):

- *Jatharagni* is active in the mouth, stomach, and gastrointestinal tract and responsible for breaking down food. Feces result from this activity.
- *Bhutagnis* are five enzymes located in the liver; they adapt broken-down food into chyle, which circulates through the blood channels, nourishes the body, and supplies the seven dhatus.
- *Dhatvagnis* are seven enzymes that synthesize the seven dhatus.

Digestive abilities are related to the strength of agni (Morrison, 1995). When agni is healthy, normal body functions occur and the individual is vital, enthusiastic, and healthy in every way. When agni is ineffective or inefficient, the individual can become unhealthy or diseased (Lad, 2004; Pai et al., 2004).

Communicating Channels: Srotas

Srotas, or bodily communication channels, are somewhat equivalent to the organ systems of the body (e.g., respiratory, circulatory, reproductive, etc.). They are additional sites where doshas can be aggravated and diseases can occur. Ayurvedic practitioners believe that nutrients and other substances move in and out of the body. For example, food passes; we breathe oxygen; and urine, feces, and sweat are formed and excreted, all through the srotas

(Pai et al., 2004). These 13 channels are also the route through which information and intelligence spontaneously flow. When the channels are open due to the body's receiving appropriate nutrients and energy, the body is healthy. When there is too much or too little of a dosha, or when the channels are blocked, diseases can result.

CAUSES OF DISEASE

According to Ayurvedic medicine, an imbalance of the doshas results in diseases, which originate in one of three ways (Warrier & Gunawant, 1997; Zysk, 2006):

- Diseases that originate within the body (such as a congenital condition, an inherited trait, or an abnormal sense organ)
- Diseases that originate outside the body (in the form of accidents, mishaps, germs, viruses, or bacteria)
- Diseases that originate from supernatural sources (like seasonal changes, planetary influences, or curses)

Diseases Originating Within the Body

Our sensory perception is influenced by:

- The five sensory organs of the body (ears, eyes, nose, tongue, or taste buds, and skin)
- The five sense faculties and perceptions (auditory, visual, olfactory, gustatory, and tactual)
- The five sense substances (ether, light, earth, water, and air)
- The five sense objects (sound, shape, smell, taste, and touch)

Stimuli that are stressful to the senses can occur in the form of overuse (e.g., too much sun exposure), disuse (e.g., reading with poor lighting), or misuse (e.g., use of a heat pack on a strain). This overuse, disuse, or misuse can result in disease that originates within the body.

Diseases Originating Outside the Body

Diseases that originate outside the body can result from any act arising out of passion or delusion that is harmful to the mind or the body. For example, restraining the urge to urinate could lead to bladder problems (Warrier & Gunawant, 1997).

Diseases Originating from Supernatural Sources

Diseases that originate from supernatural sources include seasonal excesses or deficits (such as droughts or floods) or abnormal seasons (such as a hot winter). Seasons are classified according to their predominant dosha. For example, in some parts of the world, autumn is windy, cool, dry, and largely vata, whereas winter is dark, heavy, damp, and cloudy, with kapha qualities (Lad, 1998). In addition, doshas are responsive to day and night, the intake of food, and age. For example, in India it was traditional for individuals to leave their active way of life at about age 55 and seek a more spiritual existence. They believed that attachment to material desires and a fear of illness and poverty usually accompany old age, but pursuing a spiritual path causes these fears and attachments to disappear; therefore, they achieved healthy living and balance through this enlightening experience (Warrier & Gunawant, 1997).

Contributors to Illness

Lad (1998) believes that 10 factors contribute to illness. Each provides individuals with a great deal of choice and control over whether they produce health or imbalance.

- *Like increases like:* For example, dry foods, dry fruit, running, always being in a rush, and working too hard all aggravate vata in the system.
- *Food and diet:* Eating incorrect foods creates imbalance in the doshas.
- *Seasons:* Each season affects a corresponding dosha and can aggravate it if the effect is not counterbalanced.
- *Exercise:* Overexertion, underexertion, or the wrong type of exertion for a particular dosha can aggravate that dosha and any corresponding conditions.
- *Age:* Each stage of life has its own choices that will or will not support the corresponding dosha.
- *Mental and emotional factors:* Positive and negative emotions can disturb the doshic balance.
- *Stress:* Stress disturbs the doshas and can create disequilibrium of vata, pitta, or kapha.
- *Overuse, underuse, and wrong use of the senses*: Since perceptions, thoughts, and feelings are biochemical events as well as conscious experiences, the improper use of the senses can create imbalances in the body.
- *"Knowing better":* Ignoring our own knowledge and wisdom can lead us to do things that are unhealthy for us.

- *Relationships:* Relationships between friends, parents, children, spouses, coworkers, and one's own body can affect health and create stress and a lack of balance.

STAGES OF DISEASE

Diseases are believed to proceed through six distinct stages in their pathogenesis. These stages are determined by which dosha becomes aggravated and how it moves through the channels (srotas) to produce disease (Lad, 1998; Sharma & Clark, 1998; Warrier & Gunawant, 1997; Zysk, 2006).

1. During the stage of *sanchaya* (accumulation), symptoms are vague and ill defined. In this stage, Warrier and Gunawant (1997) assert that "the doshas accumulate and stagnate in their own specific places and do not circulate freely" (p. 115). Overaccumulation is brought on by an error in diet, regimen, or thought. Seasons and emotions can also be causes. Treatment should begin as soon as symptoms appear to avoid complications.
2. During the stage of *prakopa* (aggravation), the accumulated and stagnant doshas become excited and symptoms are exacerbated. For example, an individual with a mild stomachache may eat the incorrect food and have an acute episode of intense stomach pain. Any damage that occurs to the body is still correctable in this stage, and the individual can reverse these two phases.
3. The stage of *prasara* (dissemination) is characterized by a spreading of the excited and accumulated doshas to other organs, body parts, and body systems. The accumulated doshas are said to travel to another body part, where the disease may also occur. At this stage, a purification program is needed to return the doshas to their respective states.
4. During the stage of *sthana samsraya* (localization), the wandering doshas are localized in a particular organ, tissue, or system, which becomes diseased. For example, doshas confined to the stomach may result in diarrhea, constipation, or tumors. At this stage, the individual may not feel 100% well but does not know exactly what the problem is.
5. In the stage of *vyakti* (manifestation), the symptoms of disease are fully developed. Qualitative changes and symptoms of disease may become apparent as the individual becomes sick.
6. The stage of *bheda* (disruption) is one in which the disease becomes chronic or incurable. The pathological process is fully developed and the disease completely manifested. Structural changes and complications resulting from the involvement of other organs become apparent. Disease is the most difficult to treat in this stage.

DIAGNOSTIC TECHNIQUES

In traditional Western medicine, diagnosis involves identifying a disease after it has manifested symptoms. In Ayurveda, diagnosis is a moment-to-moment monitoring of the interactions between order (health) and disorder (disease). Ayurveda considers disease processes to be responses between the bodily humors and the tissues, and symptoms are always related to tridoshas (Lad, 2004).

Ayurvedic physicians rely on their powers of observation rather than on equipment and laboratory tests to diagnose illnesses. Diagnosis includes physical observation; obtaining a thorough personal and family history from the client; palpation; and listening to the heart, lungs, and intestines. This approach is changing as Ayurvedic physicians integrate modern diagnostic methods with traditional ones (Trivieri & Anderson, 2002).

An individual who feels out of balance or ill can visit an Ayurvedic practitioner, who may employ one or several of the following diagnostic techniques:

- The *tenfold examination*, which includes body composition, pathological state, tissue vitality, physical build, body measurement, adaptability, psychic constitution, digestive capacity, capacity for exercise, and age
- The *eightfold examination*, which looks at pulse, tongue, voice, skin, eyes, general appearance, urine, and stool

Ayurvedic physicians pay special attention to the pulse, tongue, eyes, and nails. They consider the body "to be a pattern of information and intelligence. Information about the body as a whole is carried in the cardiovascular system in the form of fluid vibratory waves. Any imbalance creates a particular wave function" (Leddy, 2006, p. 178).

- *Pulse:* According to Trivieri and Anderson (2002), Ayurvedic physicians can distinguish 12 radial (wrist) pulses: six on the right wrist (three deep and three superficial) and six on the left wrist. Combining knowledge of the relationship between the pulses and the internal organs, as well as information about the dosha-organ relationship, skilled Ayurvedic practitioners can detect the strength, vitality, and normal tone of specific organs at each of the 12 sites using their index, middle, and ring fingers (Zysk, 2006). The relative strength and character of the pulsations under each finger relate to a specific dosha. For example, "a Vata pulse is compared to the motion of a snake: light, quick, rough, thin, and rapidly undulating; Pitta's pulse pattern is compared to a frog; sharp, cutting, and jerky; and Kapha's pulse pattern is compared to the motion of a swan; heavy, full, slow, soft, and graceful" (Leddy, 2006, p. 179). Pulses should not be taken after exertion, massage, eating, bathing, or sex (Lad, 2004).

- *Tongue:* The tongue, also an important diagnostic site, is the organ of taste and speech. By observing its surface and looking for discoloration and/or sensitivity in certain areas, the practitioner can assess the functional status of internal organs. For example, a black to brown discoloration can indicate a vata disturbance, and a dehydrated tongue is symptomatic of a decrease in plasma (Lad, 2004; Trivieri & Anderson, 2002).
- *Eyes:* Eyes provide the Ayurvedic practitioner with information about the tridoshas. Vata eyes are small and nervous and may blink frequently. Large, beautiful, attractive eyes indicate a kapha constitution (Lad, 2004).
- *Nails:* According to Ayurveda, nails are a waste product of the bones. If nails are dry, crooked, rough, and easily broken, vata predominates in the body. If they are soft, pink, tender, and easily bent, pitta predominates. Pale nails indicate anemia. Each finger and thumb corresponds to a specific organ in the body. For example, the ring finger relates to the kidney, and the little finger relates to the heart (Lad, 2004).

Once diseases are detected and prior to treatment, they are classified according to the sevenfold system (Warrier & Gunawant, 1997):

1. *Genetic*, such as hemophilia
2. *Congenital*, such as dwarfism or blindness
3. *Internal or constitutional*, such as somatic or psychic disorders
4. *Traumatic*, such as injuries that are external or those caused by insect or animal bites
5. *Seasonal*, such as frostbite or sunstroke
6. *Infectious and spiritual*, such as illnesses due to acts of God (earthquakes, floods, or lightning), those caused by epidemics, or those caused by sexual or body contact with others
7. *Natural tendencies or habit*, such as stroke, rheumatism, or those caused by age

AYURVEDIC TREATMENTS

According to Lad (1998), self-esteem is at the core of healing. An awareness and connection between the mind, body, and spirit are essential. Ayurveda believes that every cell is a center of intelligence and awareness and that each carries with it a sense of survival. Proper cell function and immunity cannot occur unless self-esteem, self-confidence, and self-respect promote cellular intelligence. Ultimately, a daily lifestyle in tune with nature and the doshas is essential.

The four pillars of Ayurvedic treatment consist of appropriate drugs, diet, and practices, as well as a quality physician (practitioner) who is well trained, knowledgeable, and has a "pure mind and body" (Warrier & Gunawant, 1997). The medication must be of high quality and suitable to the individual being treated, obtainable in multiple forms, abundantly available, and potent. Also necessary are a quality nurse who is skilled and knowledgeable, has compassion for the client, and is also pure of mind and body, and a good client who can appropriately describe his or her symptoms, follows instructions, has courage, and has a good memory.

Forms of Treatment

According to Ayurvedic medicine, once the four pillars are achieved, several forms of treatment can be used to reduce toxins that have accumulated in the body (Fontaine, 2000; Warrier & Gunawant, 1997; Zysk, 2006). Prior to the actual purification process, however, the body needs to be prepared so it will readily let go of the toxins. An oil massage (snehan) makes the body supple, releases stress, and nourishes the nervous system; this massage is done for 3–7 days. Sweating (swedan) is done every day immediately following the massage and serves to liquefy the toxins and speed their movement into the intestinal tract. After these processes have been completed, the doshas are said to be ripe and ready for cleansing therapies (Lad, 2004), which include the following:

- Drug therapy
- The five systems of treatment
- Dietary regimen
- Regulation of lifestyle

Drug (Herbal) Therapy

The drugs used in Ayurvedic therapy originate from vegetables, animals, or minerals and can be found in many different forms (such as pastes, powders, fresh juices, pills, infusions, suppositories, alcoholic preparations, ash residues, and oils). The drugs can be used alone or in combination with each other. The taste, effects, potency, and specific actions of each drug are specifically considered in treating a disease. Herbs also help to balance the doshas, and their use must be medically supervised.

The Five Systems of Treatment

After impurities from other parts of the body have been loosened and drawn into the abdominal tract, the five systems of treatment allow them to be more easily excreted (Sharma & Clark, 1998). These therapies are administered in a sequence over approximately 7–28 days, and the client is advised to set aside time ("retreat from the world") for them because of the profound nature of their effects (Zysk, 2006).

The five systems, collectively called pancha karma, are emesis (vomiting), purging, enemas, nasal drops, and bloodletting. These purifying techniques are used to remove toxins from different areas of the body. Since toxins are considered the root of disease, these methods of treatment remove undigested, unabsorbed, and unassimilated food (Lad, 2004; Pai et al., 2004; Trivieri & Anderson, 2002; Williams & Gunawant, 1997).

- *Emesis therapy (vamana)* is used to eliminate excessive kapha dosha, which results in diseases such as bronchitis, asthma, goiter, diabetes, poor digestion, heart disease, rhinitis, pharyngitis, and tonsillitis. Multiple glasses of licorice or salt water are taken orally, and vomiting is stimulated by rubbing the tongue. Vomiting is believed to relieve emotions that are held in the kapha area of the lungs and stomach. Chronic asthma, diabetes, chronic colds, and chronic indigestion may be treated in this manner (Lad, 2004). Of the five classical pancha karma therapies, this is the only one that needs to be performed by a qualified pancha karma specialist. It is a highly specialized procedure for treating kapha and pitta disorders (Pai et al., 2004).
- *Purgation therapy (virecana)* is the use of herbal medication to lubricate the intestines and colon. It is used to eliminate doshas that cannot be removed by emesis or through the kidneys, lungs, and sweat glands. Senna leaf tea, flax seeds, psyllium husks, or hot milk are taken to rid the body of excess pitta. Allergic rashes, skin inflammations, acne, chronic fevers, internal worms, and conjunctivitis are just some of the disorders treated with this therapy (Lad, 2004; Pai et al., 2004).
- *Enema therapy (basti)* is the treatment of choice for vata disorders, which, according to Ayurveda, are responsible for the majority of all diseases. Sesame oil, almond oil, or herbal mixtures may be given through the rectum, urethra, or vagina. This form of therapy is used to treat disorders that can manifest as constipation, rheumatism, arthritis, or selected ovulatory disorders (Lad, 2004). Ayurveda believes that routine cleansing and toning of the colon can heal and rejuvenate the entire body (Pai et al., 2004).
- *Nasal drops/administrations (nasya)* are used to treat diseases of the ear, nose, throat, head, and teeth. The nose is considered the doorway to the brain and to consciousness, and this treatment is used for certain eye and ear problems, anxiety, colds, nasal congestion, epilepsy, intestinal parasites, headaches, and thinning hair (Lad, 2004). The current practice of lavaging the nasal cavities to prevent sinus problems was used in

Ayurveda hundreds of years ago to deliver medicated nasal solutions (Pai et al., 2004).
- *Bloodletting (raktamokshana)* is used to treat skin diseases, certain tumors, gout, excessive sleepiness, alopecia, and hallucinations. Extracting a small amount of blood from a vein is believed to relieve tension due to accumulated pitta toxins. This therapy is used to treat rashes, acne, eczema, scabies, hives, and gout (Lad, 2004). In addition, when blood is removed, the bone marrow is stimulated (Pai et al., 2004; Trivieri & Anderson, 2002).

An experienced, skilled Ayurvedic practitioner should administer all of these therapies, and every one of them has specific contraindications for treatment. Many of these therapies are not suited for children, the elderly, or pregnant women and are appropriate in treating specific diseases (Zysk, 2006).

Ghee and buttermilk yogurt are often used to reestablish intestinal flora after cleansing routines (Lad, 2004). In addition, the following may be performed (Trivieri & Anderson, 2002):

- Herbs may be inserted through routes other than the mouth (the nose, anus, and skin) to ensure that stomach enzymes do not break down the medicinal qualities.
- A palliation or shaman may be used to balance and pacify the doshas. This aspect of disease management uses herbs, fasting, chanting, yoga stretches, breathing exercises, meditation, and lying in the sun for a limited time.
- Rejuvenation, or rasayana, is a program of tonification that is similar to a physiological tune-up. Special herbs, mineral preparations specific to a person's condition, and exercises (including breathing and yoga) are utilized.

Dietary Regimen

Ayurveda teaches that individuals have the power to heal themselves, so a sound diet and stable health routine are necessary to maintain or attain health (Lad, 2004). Since no two individuals have the same doshic equation and no one has a mono-doshic prakrti, the following Ayurvedic diet is only a general guideline. Only experienced Ayurvedic practitioners should prescribe specific dietary advice, and only after thoroughly assessing the individual and considering any specific health issues. When choosing a diet, they should also consider the seasons of the year as well as the quality, freshness, and taste of the food (sweet, sour, salty, pungent, bitter, or astringent) (Lad, 2004; Warrier & Gunawant, 1997). The foods shown in table 7-2 may be recommended for specific constitutions (Lad, 2004; Morrison, 1995; Warrier & Gunawant, 1997).

Table 7-2 Dietary Recommendations for Specific Constitutions

Vatika Diet		*Paittika Diet*		*Kaphaja Diet*	
Balances Dosha	**Aggravates Dosha**	**Balances Dosha**	**Aggravates Dosha**	**Balances Dosha**	**Aggravates Dosha**
Milk	Yogurt	Milk	Yogurt, cottage cheese	Apples	Milk
Okra	Cabbage and raw vegetables	Butter	Lemons	Peaches	Cheese
Eggs	Peas	Apples, coconuts, figs, mangos	Lemons or other sour fruits	Peaches, berries, mangos	Avocado
Eggs	Peas	Avocado	Papaya	Garlic	Bananas, grapes
Fish	Spinach	Melons	Papaya	Garlic	Dates
Oats	Spinach	Lettuce, green beans	Garlic	Onions	No dairy or oils
Almonds	Pepper	Spinach	Almonds	Tomatoes	Cold food
Sunflower seeds	Garbanzo beans	Eggs	Most peppers and chilis	Most peppers and chilis	Cashew nuts
Oils	Turkey, lamb, pork	Fish	Very hot, spicy food	Chicken	Peanuts
Spices	Coffee	Chicken, seafood, lamb, or pork	N/A	Fish	Most sweeteners
N/A	Cold drinks	Rice	No spices	Rice	Chicken, turkey
N/A	Dried fruits	Wheat	N/A	N/A	N/A

According to Ayurvedic medicine, a wholesome diet should also adhere to the following guidelines (Sharma & Clark, 1998; Warrier & Gunawant, 1997):

- Food should be eaten at regular mealtimes.
- Food should be eaten in a relaxed, calm atmosphere.
- Food should be warm to aid digestion.
- Food should be oily to stimulate digestion and provide the body with strength.
- Food should be in the proper quantity to promote longevity, soothe the doshas, and maintain digestion.
- The main meal should be eaten around noon, when the digestive fire is strongest.
- Food should be eaten only when a previous meal has been digested (usually about 2.5 hours).
- Food should be eaten at the proper place and at the right time (i.e., when one is not angry, grief stricken, anxious, or otherwise upset).
- Food should not be eaten in a hurry or carelessly.
- One should sit down when eating and not talk while chewing.
- Food should be eaten with awareness, when signs of hunger are present.
- Food should be beneficial to an individual's specific constitution.
- Certain food combinations should be avoided, depending on an individual's constitution.
- Fresh, wholesome foods (grown organically) are the best.
- Cold drinks should be avoided.

According to Ayurvedic medicine, an individual who lives according to the guidelines for healthy living should live 100 years (Warrier & Gunawant, 1997). Health is a state of equilibrium between the tridoshas, when digestion, metabolism, tissue elements, and excretion are normal and working properly, and the individual is physically and emotionally happy. Effective digestion is crucial to good health. Therefore, food must be taken in a "proper" way: it must be of the proper quality, in the proper quantity, and with the proper frequency (Warrier & Gunawant, 1997).

Disharmony and disease result from improper nutrition. Foods are classified according to their nature and qualities, and dietary rules are considered in relation to the time of the day and the seasons. For example, a pitta diet should not be eaten during midday when pitta activity is dominant (Warrier & Gunawant, 1997).

Lifestyle Regulation

Ayurvedic medicine proposes that if we adhere to a healthy way of living, our doshas can become and remain balanced, resulting in vitality, optimal health, and a long healthy life. This healthy way of living involves two main routines (Warrier & Gunawant, 1997):

- Daily living routines
- Seasonal routines

A *healthy daily routine* begins with rising early in the morning (preferably before sunrise) and involves the following steps (Lad, 2004; Sharma & Clark, 1998; Warrier & Gunawant, 1997):

- *Keeping the body very clean* by having excellent oral hygiene (teeth brushing, tongue scraping, and gargling with oil), regular massage (using specific oils to aid health), regular bathing (to remove impurities from the skin), and the use of perfumes, scents, and ornaments
- *Exercising regularly and properly*, depending on age, prakrti, and health condition
- *Immediately tending to natural urges*, such as urination, defecation, hunger, sleep, sneezing, eructation, yawning, vomiting, flatus, ejaculation, and panting
- *Suppressing psychological urges*, such as anger, fear, greed, vanity, jealously, malice, or an obsessive attachment to anything or anyone
- *Practicing meditation and breathing* in the morning and in the evening
- *Daily practice of mental and moral discipline* through respect for God, teachers, saints, and the elderly; the avoidance of undesirable places or people; making fearless, brave, intelligent decisions; avoiding conduct that causes stress; helping others and practicing forgiveness; and avoiding excess alcohol.

Seasonal routines are also important. According to Ayurvedic medicine, our bodies are influenced by the daily rotation of the earth as well as by its annual orbit around the sun. By adjusting one's routine to the seasons, we can keep our bodies in balance and greatly reduce the risk of disease (Sharma & Clark, 1998).

The entire year is divided into two main periods and six seasons occurring in the following continuous cycle (Warrier & Gunawant, 1997).

During the *period of dehydration,* the sun and winds absorb moisture from the body and can cause weakness.

- Late winter (sisra rtu), from January through March is a period of much strength and health.
- Spring (vasanta rtu), from March through May, is a period of moderate strength and moderate health.
- Summer (grisma rtu), from May through July, is a period of weakness.

During the *period of hydration*, water relieves the excessive heat of the earth and stimulates growth and strength.

- The rainy season (varsar rtu), from July through September, is a period of weakness.
- The fall (sarad rtu), from September through November, is a period of moderate strength and health.
- Early winter (hemanta rtu), from November through January, represents a period of much strength and health.

The seasons very much affect the tridoshas. The seasons, times of day, and life periods can be classified by the doshas as follows (Sharma & Clark, 1998; Trivieri & Anderson, 2002):

- *Kapha season* is spring through early summer (March through June). Kapha time is approximately 6–10 a.m. and 6–10 p.m. Kapha time in the life cycle is childhood, since sleep is more prevalent, and physical growth is a dominant theme of childhood. A spring (kapha) routine involves minimizing daytime sleep; exercising regularly; and avoiding cold, sweet, sour, salty, or oily foods.
- *Pitta season* is midsummer through early autumn (July through October). Pitta time is approximately 10 a.m. to 2 p.m. and 10 p.m. to 2 a.m. Pitta time in the life cycle is adulthood, with the emphasis on activity and achievement. A summer (pitta) routine involves reducing the amount of exercise; swimming; wearing a hat and sunglasses outdoors; avoiding overeating; and eating cool, sweet, bitter, astringent, and oily foods.
- *Vata season* is late autumn through winter (October through February). Vata time is approximately 2–6 a.m. and 2–6 p.m. Vata time in the life cycle is old age, since sleep occurs less frequently, and dry skin and arthritis are more common. A winter (vata) routine involves using a humidifier; avoiding drafts; and choosing warm, well-cooked sweet, salty, or sour foods.

Ayurvedic medicine prescribes other lifestyle practices that are beneficial to health and vitality. One such practice is exercise that conforms to one's dosha type. Yoga, a science and a method for achieving spiritual harmony through control of the mind and body, is one of the most effective forms of exercise for the body as well as a form of nourishment for the mind. Yoga, an essential element of Ayurveda, comes from the Sanskrit word meaning "to unite" or "to join." Yoga is believed to bring people to a naturally tranquil state and a perfect state of equilibrium. Yoga exercises have both a preventive and a curative value: they bring natural order and balance to the body's neurohormones and metabolism, and they protect the body from stress. Ayurveda indicates specific types of yoga that are suitable for each person according to their type of constitution (Lad, 2004). The most common form of yoga is hatha yoga, which incorporates postures, breath work, and meditation.

Breathing, meditation, massage, music, and purification therapies (all previously discussed) are also important elements of a healthy Ayurvedic lifestyle. Breathing exercises, called pranayama, are yogic healing techniques believed to affect creativity, provide calming, and bring joy into one's life. There are different types of pranayama depending on one's constitution. For example, a person of vata constitution should perform alternate nostril breathing (Lad, 2004; Leddy, 2006).

Other forms of treatment in Ayurvedic medicine include external medicine, such as massage, the application of pastes and powders, different types of gargles, various types of physiotherapy, surgery, and psychotherapy (Warrier & Gunawant, 1997).

Timing of Treatment

According to Ayurvedic medicine, there is a correct time to receive treatment, and the correct time is determined through an understanding of kriyakala, which literally means "treatment period" or "time for action" (Warrier & Gunawant, 1997). For a treatment to be most effective, it must be prescribed at the correct time. Just as Western medicine believes that medications are most effective when administered to optimize absorption, Ayurvedic medicine follows similar guidelines. For example, Ayurvedic medicine has 10 proper occasions for taking medications, all related to the timing of meals (Warrier & Gunawant, 1997):

- On an empty stomach
- Before a meal
- After a meal
- Between meals
- During the course of a meal
- Mixed with a meal
- At the beginning and at the end of a meal
- Repeatedly
- With every morsel of food
- With each alternative morsel of food

AYURVEDIC PRACTITIONERS IN THE UNITED STATES

Interest in Ayurveda in the United States began in the 1970s as a result of efforts by the Maharishi Mahesh Yogi's organization of Transcendental Meditation. During the 1980s, Deepak Chopra, MD, wrote *Perfect Health* and opened the eyes of many Westerners to the ancient healing science of Ayurveda. Other American pioneers who have shed light and piqued interest in Ayurveda include Dr. David Frawley of the American Institute of Vedic Studies; Vasant Lad, an Ayurvedic physician and director of the Ayurvedic Institute in New Mexico; and Dr. Robert Svoboda.

Ayurvedic medicine is a powerful form of medicine, and only skilled, properly trained practitioners should practice it. Specific medicines or diet and lifestyle recommendations can be ineffective or dangerous if not prescribed by knowledgeable practitioners.

Training and Education

In India, the duration of training for an Ayurvedic physician is similar to that of Western medical training, ranging from 4 to 6 years, with postgraduate training in the specialty areas. Education includes training in both Western and Ayurvedic concepts of anatomy, biochemistry, pathology, pharmacology, physiology, laboratory medicine, and preventative and public health. Clinical training consists of at least 3–5 years of inpatient hospital and outpatient clinical care. There are approximately 200 Ayurvedic undergraduate schools, 53 postgraduate schools, and more than 200,000 trained Ayurvedic physicians (Pai et al., 2004).

The quality of educational programs for Ayurvedic practitioners varies widely in the United States. Ayurvedic colleges have no national standards of required compliance and no national approval of licensure or state certification boards, so each institution is free to create its own guidelines for training and certifying practitioners. Most training in the United States ranges from 1- to 4-year programs (Pai et al., 2004). Some practitioners are trained in the Western medical tradition and others in a whole medical system called naturopathic medicine before or after they study Ayurveda. Many learn in India and may be trained in different aspects of Ayurvedic practice (such as massage but not herbal treatments) (Pai et al., 2004).

The programs are open to healthcare practitioners, who may include medical doctors, osteopaths, naturopaths, chiropractors, nurses, dietitians, and massage and physical therapists. After completing a training program, they can be certified as a health instructor or as an Ayurvedic specialist/consultant. This designation allows them to educate others on diet, herb use, and lifestyle/behavioral changes (Pai et al., 2004).

Some facilities offer Ayurvedic treatments by practitioners who have no Ayurvedic medical school training. Spas and salons offer services that may fall into this category. Because Ayurveda offers many types of therapies and is used for many health conditions, clients should make sure that the individual who is providing the treatment has received adequate training.

Ayurvedic Organizations

Two independent representative organizations support the growth of Ayurveda in the United States: the National Ayurvedic Medical Association (NAMA) and the California Association of Ayurvedic Medicine (CAAM). Pai et al. (2004) note that other organizations are studying Ayurveda:

> Currently, with the emerging growth of Ayurveda worldwide, private organizations (such as the Maharishi University) and governmental organizations such as the National Center for Complementary and Alternative Medicine (NCCAM) of the National Institutes of Health (NIH) are performing clinical studies to demonstrate the use and efficacy of Ayurveda. (p. 220)

In addition, the Ayurvedic and Naturopathic Medical Clinic, the Ayurvedic Institute, the Sharp Institute for Human Potential and Mind-Body Medicine, and the Canadian Association of Ayurvedic Medicine all provide information on treatments and physicians and educate individuals about Ayurveda (Trivieri & Anderson, 2002).

Practicing Ayurveda in the United States

Practicing Ayurveda in the United States is legal, depending on how it is practiced. Individuals seeking Ayurvedic treatment should check the credentials of their practitioners and/or the claims of Ayurvedic products. Currently, practitioners can receive thorough training at only a few locations in the United States. When evaluating and finding competent practitioners, be sure to investigate the extent of their education, verify their certification and that of the certifying organization, obtain proof of their competency, and meet with the practitioner.

Ayurvedic Medicines

Clinical trials, a necessity for any prescribed pharmaceutical product, provide scientific proof of the efficacy of any treatment. Not all Ayurvedic products lend themselves to this method of testing, however, because Ayurvedic medicine proposes that each individual is unique. While there have been several clinical trials for herbal products, further study is warranted. Indeed, the Centers for Disease Control and Prevention received 12 reports of lead poisoning in 2004 that were linked to the use of Ayurvedic medications. A similar report in the *Journal of the American Medical Association* in 2004 reported findings of lead, mercury, and arsenic in over-the-counter remedies (Saper, et al., 2004). The NIH is currently researching Ayurvedic practices, and the World Health Organization (WHO) is supporting research in this area as well as in the integration of the Ayurvedic healthcare system into modern medicine (Trivieri & Anderson, 2002).

KEY CONCEPTS

1. Ayurveda is the oldest complete medical system in the world, with recorded origins dating back 3,500–4,000 years to 1200–800 BC. It has been practiced in India and Sri Lanka for at least 5,000 years. Ayurvedic medicine is a highly sophisticated system of medicine that focuses on the whole individual and his or her relationship to the environment. Balance within the body and between the body and the external environment is a dynamic process that results in health, vitality, and a long life.
2. In Ayurvedic medicine, everything is composed of five elements, or panchamahabhutas, that interact, giving rise to all that exists. In humans, these five elements combine to form three doshas (tridoshas)—bioenergetic forces that determine an individual's physical constitution (prakrti).
3. Only skilled, knowledgeable practitioners should practice Ayurveda. Western healthcare professionals will find knowledge of this form of medicine helpful as they care for clients from diverse cultures.

QUESTIONS FOR REFLECTION

1. What is the history of Ayurvedic medicine?
2. How do the three doshas differ?
3. What are the five systems of Ayurvedic treatment?

REFERENCES

Basuray, J. (2002). India: Transcultural nursing and health care. In M. Leininger & M. R. McFarland (Eds.), *Transcultural nursing* (3rd ed., pp. 477–491). New York: McGraw-Hill.

Fontaine, K. L. (2000). *Healing practices: Alternative therapies for nursing.* Upper Saddle River, NJ: Prentice Hall.

Lad, V. (1998). *The complete book of Ayurvedic home remedies.* New York: Three Rivers Press.

Lad, V. (2004). *Ayurveda: The science of self-healing.* Twin Lakes, WI: Lotus Press.

Leddy, S. K. (2006). *Integrative health promotion: Conceptual bases for nursing practice* (2nd ed.). Sudbury, MA: Jones and Bartlett.

Morrison, J. H. (1995). *The book of Ayurveda.* New York: Fireside.

Pai, S., Shanbhag, V., & Archarya, S. (2004). Ayurvedic medicine. In B. Kligler & R. Lee, *Integrative medicine* (pp. 219–240). New York: McGraw-Hill.

Qutab, M. A (2002). Ayurveda. In M. A. Qutab, *Holistic health and healing.* Philadelphia: F. A. Davis.

Saper, R. B., Stefanos, N. K., Paquin, J., Eisenberg, D. M., Davis, R. B., & Phillips, R. S. (2004). Heavy metal content of Ayurvedic herbal medicine products. *Journal of the American Medical Association, 292*, 2868–2873.

Sharma, H., & Clark, C. (1998). *Contemporary Ayurveda: Medicine and research in Maharishi Ayurveda.* Philadelphia: Churchill Livingstone.

Shealy, C. N. (Ed.). (1996). *The complete family guide to alternative medicine: An illustrated encyclopedia of natural healing.* Shaftesbury, Dorset, UK: Element Books.

Trivieri, L., Jr., & Anderson, J. W. (Eds.). (2002). *Alternative medicine: The definitive guide* (2nd ed.). Berkeley, CA: Celestial Arts.

Warrier, G., & Gunawant, D. (1997). *The complete illustrated guide to Ayurveda.* New York: Element Books.

Zysk, K. G. (with Tetlow, G.). (2006). Traditional Ayurveda. In M. S. Micozzi (Ed.), *Fundamentals of complementary and integrative medicine* (3rd ed., pp. 494–507). St. Louis, MO: Saunders Elsevier.

CHAPTER 8

Humor and Health

A smile is the shortest distance between two people.
—Victor Borge

LEARNING OBJECTIVES

1. Explain the historical perspective of humor.
2. Define *humor, laughter, play,* and *gelotology.*
3. Describe the four components of humor.
4. Describe the types of humor.
5. Explain the theories of humor.
6. Describe the psychological and physiological effects of humor.
7. Explain the use of humor in health care, including the use of therapeutic humor.
8. Describe ways to develop a sense of humor.

INTRODUCTION

Imagine a prescription that reads: "Take two doses of Lily Tomlin, followed by one dose of Charlie Chaplin, and rinse with an episode of *I Love Lucy.* Repeat as necessary and call me in the morning." That is exactly what political journalist Norman Cousins decided to prescribe for himself during his treatment for a life-threatening disease.

Perhaps one of the most influential proponents of the healing effects of humor and laughter therapy, Cousins was diagnosed in 1964 with an advanced case of ankylosing spondylitis, a rare rheumatoid disease that causes progressive deterioration of the body's connective tissue. He was given a poor prognosis for recovery: roughly 1 in 500. His unique approach to recovery included watching TV shows like *Candid Camera* and movies with Laurel and Hardy and the Marx brothers. Cousins found that 10 minutes of laughter allowed him

2 hours of pain-free sleep. Through the use of laughter and high doses of vitamin C, he recovered and spent the remaining 12 years of his life as an adjunct professor at the University of California, Los Angeles Medical School, where he established what he called a humor task force to coordinate and support clinical research into laughter (Wooten, 2005). Cousins emphasized that humor is not a cure-all, nor does it substitute for competent medical treatment. Humor, he believed, is a powerful therapeutic element that interrupts the panic cycle of illness. When this cycle occurs, blood vessels constrict and negative biochemical changes occur.

Patch Adams (1998), whose book was the basis of the Hollywood movie *Patch Adams*, also extols the health benefits of humor. He wrote, "Health is based on happiness—from hugging and clowning around to finding joy in family and friends, satisfaction in work and ecstasy in nature and the arts" (p. 1).

Humor is a universal experience that involves three basic elements: the stimulus (a funny joke or humorous situation), an emotional response (mirth), and the accompanying behavior (laughter, smiling, giggling, etc.). Nearly everyone knows how it feels to experience something humorous. Someone tells a joke, makes a witty comment, draws a funny cartoon, or has a slip of the tongue, and bystanders are suddenly struck by how funny it is. They smile, chuckle, burst out laughing, or experience a sense of pleasant well-being. Humor is such a commonplace occurrence for most people that it may seem strange to explore it.

Although humor is often lighthearted, it also serves a serious social, emotional, and cognitive function (Martin, 2007). Humor adds perspective to life, helping people deal with stressors from minor irritations such as being cut off in traffic to more challenging difficulties like life-threatening illnesses. Attracting all types and kinds of people, it breaks through barriers when mere words cannot. Humor and laughter connect people and help build relationships. Laughter is also great exercise. It uses the breathing muscles, can increase heart rate and oxygenation, and can cause distraction, thus promoting relaxation. Nearly all of us have laughed until our sides hurt or until we collapsed in a giggling fit over a silly experience.

Laughter makes people feel alive. His Holiness the Dalai Lama has said, "Our business is to be happy" (Shimoff, 2008, p. 275). As long as people choose to laugh, it means they have affirmed life, no matter how burdensome it becomes. Although laughter is short lived, its effects are long lasting. As Blumenfeld and Alpern (1994) note, "The real fountain of youth is humor, and its sound is bubbling laughter" (p. 6).

AN OVERVIEW OF HUMOR

Humor is a complex phenomenon and an essential part of human nature. Seaward (2006) describes it as a give-and-take experience that is first absorbed or experienced by internalizing the perception cognitively and then expressed externally through an effort to share it with others.

Historical Perspectives

Anthropologists have never found a culture or society at any time in human history that did not include humor (Martin, 2007; Wooten, 2005). Comic relief has been around since the beginning of humanity. It provides a powerful person-to-person connection that requires a stimulus and a response to be effective (Blumenfeld & Alpern, 1994).

The ancient Greeks believed humor was a virtue. Plato believed it nurtured the soul, and he advocated using it as a healing practice. Aristotle believed that laughter arose from the enjoyment of the misfortunes of others. Other philosophers viewed laughter as a valuable asset in correcting the foolishness of society (Wooten, 2005). Adams et al. (2006) note that people who lived during Old Testament times lived by the biblical saying, "A merry heart doeth good like a medicine" (p. 355).

The word *humor* comes from the Latin *humorem*, which means "fluid" or "moisture" (Wooten, 2005). In medieval physiology, humor referred to the four basic fluids of the body:

- *Blood:* Associated with a happy, cheerful spirit
- *Cholor:* Yellow bile produced by the gallbladder that allegedly made one depressed and sad
- *Phlegm:* Produced by the respiratory system and responsible for apathy and sluggishness
- *Black bile:* Produced by the kidneys or spleen and responsible for anger and hostility

The predominant fluid determined the individual's mood or temperament. A good balance meant that the person was in "good humor" (Martin, 2007; Robinson, 1991; Seaward, 2006; Wooten, 2005). Hippocrates, the fourth-century Greek physician considered to be the father of medicine, believed that good health depended on the balance of the four humors (Martin, 2007).

In AD 1260, a progressive French physician, Henri de Moundeville, found that his clients healed faster when their friends and family cheered them up and joked with them. European monarchs also saw the importance of laughter and used jesters to add joy to their castle courts. Richard Tarlton, one of the most famous court jesters, is believed to have kept British Queen Elizabeth I (1533–1603) in better health than her physicians (Seaward, 2006).

In the 15th century, the meaning of humor continued to evolve and described an unbalanced temperament or personality trait that deviated from social norms; in other words, *humor* referred to an odd, eccentric, ridiculous, or peculiar person who was the object of laughter or ridicule. Eventually, the odd person became known as the humorist. It was not until the mid- to late 19th century that the term *humorist* meant someone who created a product called humor to amuse others. Mark Twain was viewed as one of the first humorists in this modern sense (Martin, 2007).

Laughter has not always been considered a good thing. Most biblical references associate laughter with scorn, derision, or contempt. Europeans and Puritans in North America considered laughter the work of the devil, and people caught laughing out loud were often denounced as witches or believed to be possessed by Satan. Many Christian denominations considered laughter a sin and indecent. A review of portraits of European nobility over a period of several hundred years revealed very few who were smiling (Seaward, 2006). During the 18th century, the word *humor* was used in the same way we use the word *ridicule* today: with a negative and aggressive connotation. The change from that perspective to today's perspective of humor as laughter did not occur until middle-class British society emphasized the importance of benevolence, kindness, and sympathy in people of refinement (Martin, 2007). It was not until the 20th century that people began smiling for their photographs (Seaward, 2006).

In the past, humor was neglected by researchers because it is difficult to interpret in experimental procedures and challenging to measure and control (Blumenfeld & Alpern, 1994). Only in recent years have humor and laughter been considered healing therapies. One of the earliest and most extensive reviews of humor and its use by health professionals was completed in the 1970s by Vera Robinson, a nurse educator who was completing her doctoral thesis (Wooten, 2005).

The past several decades have seen many studies, research, and educational programs on humor. There is now a humor movement, as well as studies, research, and education on the subject. Two reasons for this interest are the increased stress of living in today's world and the increasing interest in health, wellness, integrative health care, and self-care (Robinson, 1991). As more individuals learn about the benefits of proper nutrition, exercise, a positive attitude in life, healthy behaviors, and stress management, they adopt these practices. Humor, laughter, play, and self-care become part of their behavior.

In 1975, the Workshop Library on World Humor was started in Washington, D.C., to examine the use of humor. By 1989, the Seventh International Conference on Humor was held in Hawaii. The *International Journal of Humor Research* and the International Society for Humor Studies were started in 1989. Since then, many conferences, seminars, and workshops have taken place to educate the public on the health values of humor (Robinson, 1991).

In 1999, Dr. Candace Pert documented the mind-body-happiness link in her book, *Molecules of Emotion*. Shimoff (2008) states that more than 100,000 chemical reactions take place in the brain every second. Endorphins (the body's natural painkillers), serotonin (a vasoconstrictor that calms anxiety and relieves depression), oxytocin (the bonding hormone), and dopamine (which promotes alertness and a feeling of enjoyment) are just a few of the chemicals that cause these reactions.

Helpful Definitions

What is humor? What makes us laugh? Why do we even need to laugh? Humor is a universal, natural, and complex phenomenon for which there is always a need. Robinson (1991) sums it up nicely: "Humor has been described as a pleasure upon which man pounces at the slightest excuse to indulge in it" (p. xi).

While humor has been around as long as human beings have existed, there is no consensus about its definition, nature, causes, effects, purposes, and usefulness. The following definitions, however, may be helpful (Kruse & Prazak, 2006; Martin, 2007; Rankin-Box, 1996; Robinson, 1991; Seaward, 2006; Wooten, 2005):

- *Humor:* A quality of perception, perspective, and attitude toward life that enables an individual to experience joy even when faced with adversity; a perception of the absurdity or incongruity of a situation; a cognitive experience. Humor is a uniquely personal experience and what is humorous to one person may not be humorous to another. It is a form of communication.
- *Laughter:* A physical expression of humor; a distinctive, stereotyped pattern of vocalization that is easily recognized and unmistakable; the physical behavior that occurs in response to something perceived as humorous, amusing, or surprising. This behavior engages most of the muscle groups and organ systems of the body. Laughter is often preceded by physical, emotional, or cognitive tension. It is indistinguishable from one culture to another and it is innate: even children who are born deaf and blind have laughed without ever hearing the laughter of another person.

- *Play:* A spontaneous or recreational activity performed for sheer enjoyment rather than to reach a goal or produce a product. Playfulness is a mood or attitude that infuses the individual with a sense of joy and positive emotions.
- *Gelotology:* The science of laughter; the stimulus of humor with subsequent emotional and behavioral responses.
- *Humor and laughter therapy:* A humorous or amusing intervention used by the healthcare professional or client and designed to benefit to the client.

Kruse and Prazak (2006) define humor as a perceptual event connected with one's sense of self, an expression of a uniquely human capacity to adapt to experiences and situations that may be possible sources of humor. Mallett (1996) defines it as "communication (verbal and non-verbal) intended to cause amusement" (p. 109).

According to Adams et al. (2006), humor is *not* the equivalent of laughter and it may or may not stimulate laughter. Humor can be a quiet smile or an inner glow of delight, and it may accompany aggression, surprise, or even grief. It is not a form of therapy. It does not cure cancer, baldness, or major depression, but it is a wonderful adjunct to the overall approach to one's psychological and spiritual life. Joking is not a major part of humor. Only about 4% of the adult population can remember and tell jokes well, while about 90% consider themselves to have a good sense of humor. Humor is conveyed relatively nonverbally, such as in a smile or with the twinkle of an eye.

Mallett (1996) calls humor and laughter therapy an "amusing intervention used by the healthcare professional or patient to produce a beneficial response in the patient" (p. 109). The context is important, and humor shared by clients and nurses is often used to maintain a friendly relationship, especially when discussing potentially difficult or embarrassing issues. Humor can be used to convey anger, frustration, fear, and anxiety.

In some instances, laughter is inappropriate. According to Mallett (1996), inappropriate laughter can result from poisoning or disease. One example of the latter is the Fore tribe of New Guinea, who suffer from a viral disease called Kuru ("laughing death") caused by the ingestion of brain tissue. During the terminal stage of the disease, the individual suffers from uncontrollable, hilarious, and uproarious laughter. Mallett also discusses "sick joke cycles (e.g., following the Chernobyl disaster—'What has feathers and glows in the dark? Chicken Kiev.')" (p. 110). This type of humor allows for a collective mental defense in which individuals can articulate and cope with the worst types of disasters.

Humor is a social relationship and occurs in a social environment. It promotes group cohesion, initiates relationships, relieves tension during social conflict, and can be a means of expressing approval or disapproval of social action (Wooten, 2005). The culture, society, or ethnic group in which humor occurs influences its style and content as well as the situations in which it is used and considered appropriate (Ziv, 1988).

Four Components of Humor

According to Martin (2007), humor has four essential components:

- *A social context:* This context stems from the perspective that humor is basically a social phenomenon since people laugh and joke more often when they are with others than if they are by themselves. The social context is one of play. During play, people are not serious about what they do or say; they carry out activities for their own sake. The playful state of mind associated with humor is called the *paratelic mode* versus the more serious *telic mode* (from the Greek *telos* which means "goal"). Individuals can often switch back and forth between these modes.
- *Cognitive-perceptual processes:* Humor is also characterized by particular cognitive-perceptual processes. To mentally process information from their environment, memory, ideas, words, or actions, people generate witty comments or comical physical actions that others perceive as funny. Because much humor evolves from incongruous, odd, unusual, unexpected, or surprising events, ideas, and images, and because people need to be in a playful state of mind, their cognitive-perceptual processes perceive the humor.
- *Emotional responses:* Although the word *mirth* is closely associated with joy, a feeling of invincibility, and an element of exultation, it seems to be a term that effectively denotes the emotion of humor (Martin, 2007). Humor activates the brain's limbic system and causes people to respond in emotional ways. The usual response is pleasant, described as amusement, mirth, merriment, cheerfulness, or hilarity. The funnier the images, the more strongly they activate these parts of the brain. The biochemical response is also activated by pleasurable states such as eating, listening to enjoyable music, sexual activity, and using mood-altering drugs; in all these situations, people seek out humor to achieve the same biochemical response. Because of the resultant biochemical changes in the brain, autonomic nervous system, and endocrine system—all involving a variety of molecules such as neurotransmitters, hormones, opioids, and neuropeptides—humor has been linked with potential health benefits. The exact nature of these changes and their effects on health is still being researched.

- *An expressive component:* Finally, the mirthful pleasure accompanying humor has the expressive component of laughter and smiling, which can range from mild, faint grins to loud, raucous laughter where our faces become red, we throw our heads back, we slap our thighs, and go through other bodily reactions. Laughter is fundamentally a social behavior that has specific, distinct, recognizable sounds and that rarely occurs in social isolation.

Types of Humor

There are many types of humor, both adaptive and maladaptive. Adaptive styles (Kruse & Prazak, 2006) include self-enhancing and affiliative styles that protect the self. Maladaptive styles include those that are self-defeating and aggressive, employed to hide feelings and avoid dealing constructively with problems.

Another type of humor, therapeutic humor, has a beneficial effect on the body-mind-spirit. It is life affirming, it increases the cohesion between individuals, it is interactive, and it reduces stress (Kruse & Prazak, 2006). Although a lot has been written about using humor as a therapeutic tool, humor physiology is still a relatively young science (Adams et al., 2006; Kruse & Prazak, 2006).

Humor may be difficult to classify because so many types of humor and nuances can be internalized or expressed. These types are not easily separated and can often overlap. Seaward (2006) and Martin (2007) provide two of the most extensive analyses of the types of humor. They posit that there are several classifications of humor, and they are not mutually exclusive but rather follow in a particular order that relates to their efficacy in coping with stress (Seaward, 2006).

Hoping and Coping Humor

- *Hoping humor* involves the ability to hope for something better, and it enables individuals to cope with difficult situations. Hoping humor accepts life with all its dichotomies, contradiction, and incongruities. It gives individuals the courage to withstand suffering. Humor has a force of its own and can transform a person's perspective (Adams et al., 2006; Klein, 1998; Kruse & Prazak, 2006; Wooten, 2005).
- *Coping humor* involves laughing at hopeless situations. It provides a detachment from the problem and makes it possible to release tension, anxiety, and hostility. It helps individuals change their thinking and regain a sense of control. For example, a euphemism for death such as

"he bit the dust" or "he called home" can provide levity for a serious subject (Adams et al., 2006; Klein, 1998; Kruse & Prazak, 2006; Wooten, 2005).

Parody and Satire

- *Parody* is a type of humor that closely imitates something or someone for a comical effect. It is usually a verbal or physical expression of humor that highlights imperfections to exaggerate behaviors and personality traits. This type of humor is considered one of the best types in dealing with stress. Examples include celebrity roasts and the music of pop satirist Weird Al Yankovic (Seaward, 2006).
- *Satire* is similar to parody but it is the written or dramatic expression of personal, political, and cultural quirks and flaws. It is aggressive humor that pokes fun at social institutions or social policy. Writers Erma Bombeck, Dave Barry, and Art Buchwald are some of America's best-known satirists. The TV show *Saturday Night Live* offers examples of dramatic satire, and the cartoon movie *Shrek* is an example of a satire of a classic fairy tale (Martin, 2007; Seaward, 2006).

Slapstick Comedy and Absurd or Nonsense Humor

- *Slapstick comedy* is a type of humor that was common in the days of American vaudeville, when physical farces generated laughs. Slipping on banana peels and getting hit with a pie in the face, all to the accompaniment of generated sound effects, are typical examples. Individuals who are considered experts in this area include comedians Lucille Ball, the Three Stooges, Abbott and Costello, the Marx brothers, and Laurel and Hardy. Some scholars believe this type of humor is aggressive and allows the audience to release latent anger in a cathartic way by watching someone else give and get physical, though harmless, blows (Seaward, 2006).
- *Absurd or nonsense humor* unites two or more concepts resulting in a ludicrous or ridiculous perception. Cartoonist Gary Larson's *Far Side* is a great example when it depicts cows driving cars or cheetahs using vending machines on the Serengeti plains. Monty Python's popular movies and TV shows are other examples of this form of humor (Seaward, 2006).

Transformation of Frozen Expressions and Double Entendres

- The *transformation of frozen expressions* involves transforming well-known sayings, clichés, or adages into novel statements. For example, a bald man complains, "Hair today, gone tomorrow" (Martin, 2007).

- The *double entendre* is a type of wordplay whose expression has two meanings, usually of a sexual nature. James Bond movies are famous for this type of humor, as are Disney movies, which are often discreetly written at two levels: one for children and one for adults (Martin, 2007; Seaward, 2006).

Black (Gallows) Humor

Black, or gallows, humor is not a type of ethnic humor but rather a kind of humor that provides protection from the emotional impact of witnessing tragedy, disgusting or intolerable aspects of a situation, death, and disfigurement. Much of the comic humor in the movie and TV show *M*A*S*H* is an example.

Caregivers often use gallows humor as a means of maintaining some psychological distance from their suffering clients, thus protecting themselves from a sympathetic nervous system response to the suffering. Healthcare workers who often face death, tragedy, and crises (such as those in the intensive care unit [ICU], emergency room, or operating room) use this type of humor. Much of it is risqué or obscene, and the jokes are about the tragedy or suffering.

This term is purported to have originated from two brothers who were to be hanged. On the gallows, one brother had already been hanged when the other said, "Look at my brother there, making a spectacle of himself. Pretty soon we'll be a pair of spectacles" (Adams et al., 2006; Klein, 1998; Kruse & Prazak, 2006; Seaward, 2006; Wooten, 2005).

Irony and Dry Humor

- *Irony* is described as consisting of two concepts or events that, when paired, mean or expose the opposite of the expected outcome. Examples are buying a diet soft drink and a candy bar or using oxymorons such as "alone together," "jumbo shrimp," "found missing," "honest politician," or "plastic glasses" (Martin, 2007; Seaward, 2006).
- *Dry humor*, or quick-witted humor, can also be described as clever, esoteric wit that may involve double entendres. It can also consist of nonsensical replies to a statement or question that was meant to be serious. Comedians Will Rogers, Groucho Marx, and Garrison Keillor of the *Prairie Home Companion* are examples of this type of humorist. Comedians George Carlin and Click and Clack of NPR's *Car Talk* are also famous for their quick wits (Martin, 2007; Seaward, 2006).

Stock Conversational Witticisms, Teasing, and Self-deprecation

- *Stock conversational witticisms* are routinely or recurrently used humorous sayings or expressions. Examples include "faster than greased lightening" or funny or exaggerated facial expressions, odd ways of walking, or bodily mannerisms (Martin, 2007).
- *Teasing* occurs when humorous remarks are directed at the listener's personal appearance or foibles. Unlike sarcasm, the intention is not to seriously insult or offend the listener (Martin, 2007).
- *Self-deprecation* is a type of humor in which the remarks are directed at oneself to demonstrate modesty, put the listener at ease, or ingratiate oneself with the listener (Martin, 2007).

Puns, Bathroom Humor, and Sarcasm

- *Puns* are plays on words that use one word to evoke a second meaning, usually based on a homophone (a word with a different meaning that sounds the same). Some consider puns to be the lowest form of humor because they border on the silly or inane but they do not usually have any malicious intent (Martin, 2007; Seaward, 2006). Example of puns include, "California smog test: Can UCLA?" and "Egotist: One who is me-deep in conversation."
- *Bathroom humor* is also described as vulgar, ruthless, crude, and irreverent because many bodily functions are chosen to get cheap laughs. Movies like *There's Something about Mary*, *Dumb and Dumber*, and *South Park* showcase this type of humor (Seaward, 2006).
- The word *sarcasm* is derived from Greek and French words that literally mean "to tear flesh." Sarcasm often demonstrates clever wit, is aggressive, and targets an individual rather than an institution. Sarcasm can reveal latent anger, be an attempt to get verbal revenge, and be a socially acceptable way of expressing hostile feelings without becoming physically aggressive. Although sarcasm can be followed by a remark such as "I'm just kidding"—to alleviate the sting of the comment—it can hurt the listener as much as physical aggression. Sarcasm is considered the lowest form of humor because it induces rather than reduces stress. One example occurred when a dignified lady told Winston Churchill, "Sir, you are drunk," and he replied, "Yes, and you are ugly. But tomorrow I shall be sober and you shall still be ugly" (Martin, 2007; Seaward, 2006).

THEORIES OF HUMOR

For ages, people have tried to understand what makes someone laugh. Although no one has been successful at identifying just one reason (probably because human beings differ in so many ways), there are several major theories of humor, including (Kruse & Prazak, 2006; Martin, 2007; Robinson, 1991; Seaward, 2006; Wooten, 2005):

- Superiority (disparagement) theory
- Incongruity (surprise) theory
- Play theory
- Release (relief) theory
- Divinity theory
- Biological and instinct theories
- Philosophical perspectives
- Psychoanalytical perspectives
- Psychological perspectives
- Anthropological perspectives
- Sociological perspectives

Superiority (Disparagement) Theory

Believed to have originated with Plato, superiority theory is considered the oldest theory for explaining people's affinity for the ridiculous. Proponents of this theory believe that laughter comes from the enhanced feelings of self-esteem (superiority) that occur in response to situations of others less fortunate. In other words, people feel better when they view someone else as more inferior, stupid, or unlucky. Pies in the face; someone slipping on a banana peel; and the comedy of Charlie Chaplin, Laurel and Hardy, and the Keystone Kops reflect this theory.

Ancient writings link laughter to scorn and mockery. Laughter of this type gives people a sense of control over a situation and may be a key element in survival and coping.

Some believe this type of humor actually expresses warmth and empathy, since it encourages people to laugh at themselves. Others believe it is the reason for offensive and negative humor. For one moment, individuals feel superior but they know that "this could happen to us!" Some describe humor as a continuum: We laugh at no one (puns, nonsense); we laugh at someone or a group (moron jokes, ethnic jokes); we laugh in general at humanity's foibles; and finally, we laugh at ourselves (the most therapeutic aspect). The greater the dignity of the object, the bigger the laugh—as in sarcasm or in ethnic, sexist, racist, and even blonde jokes.

Superiority or disparagement theory is considered to be one of the classic, traditional theories of humor, and some believe it to be an element in all humor.

Incongruity (Surprise) Theory

Incongruity theory is also considered a classic theory of humor. Laughter in this type of humor occurs when a sudden shock, surprise, or conflict occurs. We just don't expect the outcome. In this type of humor, a sudden and surprising shift in cognitive processing brings together two concepts, normally considered remote from each other, to reveal their similarities (e.g., the surprise ending of a joke). There must be an ambivalence or conflict of ideas or emotions that produces an absurdity, resulting in a burst of laughter.

According to Robinson (1991), this theory is based on Gestalt psychology, which involves perception of the whole. People order their perceptions, as they are presented, in a reasoning fashion. Unexpected configurations produce a surprise that can appear ludicrous. The appreciation of the joke, or getting the point, occurs when this shift in perception occurs. Oxymorons are an example of this type of humor.

There are two types of incongruity humor. The ascending (or aha) type produces wonder and awe; the descending (or ha-ha) produces humor. Many theorists believe that the concept of surprise is essential to humor.

Play Theory

Humor has been described as an aspect of play, and the playful nature of humor and laughter is central to most theories about humor. Some theorists believe humor is enjoyable because it stimulates a playful mood, a sense of fun, and a refusal to take the situation seriously. A sense of humor develops as a result of an individual's social, emotional, intellectual, and physical development.

Release (Relief) Theory

This theory suggests that laughter occurs when the tension of anxiety, frustration, or anger needs a release (e.g., nervous laughter or hostile humor). The relief can be cognitive (such as an escape from reality or reason), emotional (such as an escape from anxiety, fear, anger, embarrassment, or social conflict), or physical (such as the release of nervous energy).

This theory is credited to Sigmund Freud, who asserted that the act of laughter is a physical release or expression of sexual and hostile impulses suppressed by the conscious mind. The greater the suppression, the greater the laughter. Often the subject matter includes taboo subjects that are not socially acceptable in professional or mixed company, sexual references, or social taboos such as illegal drugs and questionable behavior. Freud believed that humor was a precious gift and the most advanced defense mechanism (Seaward, 2006).

Divinity Theory

Relatively new, divinity theory posits that humor strengthens the spiritual nature of humanity, is a gift from God, reveals the raw truth about subjects, and connects and bonds people together. This theory states that humor is God's (or the higher power's) way of telling people they're not perfect.

A connection between clowns and a divine presence is apparent in many cultures. For example, medicine men and shamans dress in "funny" outfits and act in outrageous ways. Even though what is deemed funny is culturally specific, such outfits are often excessive and bold in color or design, and the performers often exaggerate behaviors in a way designed to make their audiences laugh. With the mystical power to heal, medicine men and shamans wear clothing and exhibit behaviors that are often interpreted as having a special meaning. Clowns also have been used as a form of entertainment for centuries to poke fun at attitudes and behaviors—with androgynous face masks or makeup that is neither male nor female. Clowns are used in hospital wards today, especially to help children heal (Seaward, 2006).

Biological and Instinct Theories

These theories view humor and laughter as a healthy mechanism for the body because laughter and humor produce a sense of well-being and euphoria that has biological survival value. Since humor and laughter also serve a social function, they help people connect with each other and laugh at their own misfortunes. Some describe laughter as a physiological reaction that is similar to tears. Others describe it as a way to communicate to other human beings that they can relax (Robinson, 1991).

Philosophical Perspectives

Philosophical perspectives are primarily concerned with humor as a reflection of the human nature and the issues of good and evil. Plato and Aristotle felt that humor was the result of others enjoying someone's misfortune and that comedy was an imitation of humans at their worst. Others felt that humor was a weapon against evil and that it helped correct the small, foolish aspects of society.

Psychoanalytical Perspectives

The psychoanalytical perspectives originated with Freud, who became interested in jokes when he studied the relationship between dreams and jokes. Since members of a civilized society repress many of their basic impulses, Freud says, joking becomes a socially acceptable way of satisfying these needs, and laughter becomes a way to release nervous energy. Freud recognized four types of purposeful jokes: the sexual joke, the aggressive or hostile joke, the blasphemous joke, and the skeptical joke. He developed the theory of laughing at death and tragedy (gallows humor) and believed that humor was liberating and provided a release from the stress of reality. Freud felt that people enjoyed jokes so much because jokes provided moments of illicit pleasure derived from releasing primitive sexual and aggressive impulses. He drew a sharp distinction between humor (the benign and sympathetic amusement at the ironic aspects of life) and wit (aggressive and less clearly psychologically healthy). Freud's theories have provided the basis for many other theories of humor.

Psychological Perspectives

The psychological perspectives of humor deal primarily with why one individual finds something humorous and another does not. These perspectives look at individual traits, such as aggression, sex, creativity, and intelligence, and they examine how a sense of humor develops. They view humor as a psychologically liberating experience that releases people from the restrictions of their daily lives and, in so doing, makes them joyful. Humor reduces stress. Humor and laughter help people maintain their psychological and physiological health in the face of life's difficulties.

Anthropological Perspectives

These perspectives view humor from the perspectives of cultures or ethnic groups. They see humor as a kind of permitted disrespect or a combination of aggression and friendliness. While humor is universal, it cannot occur in a vacuum. It must exist in some kind of cultural framework that allows individuals to express socially taboo subjects or ideas.

Sociological Perspectives

The sociological perspectives view humor as a way of socially correcting rigid, automatic, unadaptive behavior and thus socializing individuals within a society's group or groups. Seen through these perspectives, humor produces group cohesion and is a way of initiating friendships and social connections. It provides an acceptable way of expressing disapproval, reinforcing the norms of the group (via the scapegoat or fool), and relieving social tension. Sociology is the most recent discipline to explore the effects of humor on individuals.

MYTHS ABOUT HUMOR AND LAUGHTER

Dr. Patch Adams describes three myths about laughter that keep people from laughing or developing a sense of humor (Adams et al., 2006). These myths are important for healthcare providers to overcome if they are to develop and use humor to heal.

1. *People need a reason to laugh, and, when they do laugh, it must be for a good reason.* If someone asks them why they're laughing, they can explain and the listener will also laugh. If someone doesn't laugh, has a puzzling expression on his or her face, or says something like, "Boy, you have a weird sense of humor," people unconsciously censor their laughter. Yet, as Adams explains, laughter is unreasonable, illogical, and irrational. The truth is that people do *not* need a good reason to laugh.
2. *People laugh because they're happy.* Dr. Adams believes the opposite—people are happy because they laugh. He states that if laughter resulted from happiness, people would not feel better after laughing because they already felt good. Most people do not know what happiness *is*, so they seek some outward sign to validate its presence. Those who have laughed until they cried know that, in the middle, they often don't know which is which. People don't laugh because they're happy or cry because they're sad. Either expression occurs because people are tense, stressed, or in pain. Adams states that "laughter and tears rebalance the

chemicals our bodies create when these distressed states are present, so we feel better after we have laughed or cried" (p. 364).

3. *A sense of humor is the same as laughter.* Although people often use humor and laughter interchangeably, the two are very different. People don't need a sense of humor to laugh. For example, babies laugh but have not developed a sense of humor. Laughter is innate, but a sense of humor is learned.

Humor and laughter are healing in many ways. Just two days after comedian Bill Cosby's only son, Ennis, was gunned down and killed at the age of 27, Cosby resumed taping his television show and did two live performances in Florida. While he was onstage, he shared personal details of his son's funeral. Some thought he was returning to work too soon, but even in his grief, one of America's most loved entertainers said that "we have to laugh—we've got to laugh" (Klein, 1998).

EFFECTS OF HUMOR AND LAUGHTER

Humor is an adaptive coping mechanism that increases pleasure and reduces pain—all at the same time. As Seaward (2006) says, "In its simplest terms, the use of humor is a defense mechanism. Yet, unlike other conscious or unconscious defense strategies to protect the ego, such as rationalization and projection, humor seems to dissolve the walls of the ego rather than intensity them" (p. 269).

Psychological Functions of Humor and Laughter

While humor is a form of social play that allows people to have fun and receive emotional pleasure from nonserious incongruities, it also serves several serious functions that have probably contributed to our survival as a species. Three broad psychological functions of humor are (Martin, 2007; Robinson, 1991):

- Cognitive and social functions
- Social communication
- Relief from stress and adversity

Cognitive and Social Functions

The cognitive and social functions of humor provide important adaptive roles. While emotions like fear and anger help people focus attention, mobilize energy, and take action, emotions like joy and mirth do not seem to evoke similar actions.

In recent years, researchers have found that laughter brings people closer together. When people experience positive emotions (Martin, 2007):

- They are more cognitively flexible and creative than normally.
- They are capable of more effective thinking, planning, and judgment.
- They have higher levels of social responsibility and prosocial behaviors (such as helpfulness and generosity).
- They are able to build more solid social relationships.

Humor and laughter also affect how people perceive and respond to change and may influence the mind by enhancing the ability to learn. For example, healthcare professionals spend a great deal of time educating clients about drugs, diet, lifestyle change, and treatment benefits. By using humorous communication methods to deliver the information, healthcare professionals may find that they are better able to capture the attention of learners, enhance their retention of the material, and help release tension that blocks learning (Wooten, 2005).

Social Communication

A form of social communication, humor conveys implicit messages indirectly. It is useful when situations are serious and when direct confrontation may be potentially embarrassing or risky. It can smooth over conflicts and tensions between people and allow individuals to save face or to test the waters to see how others will respond. This form of humor most commonly occurs between two people.

The social functions of humor can also be aggressive, coercive, and manipulative. These functions often involve more than two people (the speaker, the listener, and the target of the humor). Since most people do not like to be at the receiving end of aggressive humor, it can serve to force them to conform to the desired behaviors.

Humor can serve to exclude individuals from groups as well as to reinforce power and status differences (Martin, 2007).

Relief from Stress and Adversity

Humor can provide relief from life's stress and adversity (Martin, 2007). It can diffuse anger and anxiety, relieve depression, and act as a buffer to decrease the impact of stressful experiences (Seaward, 2006). When stress or anxiety is too high, humor may fall flat or be inappropriate. However, it can also become a healthy escape from reality and can ease the way to facing the seriousness and threats of illness or tragedy (Robinson, 1991).

Healthcare professionals work in chaotic and stressful environments. Humor and laughter are excellent tools for helping them cope with clients and staff situations. These tools can prevent caregiver burnout, reduce social conflicts, and help healthcare professionals survive the constantly changing healthcare environment (Blumenfeld & Alpern, 1994; Wooten, 2005). For healthcare professionals, humor is a major relief mechanism, it reduces anger, and it is a healthy outlet for anger and frustration resulting from the heaviness of crises, tragedy, and death. Finally, it provides a wonderful tool to use when working with clients. When staff can laugh and joke with clients, *in the right time, the right place, and the right amount* (just like a judicious dose of medicine), the clients often interpret the humor as "caring" (Adams et al., 2006).

Sometimes caregivers experience *compassion fatigue*—a sense that they have very little to give—because they are sensitive, caring individuals who work with people who are suffering. Humor is an excellent tool to prevent compassion fatigue. As noted in Adams et al. (2006), "Humor is a perceptible quality that enables us to experience joy even when faced with adversity" (p. 367).

By allowing individuals to laugh at the fundamental absurdities of life, humor lets them refuse to be overcome by people and situations, both large and small, that threaten their well-being. Humor therefore contributes to both physical and mental health (Martin, 2007). When people focus on what makes them happier, they experience more happiness (Shimoff, 2008).

Physiological Responses to Laughter

Can laughter actually help people heal? Can the benefits of humor protect people from or prevent disease? Research seems to say yes. In his book *Love, Medicine, and Miracles*, noted medical author Bernie Siegel, MD, discusses the concept that thoughts are chemicals that are released into the body and can either kill or cure. The brain quickly transforms thoughts and perceptions into chemical reactions that affect the entire body. Negative thoughts trigger the release of stress hormones and suppress the immune system. Positive thoughts induce the release of special neuropeptides (such as endorphins, interleukins, and interferons) from the pituitary gland and other tissues and strengthen the immune system.

Laughter is actually good for health. Like a form of internal jogging, laughter exercises the body and stimulates the release of beneficial brain neurotransmitters and hormones. Peptides are found throughout the body, including the brain and immune system. The brain also contains more than 60 different neuropeptides; they are formed from amino acids and they carry messages to the brain and body. Emotions trigger the brain to release neuropeptides, which enter the bloodstream, plug into receptor sites on the surfaces of immune cells, and alter (either positively or negatively) the cells' metabolic activity. Viruses use the same receptor sites. The amount of natural peptide available for that receptor determines whether the virus has an easier or harder time getting into the cell, so a person's emotional state affects whether he or she will get sick from the same loading dose of a virus (Wooten, 2005). It is interesting to note that although children laugh about 400 times a day, adults laugh only about 15 times per day—the same number of times they get angry (Seaward, 2006).

The ability to laugh does not belong solely to human beings. Many primates (such as chimpanzees, bonobos, orangutans, and gorillas) have been observed laughing, and some evidence suggests that they even have the capacity for a sense of humor. Laughter in primates appears to have originated in social play and to be derived from play signals (Martin, 2007).

Although humor is a perceptual process, laughter is a behavioral response (Wooten, 2005). Martin (2007) describes the physiological process of laughter as follows:

> . . . boisterous laughter comprises a very strange set of behaviors. A hypothetical alien from outer space would certainly be struck by the oddity of this behavior, noting the loud, barking noises that are emitted, the repetitive contractions of the diaphragm and associated changes in respiration, the open mouth and grimaces caused by contractions of facial muscles, the flushing of the skin, increased heart rate and general physiological arousal, production of tears in the eyes, loss of strength in the extremities, and flailing body movements. (p. 154)

Laughter's Effects on the Body

Laughter creates predictable, physiologic changes in the body that occur in two stages (Wooten, 2005): the arousal stage, in which physiologic parameters increase, and the resolution stage, in which physiologic parameters return to resting values or lower.

During laughter, many muscle groups become active, including:

- The diaphragm
- The abdominal, intercostal, respiratory accessory, and facial muscles
- Sometimes muscles in the arms, legs, and back

During vigorous, sustained laughter, the heart rate is stimulated, normal respiratory patterns become chaotic, respiratory rate and depth are increased, and residual volume is decreased. Conditions such as asthma or bronchitis may actually be aggravated by vigorous laughter (Wooten, 2005).

A lot has been written about using humor as a therapeutic tool, but humor physiology is a relatively young science (Kruse & Prazak, 2006). Current research in the areas of psychology, physiology, and psychoneuroimmunology is defining the specific changes produced by mirthful laughter, which has been shown to have clear short- and long-term effects on the body (Adams et al., 2006; Berk, 2004; Huelat, 2003; Kruse & Prazak, 2006; Mallett, 1996; Shimoff, 2008; Wooten, 2005). Mirthful laughter:

- Increases the number and activity of natural killer cells, which attack viral infected cells and some types of cancer cells
- Increases the secretion of catecholamine endorphins
- Decreases cortisol secretion
- Facilitates digestion
- Lowers the sedimentation rate
- Increases the levels of complement 3, which helps antibodies pierce infected cells
- Increases tolerance to pain and reduces the amount of pain medication used
- Increases the number of activated T cells (these cells are considered to be turned on and ready to fight infections)
- Increases oxygenation of the blood
- Improves mood, lifts spirits, and helps people feel peaceful and satisfied with life
- Increases the level of the antibody IgA, which fights upper respiratory tract infections
- Increases the levels of gamma interferon (a lymphokine that activates many immune components)
- Exercises the diaphragm and cardiovascular system (initially raising heart rate and blood pressure but after a short time causing a longer lasting decrease in heart rate and blood pressure as the relaxation response takes over)
- Stabilizes blood sugar, massages vital organs, and contributes to homeostasis.

Mirthful laughter consists of four individual notes or calls. The frequency (pitch) of male laughter is lower than that of female laughter. "Ha-ha" laughs are more common than "ho-ho" and "he-he" laughs. Laughter is also characterized by a distinctive facial display (called the Duchenne display, after the French anatomist who first identified it in 1862) that closely resembles smiling. The display involves symmetrical, synchronous, and smooth contractions of the mouth and eyes, resulting in wrinkling of the outside of the eyes and crow's feet (Martin, 2007).

Laughter produces tears that are believed to rid the body of stress-related toxins, suggesting that physical expressions such as laughter and crying are natural and healthy (Seaward, 2006). Laughter has been shown to aid in recovery from surgery, help cure depression, release tension and restore equilibrium, help digestion, and stimulate internal organs (Mallett, 1996). While there is no research that conclusively shows a release of endorphins with mirthful laughter, the anecdotal literature about laughter's ability to reduce pain is enormous (Adams et al., 2006). Norman Cousins (1979) discusses this effect at length in his book.

Pathological Laughter

Pathological laughter can be categorized in three ways (Martin, 2007): excessive laughter, forced laughter, and gelastic epilepsy.

- *Excessive laughter* involves emotional lability, euphoria, the inability to inhibit laughter, and a lack of insight into the abnormality of laughter. It is associated with schizophrenia, mania, and dementia, which are affected by the parts of the brain involving emotion (the limbic system and frontal lobes).
- *Forced laughter* occurs in individuals who experience involuntary outbursts of explosive, self-sustained laughter, accompanied by the autonomic disturbances in heart rate, vasomotor control, and sphincter tone. While they may appear mirthful, people experience forced laughter as unpleasant and embarrassing. These individuals also often experience uncontrollable crying. Forced laughter is associated with Parkinson's disease, multiple sclerosis, and amyotrophic lateral sclerosis, as well as various brain tumors or lesions.
- *Gelastic epilepsy* is a relatively rare condition in which seizures predominantly take the form of bouts of laughter, possibly accompanied by motor convulsions, autonomic disturbances, and abnormal eye movements. This condition usually begins in childhood.

Humor and Stress

The harmful effects of stress on an individual's health are well known. Diseases such as hypertension, insomnia, ulcerative colitis, and coronary disease are, in part, the result of prolonged stress (Wooten, 2005). Stress and negative emotions have been associated with immunosuppression and partially altered by increased epinephrine and cortisol blood levels.

One way to reduce the effects of stress is to play. When children play, they use their imaginations to invent a new reality that meets their needs. As people grow older, they tend to lose their ability to be spontaneous and open to moments of playfulness. Yet research on animals has shown that play is crucial in brain development. Play occurs when the brain is rapidly forming its synaptic connections. These connections create a dense array of neural connections that pass electrochemical messages from one part of the brain to the next. Proper motor development is one result of intense sensory and physical stimulation. Play also provides a place for humans to socialize, mimic cultural rituals, build trust, and create connections with each other. Creative people are playful, experimental, willing to take risks, and more adaptable. In serious situations, such as those involving illness or disease, the ability to adapt can mean the difference between life and death (Wooten, 2005).

Humor helps people adapt to the stresses in their lives. Stress does not result from a specific event; rather, a person's perception of the event causes stress. A sense of humor helps people view their circumstances or events in a less stressful way. Hardiness can increase a person's resilience to stress and is affected by a commitment to oneself, by the belief that one is in control of one's life, and by a view of change as challenging rather than threatening (Wooten, 2005).

The pleasant feelings associated with mirthful laughter may modify some of the neuroendocrine components of the stress response. Humor can stimulate the immune system, enhance perceptual flexibility, and renew spiritual energy (Wooten, 2005). Research supports the theory that people experience a general decrease in the stress hormones that constrict blood vessels and suppress immune activity after being exposed to humor (Berk, 2004).

HUMOR IN HEALTH CARE

For years, human experience has shown that laughter is good for people. The 18th-century French writer and philosopher Voltaire is credited with saying, "The art of medicine consists of amusing the patient while nature cures the disease" (Berk, 2004, p. 46), and there are many such comments on humor and laughter from philosophy, religion, and the arts. Even a literary mainstay like *Reader's Digest* has a section called "Laughter, the Best Medicine." Recent studies demonstrate the effects of humor and laughter on health as well as on the psyche. This was not always the case; much of the history of laughter used as therapy is only being made now (Adams et al., 2006).

One explanation for the growth of humor in healthcare settings has to do with the current evolution in health care and the increased focus on holistic care, integrative practices, and complementary and alternative practices. Humor has long been used in health care to establish and maintain collegial relationships and to improve team productivity and group solidarity. This section addresses how humor can also be used to support client care.

Therapeutic Humor

What is humor therapy? Adams et al. (2006) define it as "whatever one does to put mirth into a patient encounter or hospital setting" (p. 358). Others have described it as the intentional and spontaneous use of humor techniques by healthcare professionals that can lead to enhanced self-understanding by clients (Martin, 2007). According to Wooten (2005), therapeutic humor can improve client smiles and increase client laughter by incorporating humor and laughter into the clinical setting.

Therapeutic humor can be used in group or individual counseling sessions, and clients can be provided with many opportunities to laugh. Humor carts, lively rooms with humorous items, and humorous individuals (such as clowns and staff who use their sense of humor) are examples. Therapeutic humor can be used to reduce stress, boost immunity, relieve pain, decrease anxiety, stabilize mood, rest the brain, enhance communication, inspire creativity, maintain hope, and bolster morale (Huelat, 2003; Wooten, 2005).

Since humor is a uniquely personal experience (Kruse & Prazak, 2006), individual preferences must be considered when using humor as a therapeutic tool. Exposure to material that an individual does not find funny can have deleterious effects, especially in psychotherapy. Studies have demonstrated that insensitive joking by healthcare professionals can be offensive and distressing. Clients with life-threatening illness can show many responses to humor; therefore, humor should be used carefully with them (Adams et al., 2006; Penson et al., 2005).

Choosing and Using Therapeutic Humor

Humor as a deliberate therapeutic tool should be carefully understood, considered, and administered. Before introducing an intervention, healthcare professionals should assess the client carefully to ensure that the humor is appropriate. When using humor to help a client or family member who is dealing with death, for example, healthcare providers need to wait until after the shock of the death subsides. They may have to put the humor on hold until the individual understands, in some small way, that eventually everything will be all right. However, laughter in the face of death allows people to poke fun at death and helps them feel empowered and defiant, gain perspective, and affirm life (Klein, 1998).

The types of laughter vary with age, gender, and culture. For example, young people think laughter should be strong, active, uninhibited, and loud (Kruse & Prazak, 2006). Older adults are less tolerant of sarcasm, tend to be more concerned with social appropriateness, and feel more comfortable with a relatively gentle, less active laughter (Robinson, 1991). Females laugh and smile more than males (Mallett, 1996). Eskimos reportedly use humor to resolve quarrels by insulting their opponent—whoever wins the most laughter during the insults wins the argument. Navajos have a keen sense of humor with a whimsical quality that is seldom cruel. Clowns are an important part of the Navajo culture and religious rituals; religion and illness are closely related, and medicine or treatment can be administered by clowns who are impersonating the gods (Robinson, 1991).

In addition, healthy individuals use humor differently from those with medical conditions. Kruse and Prazak (2006) add that, "People who recognize humor more readily in their surroundings have a different perspective and take themselves and others less seriously, resulting in more positive attitudes and less fear abut physical health and illness" (p. 192). An example of this is the joke, "What's the benefit of Alzheimer's? You get to make new friends every day!"

Although humor can help, it can also hurt. Humor can separate people as easily as it can bond them. It can cut off communication as easily as it can enhance it. Laughing at someone else's expense is never helpful, and it creates animosity and stress. Blumenfeld and Alpern (1994) note that this type of humor includes humor that:

- Pokes fun at other people's shortcomings
- Reflects anger
- Divides a group by using put-downs
- Gives license to hurt someone
- Uses stereotypes to denigrate a person or group
- Creates a cruel, abusive, or offensive atmosphere
- Offends with the inappropriate use of profanity or sexual references
- Is insensitive to what causes others pain

As times change, so does the concept of what is considered humorous or socially acceptable. If someone directs stress-producing humor toward you, you can deal with it in various ways. You can decide not to laugh, or you can say "I don't think that's funny." Or, if you want to allow the offender to save face, you can say something like, "I'm sure you're not aware of how cruel that joke makes you sound, but many people find that humor offensive and I would appreciate your not repeating it." These conversations can be held publicly or privately (Blumenfeld & Alpern, 1994).

Humor can also be used too much or as a cover-up for dealing with important issues. One of the characters in the movie *One Flew Over the Cuckoo's Nest* says, "Man, when you lose your laugh, you lose your footing." While that is true, humor needs to be used for balance.

Mallett (1996) identified three criteria that can be used to determine whether humor will be helpful to a client:

- *Timing:* For example, not using humor at the height of a crisis
- *Receptiveness:* What might be funny at one time to a client might not be funny at another time
- *Content:* Adults and children, for example, have different opinions about what is funny

Adams et al. (2006) suggest that a practitioner applying humor in a healthcare setting must do so with kindness, compassion, and empathy. The humor should take the form of a smile, eye twinkle, and only rarely, jokes. Further, Adams believes that a relationship, rapport between practitioner and client, setting, and timing are necessary elements to the successful communication of humor in a healthcare setting.

Wooten (2005) offers these suggestions for the use of humor in healthcare settings:

- Offer a brief explanation of the health benefits of humor so clients do not think you are unprofessional.
- Establish your competence first, and then let your sense of humor emerge.
- Shared humor never replaces concern, care, and respect.
- If a client's humor is offensive, be honest and say that you do not enjoy that type of humor.
- Be sensitive to whether clients are responding positively or negatively to humor, and don't force your humor on them if they are not receptive.
- Humor is like medication. You need to administer the right type, in the right amount, at the right time to achieve the greatest therapeutic benefit. Just as some clients are allergic to certain medications, it is helpful to be aware of potential "humor allergies."
- Clients may not be receptive to humor until they have come to terms with the realities of their illness or disease, and some just don't feel like laughing. Others may have religious convictions that stress reverence for the seriously ill.
- Humor is not appropriate when the client needs time to cry, rest, be quiet, contemplate, or pray. Humor is not appropriate when clients are trying to communicate something important to you, when they are coming to terms with an emotional crisis, or when the person in the next bed is very sick or dying.

Humor Therapy Examples

One form of therapy practiced by Patch Adams (Adams et al., 2006) is called "laughing spirit listening circles." Groups of 6–10 individuals get equal time receiving absolute, positive, silent attention, first for 3 minutes, and then for 5 minutes. The individuals are told to "dare to be boring." They do not have to speak, but if they choose to do so, they have to tell the truth without trying to be funny and to stay connected with each other. The goal is to receive support rather than give it. Usually, the first time around the circle is serious or grave, but as the relationships between individuals build and integrity and safety are established, the laughter and tears abound.

The Big Apple Circus Clown Care Unit (CCU) is a community outreach program of the Big Apple Circus. This not-for-profit performing arts organization uses classic circus arts to help in the care and healing of hospitalized pediatric clients, their parents, and caregivers. Created in 1986 by Michael Christensen, director of clowning, in cooperation with the medical staff at Babies and Children's Hospital of New York at Columbia-Presbyterian Medical Center, the program has received numerous awards, including the Red Skelton Award and the Northeast Clown Convention's annual Gold Nose Award. The hospital room becomes the circus ring, the physician is the ringmaster, and all the "rules, charts, formulas, procedures, machines, and straight-laced, white-washed corridors of the hospital become the source of endless parody" (Adams et al., 2006, p. 359). Specially trained doctors of delight, as they are called, bring joy and excitement to the hospitalized children. Clients are often anxious, frightened, and alone much of their time in the hospital. Humor opportunities are a wonderful way to provide them with a spirit boost and an opportunity to laugh away their concerns—even if only for a moment.

Another example of humor used in healthcare settings is the Duke Humor Project at Duke University Medical Center in Durham, North Carolina, where oncology clients come for various cancer treatments and often cannot leave their rooms. The Laugh Mobile brings humorous media to their bedsides and initiates a humor intervention: "a plan to promote joy and laughter in the treatment program for patient care" (Adams et al., 2006, p. 365). Yo-yo demonstrations, guitar playing, and practical jokes (such as whoopee cushions or water guns) may be used. Staff members are involved in the project and provide information about which clients might be the most receptive to humor.

Comic relief is currently used in many rehabilitation programs that treat alcoholism and drug addiction.

Senses of Humor

Just as there are several types of humor, there are also several senses of humor. The sense of humor developed by individuals usually results from exposure to their family's culture, traditions, religious background, and environment. One sense of humor tends to be dominant, but a person can have the makings for all types. Consequently, it is challenging to advise individuals on how to best develop their senses of humor.

Seaward (2006) identifies four senses of humor:

1. *Conventional sense of humor:* Two or more people find a common ground by sharing a similar humorous perspective and laughing at the same thing. The laughing occurs with someone, not at someone.
2. *Life of the party sense of humor:* This style of humor is best exemplified by people who like to wear a lampshade on their heads at a party, always remember punch lines, and can tell any story and make it funny. These people are quick-witted and creative.
3. *Creative sense of humor:* These people often make their living writing jokes. They can find something humorous in almost anything and are easily entertained. They usually prefer to let someone else tell the joke.
4. *Good-sport sense of humor:* This sense of humor is demonstrated by people who can laugh at their own imperfections and mistakes and who can take a practical joke.

Developing a Sense of Humor and Initiating Humor Therapy

Despite much discussion about what constitutes humor, how does one go about cultivating a sense of humor so that it can be incorporated into healing and helping the therapeutic process? You can take steps to cultivate a sense of humor.

- *Understand the concepts of humor, its nature, theories, functions, and purposes.* Understanding allows you to review your attitudes toward humor, accept its value, and acknowledge its attributes. Once you gain this understanding, the next step is to change your own behavior by developing your own sense of humor, recognizing its therapeutic value for yourself and your clients, and then applying it to your life and work (Robinson, 1991). Start by not taking life too seriously. See yourself as more than your work. People who laugh at themselves and their mistakes are more emotionally healthy than those who become distressed at the slightest hint of imperfection (Seaward, 2006).

- *Develop your own style.* Look for the ludicrous. Find one humorous thing a day to laugh about. Take time to read the cartoons in newspapers. Expose yourself to funny stories and movies. Begin to collect one-liners that make you laugh (Eliopoulos, 2004; Klein, 1998).
- *Develop what is called aikido humor.* This type of humor uses the momentum of the situation to roll with the punches (Eliopoulos, 2004).
- *Give yourself permission to laugh.* Plan to laugh more, be open to all forms of humor, and actively pursue more humor in your life. See what tickles your funny bone. If you can't laugh, try smiling.
- *Keep a humor journal.* Use a notebook, a scrapbook, a file, index cards, or a drawer with funny items that appeal to your sense of humor (Blumenfeld & Alpern, 1994). Watch for funny bumper stickers, odd newspaper headlines, humorous billboards, signs, puns, and oxymorons. When you hear something funny, write it down. Once you put your energy in this direction, you will be surprised at the wealth of humorous experiences and examples you see every day.

Developing your comic vision and sense of humor can be fun. Try the following (Eliopoulos, 2004; Robinson, 1991):

- Laugh at yourself, and give yourself permission to be human and make mistakes. None of us is perfect, and when we laugh and gently poke fun at ourselves, we lighten up and learn to be less serious.
- Visit a comedy club or listen to humorous CDs on the way to work.
- Pay attention to your own self-talk and replace your negative thoughts with positive ones.
- Collect funny material from comedy writers and comedians.
- Tell secondhand jokes or stories.
- Focus on being with funny people and on being someone others like to be with because you are pleasant.
- Read more books (fiction and nonfiction) and watch less television.
- Write a story, fable, or poem every now and then to improve your imagination and creativity.
- Share your vision to make others laugh. Laughter is contagious and is needed in all lives. Humor shared is humor doubled.
- Learn to hyperexaggerate when describing a situation or story.
- Develop a humor kit or tickler notebook with funny notes, letters, and love poems so you have a humor capsule of things that make you laugh or smile.
- Plan to play. A part of the richness of life, play enables people to live and grow. Infants and children play to learn. Many animals play at least some time in their lives. As adults, we play to relax, to interact with others, to

gain a perspective on our lives, and to grow. When we truly play, we seek to impress no one, and we produce no product. We just enjoy being in the moment, being spontaneous, and laughing. Have fun with toys.

How can you increase your creativity and play time? Put leisure activities on your calendar. Spend time doing nothing but looking at the sky, playing a game, or taking time to just be. Go to a museum or a concert. Wear a wild hat or shirt. Draw, paint, or make something out of clay. Wander through a beautiful store. Play miniature golf, go bowling, dance, take a new class at your local community college, or find a new recipe and try it. Start a joy box, filled with cards, notes, and things that bring a smile to your face. Open it, and go through the items when your spirit needs a lift (Eliopoulos, 2004).

Healthcare staff can develop many of the same options to help them laugh at work. In addition, they can offer clients humor opportunities in various formats (audio, video, reading, visual, and tactile). These formats can involve:

- Discussing new research showing that humor and positive emotions facilitate recovery and enhance immune system function
- Telling jokes (as long as the material is tasteful and appropriate for the client's age, gender, and culture, and you avoid sexual, religious, or ethnic jokes)
- Sharing cartoons and creating a scrapbook
- Creating a bulletin board and posting cartoons, bumper stickers, and funny signs
- Developing a file of funny jokes, stories, cards, bumper stickers, poems, and songs
- Wearing a funny button, nose, or hat
- Creating a humor journal or log to record funny encounters or humorous discoveries
- Collecting funny books, videotapes, and audiotapes of comedy routines and creating a lending library
- Creating a well-stocked costume and prop room
- Providing space for performing artists
- Offering humor classes
- Forming an interdisciplinary humor committee of interested people who appreciate and use humor

Healthcare providers can also subscribe to a humorous newsletter or journal to collect new ideas and inspiration. They can educate themselves about therapeutic humor by attending conferences, workshops, and conventions. They can also commit to using themselves as tools. Communication studies have shown that people remember 7% of what is said, 38% of how it is said, and 55% of nonverbal signals sent when someone is saying something. Because clients remember less than 10% of your words, you need to choose them carefully. Think about how you say something. Try to change the tone and pace of your voice, and watch your facial expressions, physical gestures, costuming, and props if you are trying to use humor (Wooten, 2005).

A humor kit or basket (a small collection of funny toys, gadgets, or props) or a comedy cart (a mobile unit with comedic supplies) is one way to introduce humor into healthcare environments. Some call their carts by clever names such as Laughmobile, Jokes on Spokes, Humor on a Roll, or Humor à la Cart. The kit or cart can include (Huelat, 2003):

- Joke books
- Soft modeling clay
- Games
- Puzzles
- Whimsical hats
- Clown noses and other wild noses
- Children's games, such as wooden paddle and ball, pickup sticks, coloring books and crayons, and finger paints
- A lapel button with funny one-liners
- A magic wand
- Funny stickers
- Bubble gum for a brief bubble-blowing contest for staff stress relief
- Bubbles (small bottles, bubble bottles in necklaces, or wands that make giant bubbles to make others laugh and appreciate the small wonders in life)
- Funny movies, books, and audiotapes in all the waiting rooms
- Cartoons and funny pictures in high-stress areas like radiology and mammography dressing rooms, exam room ceilings, and diagnostic rooms

The Future of Humor Therapy

Some hospitals have developed humor therapy rooms that provide humorous books, records, movies, games, song fests, and entertainment for clients and families. The staffs at these hospitals believe that humor is a great adjunct therapy to other forms of medical treatment and can be as effective as a pill in treating pain and anxiety during periods of crisis. Prototypes have included the Living Room at the William Stehlin Foundation for Cancer Research and St. Joseph's Hospital in Houston, Texas, and the Lively Room at DeKalb General Hospital in Atlanta, Georgia (Blumenfeld & Alpern, 1994).

Hospitals that deal with long-term care clients have found that equipment such as wheelchairs and intravenous (IV) poles can be decorated to cheer clients. Ideas include reflector lights, tourist tags of places visited, slogans, college pennants, and sports team insignias.

The Association of Therapeutic Humor is creating a practice to introduce humor as therapy. Patch Adams and his Gesundheit Institute are planning to build a teaching center and clinic on their land in West Virginia—the country's first hospital to incorporate humor in all aspects of care. According to Dr. Adams:

> Science and art play different roles in the healing interaction. Medical science works at tackling the disease . . . the "art of medicine" is concerned with how disease affects the patient, the family, and their society . . . the art of medicine comes from the intuition and inherent magic found in compassion, love, humor, wonder, and curiosity. (Adams et al., 2006, p. 357)

KEY CONCEPTS

1. Humor is a complex phenomenon and an essential part of human nature. Anthropologists have never found a culture or society, at any time in human history, that did not have humor.
2. There are numerous types of humor, and they are not mutually exclusive. Some reduce stress while others actually increase stress.
3. Developing a sense of humor and an awareness of its uses and effectiveness is an important step in utilizing humor in a therapeutic manner.

QUESTIONS FOR REFLECTION

1. Why do you think humor exists, and how does it effectively manage stress?
2. How does laughter affect people both physiologically and psychologically?
3. In what ways can you introduce humor, play, and laughter into your life or workplace?

REFERENCES

Adams, P. (1998). *Gesundheit!* Rochester, VT: Healing Arts Press.

Adams, P., Fry, W. F., Glickstein, L., Goodheart, A., Hageseth, C., III, Hamilton, R., et al. (2006). Humor. In M. S. Micozzi, *Fundamentals of complementary and integrative medicine* (3rd ed., pp. 351–371). St. Louis, MO: Saunders Elsevier.

Berk, L. S. (2004). Mind, body, spirit: Exploring the mind, body, and spirit connection through research on mirthful laughter. In S. Sorajjakool & H. Lamberton (Eds.), *Spirituality, health, and wholeness: An introductory guide for health care professionals* (pp. 37–48). New York: Haworth Press.

Blumenfeld, E., & Alpern, L. (1994). *Humor at work: The guaranteed, bottom-line, low-cost, high-efficiency guide to success through humor.* Atlanta, GA: Peachtree.

Cousins, N. (1979). *Anatomy of an illness.* New York: Bantam Books.

Eliopoulos, C. (2004). *Invitation to holistic health: A guide to living a balanced life.* Sudbury, MA: Jones and Bartlett.

Huelat, B. J. (2003). *Healing environments: Design for the body, mind, and spirit.* Alexandria, VA: Medezyn.

Klein, A. (1998). *The courage to laugh.* New York: Penguin Putnam.

Kruse, B. G., & Prazak, M. (2006, September). Humor and older adults: What makes them laugh? *Journal of Holistic Nursing, 24*(3), 188–193.

Mallett, J. (1996). Humour and laughter therapy. In D. F. Rankin-Box (Ed.), *The nurses' handbook of complementary therapies* (pp. 109–117). Edinburgh: Churchill Livingstone.

Martin, R.A. (2007). *The psychology of humor: An integrative approach.* Burlington, MA: Elsevier Academic Press.

Penson, R. T., Partridge, R. A., Rudd, P., Seiden, M. V., Nelson, J. E., Chabner, B. A., et al. (2005). Laughter: The best medicine? *Oncologist, 10,* 651–660.

Rankin-Box, D. F. (Ed.). (1996). *The nurses' handbook of complementary therapies.* Edinburgh: Churchill Livingstone.

Robinson, V. M. (1991). *Humor and the health professions: The therapeutic use of humor in health care* (2nd ed.). Thorofare, NJ: Slack.

Seaward, B. L. (2006). *Managing stress: Principles and strategies for health and well-being* (5th ed.). Sudbury, MA: Jones and Bartlett.

Shimoff, M. (2008). *Happy for no reason: Seven steps to being happy from the inside out.* New York: Free Press.

Siegel, B. S. (1986). *Love, medicine, and miracles.* New York: Harper and Row.

Wooten, P. (2005). Humor, laughter, and play: Maintaining balance in a serious world. In B. M. Dossey, L. Keegan, & C. E. Guzzetta, *Holistic nursing: A handbook for practice* (4th ed., pp. 497–520). Sudbury, MA: Jones and Bartlett.

Ziv, A. (1988). *National styles of humor.* Westport, CT: Greenwood.

REFERENCES

CHAPTER 9

Music Therapy and Sound Healing

After silence, that which comes nearest to expressing the inexpressible is music.
—Aldous Huxley

LEARNING OBJECTIVES

1. Discuss the principles of sound.
2. Define *music therapy.*
3. Describe the areas of sound healing.
4. Examine music therapy interventions.
5. Describe examples of the therapeutic uses and benefits of music.
6. Explain music therapy modalities.
7. Describe the physiological and psychological responses to music.
8. Discuss evidence-based practice in music therapy.

INTRODUCTION

Music and sound have been used in healing practices throughout history, and the historical records of different cultures cite many examples of their healing powers (Cantello, 2004; Wigram, Pedersen, & Bonde, 2004). Sound as a healing modality is probably as old as the first sound made by man or woman. Early humans used sounds in sacred and ritualistic ways to promote fertility, accept death, grow crops, and commemorate events (Goldman, 2002). Pythagoras taught his students to change their emotions of worry, fear, sorrow, and anger by singing and playing a musical instrument daily. Other Western philosophers, such as Plato, Aristotle, Augustine, and Nietzsche, considered the practical and theoretical role of music in relation to a person's health. Plato discussed the influence of music on the human mind.

Today more people listen to music than ever before in the history of the world, and there are more avenues for experiencing music than anyone could have predicted years ago (Storr, 1992). Many believe that music has the power to heal the body, mind, and spirit.

In an age when people increasingly turn to holistic methods of healing, music therapy has developed into a powerful and nonthreatening medium that can be used successfully with individuals of all ages and disabilities. For example, music therapy often complements the treatment provided for individuals with neurological conditions, including brain injury, stroke, and Parkinson's and Alzheimer's diseases. Sound healing is used to help people recover from stroke and head injuries, it is effective in controlling nausea and pain (especially for the side effects of chemotherapy), and it is used in operating rooms to help relax clients and often reduce the amount of anesthesia needed.

Sound healing and music therapy have greatly expanded in recent years. They have entered mainstream health care, with Medicare often covering them for clients who have Alzheimer's disease, are recovering from strokes, or are learning to walk again.

HEALING WITH SOUND AND MUSIC

The healing power of music and sound is widely recognized by health professionals. Music therapy and sound healing are used in psychiatric hospitals, rehabilitation facilities, general hospitals, outpatient clinics, daycare treatment centers, residences for people with developmental disabilities, community mental health centers, drug and alcohol programs, senior centers, nursing homes, hospice programs, correctional facilities, halfway houses, schools, and private practice.

Profound scientific, medical, psychological, and spiritual connections are involved in the power of music. Healing with music combines music experiences with the inherent universal forms in music to heal the body, mind, and spirit. Like a tuning fork for the brain, music can stimulate specific regions to soothe emotions, boost the capacity for learning, and unlock creative genius (Borysenko, 2001). Music has been shown to reduce psychophysiological stress, anxiety, and isolation; reduce overt reactions to pain; decrease the amount of pain-relieving medications needed by clients; increase cognitive performance; and reduce the nausea and vomiting associated with chemotherapy. It has been used in neonatal intensive care environments to reduce arousal states, shorten lengths of stay, and increase weight and caloric intake in low-birth-weight infants (Cabrera & Lee, 2000). It has also been suggested that listening to complex music can produce the Mozart effect, which serves as a type of mental exercise; can facilitate the firing patterns of neurons in the cerebral cortex; and can improve concentration, intuition, intelligence, and healing.

Music is a source of energy influencing every cell in the body (Cabrera & Lee, 2000; Campbell, 2006; Keegan, 2005). Opening oneself to the vibrations of musical sound can bring about a transcendent experience. Cantello (2004) notes, "The music we each find deeply appealing is a reflection of the individual person, shaped by culture, experience, and sense of self" (p. 11). Communing with music (an innovative and thorough method that teaches how to enhance one's life with the power of music) takes one on a journey that takes place on many levels. The journey can help awaken an awareness and appreciation of music and sound and enhance well-being (Cantello, 2004).

Music therapy, music psychology, and psychoacoustics (the study of the perception of sound, including how we listen, our psychological responses, and the physiological impact of music and sound on the human nervous system) are being used to integrate positive sound into people's daily lives. Consider the following examples (Campbell, 2006):

- In a coronary care unit in Maryland, listening to half an hour of music produced the same effect in a patient as 10 milligrams of Valium.
- Researchers in Russia and India demonstrated that plants exposed to music produced better yields.
- According to Canadian researchers, wheat seedlings grew up to three times longer when treated with musical tones.
- In French monasteries, monks noted that playing music and chanting to their cows caused the cows to produce more milk.

The Principles of Sound

Understanding the principles of sound is key to appreciating its capacity to produce therapeutic psychophysiologic outcomes. Sound is best understood as being vibration (Goldman, 2002). Everything in the universe is in a state of vibration. Vibration is energy itself, moving through matter (Emoto, 2006). According to Leeds (2001), "sound is vibratory energy" (p. 10).

In addition to understanding vibration, it is important to understand three additional principles of sound: frequency, resonance, and entrainment.

Frequency

Sound is produced when an object vibrates in a random or periodic repeated motion (Guzzetta, 2005). The frequency at which an object vibrates is its resonant frequency. Everything has a resonant frequency, whether we can hear it or not.

The human ear can hear sound when its frequency, or pitch, ranges from 20 to 20,000 hertz (Hz). However, sound is heard not only through the ears but through every cell in the body (Gaynor, 2002). It is perceived through skin and bone conduction as well as through the other senses, such as sight, smell, and touch, and it allows us to perceive an even wider range of vibrations than by hearing alone (Guzzetta, 2005).

Resonance

The healing properties of sound and the vibration of homeostasis are identical to the vibration known as the *Schumann resonance*—a mathematical number of oscillations calculated at 7.8 Hz. This frequency is the same frequency detected in many sounds of nature, such as whale or dolphin songs and waterfalls.

Entrainment

The study of patterns of shapes evoked by sound is called cymatics. Matter assumes certain shapes or patterns based on the vibrations, or frequency, of the sound to which it is exposed. For example, a snowflake may take on its shape because it responds to sounds in nature. The human body is a system of vibrating atomic particles acting as a vibratory transformer that gives off and takes in sound from the environment. Music can act as an environmental pacemaker by speeding up or slowing down heart rate, brainwaves, and respiration. The result is a gradual entrainment (or synchronization) of the body's vibrations with those of the music, along with a change in an individual's psychophysiologic state (Guzzetta, 2005).

Coined by Christian Huygens, the term *entrainment* refers to the phenomenon that occurs when two elements become synchronized and vibrate at the same sound frequency. In physics, this phenomenon is referred to as the law of conservation of energy. Seaward (2006) defines entrainment as the mutual phase-locking oscillations of like frequencies in the same environment. In other words, the more powerful rhythmic vibration of one object changes the less powerful rhythmic vibration of another object to synchronize its rhythm with the first object. An example in nature is the synchronous menstrual cycles of women who live or work together. Another example is the ancient shamans' use of the drumbeat to evoke entraining vibrations for healing interventions (Seaward, 2005).

When used as a relaxation therapy, music can have a rhythm that duplicates the normal pulse beat of humans, is nonsyncopated, is lyric free, and can be used to harmonize with or bring the body's own rhythms back into sync. Entrainment with relaxing music decreases pulse rate, respiratory rate, metabolic rate, oxygen consumption, and blood pressure. Entrainment has been shown to be effective in critical care and in neonatal intensive care. The most effective method for pain reduction is entrainment music, which moves a person toward a positive or pleasant mood state (Freeman, 2004). Goldman (2002) notes that "the principles of using resonance and entrainment are the fundamental concepts behind the use of sound to heal and transform. They are found in every practice that uses sound, regardless of the tradition, belief system, or culture" (p. 15).

Music Therapy Defined

An allied health service similar to occupational therapy and physical therapy, music therapy utilizes music therapeutically to address physical, psychological, cognitive, and/or social functioning. It is recognized as a viable treatment modality by the Health Care Financing Administration (HCFA), The Joint Commission, the Commission on Accreditation of Rehabilitation Facilities (CARF), and the National Rehabilitation Caucus (NRC). In 1998, the American Association for Music Therapy (founded in 1971) and the National Association for Music Therapy (founded in 1950) merged to form the American Music Therapy Association (AMTA). The AMTA establishes criteria for the education and clinical training of music therapists.

As a profession, music therapy has emerged over the last few decades from different disciplines in different countries. Arising from psychology, special education, music education, music psychology, anthropology, and medicine, music therapy encompasses such a broad scope that defining it is no simple task. Its definition, depending on the orientation and perspective of a particular group of practitioners or different cultures, may include such paradoxical descriptors as (Wigram et al., 2004):

- Artistic versus scientific
- Musical versus psychological
- Behavioral versus psychotherapeutic
- Complementary versus alternative
- Rehabilitative versus acute

To establish an all-embracing description of music therapy, the World Federation of Music Therapy (1996) provided the following definition:

> Music therapy is the use of music and/or musical elements (sound, rhythm, melody and harmony) by a qualified music therapist with a client or group, in a process designed to facilitate and promote communication, relationships, learning, mobilisation [sic], expression, organisation [sic] and other relevant therapeutic objectives, in order to meet physical, emotional, mental, social and cognitive needs. Music therapy aims to develop potentials and/or restore functions of

> the individual so that he or she can achieve better intra- and interpersonal integration and, consequently, a better quality life through prevention, rehabilitation or treatment.

According to Guzzetta (2005), music therapy is "the behavioral science concerned with the systematic application of music to produce relaxation and desired changes in emotions, behavior, and physiology" (p. 617). AMTA (2004) defines it as:

> . . . an established healthcare profession that uses music to address physical, emotional, cognitive, and social needs of individuals of all ages. Music therapy improves the quality of life for persons who are well and meets the needs of children and adults with disabilities or illnesses.

AMTA (2004) adds that music therapy interventions can be designed to promote wellness, manage stress, alleviate pain, express feelings, enhance memory, improve communication, and promote physical rehabilitation. In addition, music therapy complements traditional therapy, encourages active participation in one's own health care, and provides individuals with an integrated mind-body-spirit experience.

The Elements of Music

Leddy (2006) notes that "music therapy is based on the physics and physiology of sound" (p. 17). It is important for music therapists to know about the elements of music and its effects on both physiological functions and psychological conditions (Campbell, 1995). The principal musical elements are (Campbell, 1995):

- *Tone:* The initial sound is the tone or utterance of the sound. Every note is produced by a specific rate of vibration and produces both physical and psychological effects that cannot be expressed in words.
- *Rhythm:* Called the heart of music, rhythm structures tone and sound, giving it definition, pattern, and boundary. Rhythm includes elements such as tempo (speed) and meter (the grouping of beats). This fundamental element directly affects both the body and the emotions.
- *Harmony*: Harmony, the relationship between tones and their rhythmic pattern, is produced by the simultaneous sounding of tones that blend with each other to form chords.
- *Melody:* Melodies are produced by the combination of rhythms, tones, and accented notes or passages.

- *Timbre:* Musical instruments and the human voice give sound a certain quality that is difficult to define in words but evokes emotional responses.

Sound Healing Defined

Sound healing, a form of music therapy in which music plays an important role, is defined as the use of vibrational frequencies of sound forms, combined with music or its elements (such as rhythm, melody, and harmony), to promote healing. According to Crowe and Scovel (1996), music therapy and sound healing are two ends of a continuum spanning all forms of healing with sound and music. Whereas music therapy uses a more psychological approach, sound healing uses a neurological approach, based on the effects of sound waves on the nervous system (Leeds, 2001). The effectiveness of healing sounds is based on the ability of harmonics to create vibrational changes that may occur in the physical body or in the mental, emotional, and etheric bodies. When these changes occur, healing is initiated (Goldman, 2002).

The Six Areas of Sound Healing

Sound healing is divided into six areas (Crowe & Scovel, 1996):

- *Self-generated sound*, such as toning and overtone chants
- *Projection of sounds in the body* through such methods as cymatic therapy (a form of sound therapy that is not applied through hearing but by means of instruments that send audible sound waves directly into the body through the skin), radionics (the transmission of subtle energy fields for healing purposes), and tuning forks
- *Sounding the body*, such as the projection of overtones (the manipulation of harmonic resonances created as air travels from the singer's lungs, past the vocal folds, and out the lips to produce a melody) and low-frequency sounds
- *Listening technologies* for the improvement of hearing and sound perception
- *Healing compositions*, such as healing songs; instrumental pieces and special ethnic music; specially composed healing music; and music produced by tuning forks, drumming, singing bowls, and gongs
- *Sound environments*, such as a somatron (a device that produces a vibrotactile effect when connected to a sound source)

Sound Healing Modalities

Singing bowls, chanting, harmonics, toning, drumming, and vibrational healing through the chakras are all examples of sound healing modalities.

Singing Bowls

These ancient instruments are often used in combination with meditation, Gregorian chant, and overtone chanting (Crowe & Scovel, 1996). A type of bell that rests on its bottom side, a singing bowl is played by rubbing a mallet around its rim to produce a continuous sound. Dr. Mitchell Gaynor (2002) explained in his book, *The Healing Power of Sound,* that singing bowls became a door through which he entered into the healing effects of sound and music. He also uses chanting, listening to music, playing bells, hand cymbals, wind gongs, drums, whistles, and toning, among other modalities.

Chanting

Chanting can synchronize brain waves to achieve states of relaxation, produce the physiologic effects of an internal painkiller, and act as a healing agent in the body. Gaynor (2002) uses bija mantras, the seven single-syllable Sanskrit words that correspond to the seven chakras or energy centers of the body. The Sufis assign the following words to the corresponding energy centers (Gaynor, 2002):

- Lam—Root chakra
- Vam—Belly
- Ram—Solar plexus
- Yam—Heart
- Ham—Throat
- Om—Between the eyebrows
- All sound—Crown (encompasses all the sound frequencies in nature)

Mantras such as these are fundamental sounds that help to focus and calm the mind, are easy to pronounce and remember, and serve as an excellent introduction to the process of chanting in tune with singing bowls.

Chanting is practiced by many cultures, religious organizations, and ethnic groups. There are Native American chants, Gregorian chants, Vedic chants, and Tibetan overtone chants, among others.

Gregorian chanting, complete with audible overtones, has echoed for many centuries throughout cathedrals. Originally sung in unison, with all the monks singing the same musical line and using elongated vowel sounds, it was called plainsong (Goldman, 2002). Campbell (1995) notes that "Gregorian chant contains all of the frequencies of the voice spectrum, roughly from 70 cycles per second up to 9,000 cycles per second, but with a different envelope curve from that of normal speech" (p. 19). In Gregorian chant there is no tempo, only the rhythm of the human breath. The slow breathing is a sort of respiratory yoga, giving the impression that the person never breathes. The resulting state of tranquility leads to an awakening of the field of consciousness (Campbell, 1995).

Tibetan overtone chanting is a low-frequency guttural chant that involves clear overtones that soar above their fundamental chanted tones. In this type of chanting, called one-voice chording, a single monk can sing a three-note chord simultaneously, making an ancient sound that can seem haunting and bewildering to some people. The sound is created by a deep chanted bass note that serves as the fundamental on which a note two octaves higher and a note a fifth above that are produced simultaneously (Campbell, 1995).

Harmonics

Harmony gives the melody color, direction, and context. It is the result produced when tones are sounded simultaneously. When a string is plucked, a single note sounds, but other notes, called harmonics or overtones, also sound. These harmonics are mathematical ratios of the first note: the first harmonic vibrates twice as fast as the first note, the second harmonic vibrates three times as fast, the third harmonic vibrates four times as fast, and so on (Goldman, 2002).

Toning

Toning uses the conscious sustaining of sounds and tones produced by the voice of the client and/or therapist. Campbell (2007) defines toning as "the elongation of vowels. It can be audible yet quiet, loud and strident, or silent and mental" (p. 27). The technique can involve finding, sustaining, and exploring a specific tone (of a certain frequency and sound quality) by using different vocals, consonants, rhythms, or mouth positions, but without text or melody (Wigram et al., 2004).

Toning can be used to release tension, activate clarity of mind, and increase energy to the body. In about 3 minutes, for example, making the sound of "Ah" can modify brain waves and create balance (Campbell, 2006). Toning can also help a person be more creative, aware, and focused. By prolonging the vowel sounds in a relaxed way, toning guides the person into the balanced, awakened state of focus (Campbell, 2007).

Drumming

Drumming is good for stress reduction, exercise, self-expression, camaraderie and support, spirituality, and meditation (Fein, 2007). Researchers have found that drumming can improve motor coordination in people with Parkinson's disease and bring back long-forgotten memories in Alzheimer's clients (Leeds, 2001).

Vibrational Healing

Music is meant to be heard, but through the technique of water crystal photography, it can also be seen. By listening to a piece of music and simultaneously observing the water crystal created by the vibration of that music, clients can see the vibrational pattern of the music in the crystal and absorb the vibrations into their bodies through their eyes and ears. In one experiment, when crystal patterns were formed in frozen drops of water, the water crystals seemed to respond not only to music but also to emotions, words, and essential oils. When the water was exposed to heavy metal music, explosive patterns without crystal formation were formed. However, when the water was exposed to classical and highly symmetrical music, it formed an exquisite geometrical crystal. Since the human body is comprised mostly of water, music can have a profound effect on our cells (Emoto, 2006).

In additional experiments, Fabien Maman demonstrated that the cells in our bodies respond directly to music, and Joel Sternheimer discovered that elementary particles vibrate in accordance with musical laws. Their combined work indicates that each of the body's tissues, organs, acupuncture meridians, and chakras has a musical note. The goal of vibrational healing is to reach a perfect harmony of all seven chakras (Gardner, 2006).

MUSIC THERAPY GOALS

A referral to music therapy may be recommended for a diverse number of reasons, including managing problems, modifying dysfunctional behaviors, overcoming impairments, and coping with illness. The client's needs may be communicative, cognitive, educational, physical, psychosocial, emotional, musical, vocational, or spiritual, or they may be related to daily living, leisure, or quality of life (Hanser, 1999).

Helping the client grow and change in a positive direction is a key goal. Sample goals for improving the aforementioned conditions may be stated as follows (Hanser, 1999):

- Improve emotional issues, including expressivity, creativity, spontaneity, and mood.
- Improve the quality of life, including well-being, self-actualization, personal growth, and acceptance.

- Improve cognitive issues, including rational thinking; orientation to time, place, or person; attention to the task; and attention to the teacher, therapist, or parent.

Once the referral to music therapy is made, the first session with a client involves building rapport, which is essential for a successful relationship with the therapist, and making a mutually agreeable contract. In subsequent sessions, an assessment is conducted, objectives are set to achieve the goals, behavior is observed, music therapy strategies are formed, and a music therapy treatment plan is designed. During implementation, revisions and adaptations may be made, and progress is recorded. Evaluation of the success of the music therapy program involves a comprehensive analysis, and treatment is ended (Hanser, 1999).

MUSIC THERAPY INTERVENTIONS

A music therapy assessment is imperative in the diagnosis and treatment of physical, psychological, and emotional conditions. Conducting an assessment helps the therapist determine the appropriateness of a specific therapeutic intervention.

Music Therapy with Children

Music is an ideal intervention for challenged children. Improvements can be achieved in the areas of social skills, identity, concentration, sharing, giving and receiving, emotions, and feelings. Music therapy for children has been shown to help with communication and speech problems, autism, attention deficit hyperactivity disorder (ADHD), mental illness, cerebral palsy, and sexual abuse. It has also been shown to enhance personal growth and self-expression. When using music therapy for children, practitioners should ask what type of music the child prefers or would like to hear (Dotton & Mandleco, 2007; Kern, Wakeford, & Aldridge, 2007; Kligler, Newmark, Mehl-Madrona, Islam, & Gerik, 2004; Wigram et al., 2004).

The most frequently served children in the clinical population are those with developmental disabilities, such as mental retardation. The second most frequently served are children with behavioral disorders, such as attention deficit or disruptive behavior disorders (Hanser, 1999). Music therapists also serve the following children with special needs (in order of frequency):

- Developmentally disabled
- Behaviorally disordered
- Emotionally disturbed

- Physically disabled
- School-age population
- Speech impaired
- Autistic
- Visually impaired
- Neurologically impaired
- Healing impaired
- Substance abusing
- Abused or sexually abused

Music Therapy and Palliative Care

Music therapy has been demonstrated in the literature to improve pain, agitation, disruptive behaviors, communication, and quality of life in a home hospice environment (Romo & Gifford, 2007). Music promotes a client's physical, mental, and spiritual well-being.

Music can be particularly beneficial at the end of life, when communications often break down and a sense of isolation sets in. Music may help the dying person achieve a deep state of relaxation, promote better sleep, reduce pain and anxiety, improve mood, and uplift the individual's spirit (Marchand, 2007). The key is to find music that helps the dying person feel relaxed and at peace. Recordings of gentle environmental sounds such as ocean waves, wind, rain, or birds, as well as music from harps, flutes, or stringed instruments, may provide a sense of peace. However, not everyone likes music, so practitioners should pay attention to the dying person's preferences.

Music Therapy and Aging

As people age, their immune systems can become impaired due to a decrease in NK cell function. Music has demonstrated a significant increase in NK cell count and activity in older clients with Alzheimer's disease, cerebrovascular disease, and Parkinson's disease. Calming music reduces agitation in the elderly (Freeman, 2004). In one music therapy study, the type of music that seniors preferred to sing was popular music, followed by folk songs and songs from musicals (Vanweelden & Cevasco, 2007).

Music Therapy in Alzheimer's and Dementia Care

Music is used in long-term care facilities with elderly residents to increase their level of physical, mental, social, and emotional functioning. Music helps to elevate mood, counteract the effects of depression, promote movement for physical rehabilitation, calm and sedate, and reduce apprehension and fear (Humphrey, 2000). Music therapy has shown promising results in decreasing physical and verbal aggression in adults with different types of dementia and at different levels of cognitive impairment (Forbes, Peacock, & Morgan, 2005).

Music Therapy and Mental Health

Clients with severe psychotic disturbances need the stability and safety of predictable music because their world is so chaotic and disconnected. In an example of music therapy for a moderately severe mental condition, a 41-year-old male was referred to a psychiatric hospital with a diagnosis of personality disorder, and he received music therapy. His characteristic traits were intellectualizing, obsessive-compulsive behavior, and very little contact with his emotional life. As an outpatient, the client attended weekly 1-hour music therapy sessions for 2 years. In the various sessions:

- The therapist and the client both improvised on the piano.
- The therapist played a metallophone, and the client played the piano.
- Both the therapist and the client improvised vocally.
- The client improvised vocally by himself.
- The therapist and the client both improvised with voice and piano.

The music helped the client achieve a more normal self-identity, greater personal freedom, clearer boundaries, and a greater degree of autonomy (Wigram et al., 2004).

Music Therapy for Stress Reduction

Music is used to help relieve stress in adults (Lichtman, 2006). Music is capable of affecting every cell in the body and releasing chemical responses in the brain that affect the way individuals feel. As Campbell (2006) notes, "It's amazing that in just a few minutes, music can trigger responses in your heartbeat, emotions, and attentiveness. Almost instantly, you can be activated, awakened, and feel like dancing" (p. xix).

Therapeutic Uses and Benefits of Music

Music therapy is used in hospitals, nursing homes, and psychiatric facilities (Campbell, 2001; Guzzetta, 2005).

- In hospitals, it is used to alleviate pain in conjunction with anesthesia or pain medication; elevate clients' mood and counteract depression; promote movement for physical rehabilitation; calm or sedate clients; and often to induce sleep, counteract apprehension or fear, and lessen muscle tension for the purpose of relaxation.
- Music is used in nursing homes to increase or maintain elderly people's levels of physical, mental, and social/emotional functioning and to maintain their quality of life.
- In psychiatric facilities, music is used to explore personal feelings, make positive changes in mood and emotional states, help provide a sense of control over life through successful experiences, practice problem solving, and resolve conflicts leading to stronger family and peer relationships.

Using a planned and systematic approach for music and music activities, music therapy interventions provide opportunities for the following (Campbell, 2001; Guzzetta, 2005; Seaward, 2006):

- Anxiety and stress reduction
- The nonpharmacological management of pain and discomfort
- Positive changes in mood and emotional states
- Active and positive client participation in treatment
- Enhanced awareness of self and environment
- The development of coping and relaxation skills
- Improved emotional intimacy with families and caregivers
- Relaxation for the entire family
- Increasing or improving meaningful time spent together in a positive, creative way

MUSIC THERAPY MODALITIES

Music therapy is used to address the physical, psychological, cognitive, and social needs of individuals with disabilities and illnesses. After assessing the needs and personal preferences of a client, the qualified music therapist provides the appropriate treatment, which can include creating music, singing, moving to music, or just listening to it (Achterberg et al., 1992).

Guidelines for a Meaningful Musical Experience

For a meaningful musical experience, Lingerman (1995) provides these guidelines for clients:

- *Before beginning the music*, quiet your mind, relax your body, calm your feelings. Be grateful for the music you are about to experience. Surrender to the music and be open to what you hear.
- *While the music is playing*, release all negativity and tension, and breathe deeply. Be open to healing, and feel the music and melody entering your being. Enjoy wherever the music takes you. Move into mystery, joy, and praise. Play the music only as long as it makes you feel good.
- *When the music is over*, sit quietly for a few minutes and absorb the music. Combine the experience of the music with another activity, such as moving, dancing, or drawing.

Our musical needs and choices are influenced by many factors, including the following (Lingerman, 1995):

- Our prior experiences
- Childhood memories and earliest exposure to music
- Temperament and personality
- Exposure to others' music in the home and work environment
- Continuous learning and self-education
- Our desires, ideals, and aspirations

Modalities in Music Therapy

The following modalities are used in music therapy (Fein, 2007; Lichtman, 2006; Priesnitz, 2006).

- *Singing* helps individuals with speech impairments improve their articulation, rhythm, and breath control. Songs help elderly adults remember significant events in their lives, and singing has produced some remarkable health effects. Singing is also being used for people with dementia and Alzheimer's disease. Researchers have found that group singing may have benefits for caregiver-client communication.
- *Playing instruments* improves gross and fine motor coordination in individuals with motor impairments. For example, playing in an instrumental ensemble helps an individual with behavioral problems learn how to control disruptive impulses by working in a group structure. Drumming is good for stress reduction: cancer clients who play drums in group settings feel more relaxed and reveal higher white blood cell counts.
- *Rhythmic movement* facilitates and improves an individual's range of motion, joint mobility, agility, strength, balance, coordination, gait

consistency, respiration patterns, and muscular relaxation. For example, the rhythmic component of music helps to increase motivation, interest, and enjoyment, and it acts as a nonverbal persuasion to involve individuals socially.

- *Improvising* offers a creative, nonverbal means of expressing feelings. For example, improvising is an opportunity to make choices and deal with structure creatively.
- *Composing* develops cooperative learning and facilitates the sharing of feelings, ideas, and experiences. For hospitalized children, for example, writing songs is an effective means of expressing and understanding fears.
- *Listening* is used for many therapeutic applications, including the development of cognitive skills such as attention and memory. For example, actively listening to music in a relaxed and receptive state stimulates thoughts, images, and feelings, which can then be further examined and discussed. Listening to music while driving may reduce the chance of an accident. A recent survey found that safe drivers tended to play easy listening and classical music in their cars.

PHYSIOLOGICAL AND PSYCHOLOGICAL RESPONSES TO MUSIC

Music can produce physical as well as psychological changes. The emotional effect of music causes a corresponding physical effect, and all the physical effects of sound inevitably create a psychological effect (Wigram et al., 2004). These changes are determined by the type of music played (e.g., soothing or stimulating).

Music heals but is not prescriptive because its power varies according to the composition, the performer, the listener, the posture assumed while listening, and additional factors. To fully understand how music heals, we have to examine what it does and some of its therapeutic effects. Following are some of music's possible uses and beneficial effects (Campbell, 2001; Goldman, 2002):

Physiological Responses to Music

Physiological responses to music include the following (Priesnitz, 2006; Wigram et al., 2004):

- *Music masks unpleasant sounds and feelings.* Many dental professionals understand the effects of music; they use it to mask the sound of the drill and dispel the uncomfortable feeling created by the harsh sounds and vibrations of the instruments.

- *Music can slow and equalize brain waves.* Beta waves occur during ordinary consciousness and vibrate from 14 to 20 Hz. Alpha waves occur during periods of heightened awareness and calm; and they cycle from 8 to 13 Hz. Theta waves occur during periods of peak creativity, meditation, and sleep; they cycle from 4 to 7 Hz. Delta waves occur during deep sleep, deep meditation, and unconsciousness; they range from 0.5 to 3 Hz. Listening to certain types of music such as Baroque, New Age, and other ambient (with no dominant rhythm) music can shift consciousness from the beta toward the alpha range. Shamanic drumming can take the listener into the theta range.
- *Music affects respiration.* Breathing at a deep, slow rate is optimal and contributes to calmness. By listening to music with longer, slower sounds, breathing can deepen and slow, creating a calm, relaxed sensation. Gregorian chant, New Age, and ambient music can create this effect.
- *Music affects the heartbeat, pulse rate, and blood pressure.* Musical variables such as frequency, tempo, and volume tend to speed up or slow down heart rate. The faster the music, the faster the heart rate; the slower the music, the slower the heart rate. A slower heartbeat calms the mind, creates less physical tension and stress, and helps the body heal itself. Blood pressure can be lowered by listening to music with a frequency of 44–55 Hz.
- *Music reduces muscle tension and improves body movement and coordination.* Through the autonomic nervous system, the auditory nerve connects the inner ear with all the muscles in the body. Thus muscle strength, flexibility, and tone are influenced by sound and vibration. Music is used in recovery wards and rehabilitation clinics to restructure repetitive movements following accidents and illnesses.
- *Music affects body temperature.* Loud music with a strong beat can raise body temperature by a few degrees; soft music with a weak beat can lower it.
- *Music can increase endorphin levels.* Endorphins can lessen pain and induce what's known as a natural high. Music can stimulate the release of endorphins, which can then decrease the need for pain medication, provide a distraction from pain, and relieve anxiety.
- *Music can regulate stress-related hormones.* Listening to relaxing, ambient music may reduce the level of stress hormones in the blood, in some cases reducing or eliminating the need for medication.
- *Music and sound can boost immune function.* Insufficient oxygen in the blood may be a major cause of immune deficiency and degenerative disease. Listening to certain types of music—as well as engaging in

singing, chanting, and other vocal forms—relaxes muscles and improves respiratory effort, resulting in better oxygenation of the cells.

Psychological Responses to Music

Music therapy can produce many psychological responses:

- It can reduce anxiety and fear, as well as create relaxing, soothing sensations (Guzzetta, 2005; Lippin & Micozzi, 2006).
- Soothing music may produce a hypometabolic response, similar to a relaxation response, in which autonomic, immune, endocrine, and neuropeptide systems are altered.
- Slow, repetitive music reduces anxiety.
- Regular rhythmic music pulsating at alpha and theta brainwave rates can help maintain respiratory and heart rates during surgery.
- Melodious music has been shown to help minimize pain and speed recovery following surgery (Cabrera & Lee, 2000).
- Music mitigates nausea and emesis in chemotherapy clients, decreases preoperative anxiety in infants, and reduces visitor stress in hospital waiting rooms (Schweitzer, Gilpin, & Frampton, 2004).

EVIDENCE-BASED PRACTICE IN MUSIC THERAPY

Wigram et al. (2004) note that evidence-based practice (EBP) is increasingly being used to determine which interventions to fund. They add that EBP "can be understood as an approach to healthcare that promotes collection, interpretation and integration of valid, important and applicable patient-reported, clinician-observed and research-derived evidence. In order to meet the requirements of EBP, clinical effectiveness must be demonstrated" (p. 257).

The types of evidence used to demonstrate and support music therapy as an intervention include the following (Wigram et al., 2004):

- Direct evidence from the clinician's assessment, evaluation, and analysis of therapeutic change
- Related evidence from the literature, case studies, and an international database of clinical music therapists
- Research evidence from the literature and from qualitative and/or quantitative investigations

With an emphasis on accountability, music therapists now use tools to document and justify their work. This documentation is especially crucial at a time when cost-saving measures are a priority in health care (Hanser, 1999).

KEY CONCEPTS

1. Music and sound have been used in healing practices throughout history, with many examples of the healing powers of music in the historical records of different cultures.
2. Music therapy and sound healing are two ends of a continuum spanning all forms of healing with sound and music.
3. The types of evidence used to demonstrate and support music therapy as an intervention include direct evidence, related evidence, and research evidence.

QUESTIONS FOR REFLECTION

1. How can I use music therapy and sound healing in my personal and professional practice for health and healing?
2. What types of music and sound healing recordings completely relax me?
3. How can I best evaluate which types of music and sound healing recordings are the most suitable for my clients?

REFERENCES

Achterberg, J., Dossey, L., Gordon, J. S., Hegedus, C., Herrmann, M. W., & Nelson, R. (1992). Mind-body interventions. In *Alternative medicine: Expanding medical horizons*. A report to the National Institutes of Health on alternative medical systems and practices in the United States. Chantilly, VA: U.S. Government Printing Office.

American Music Therapy Association. (2004). *What is music therapy?* Retrieved January 31, 2008, from www.musictherapy.org

Borysenko, J. (2001). *Inner peace for busy people*. Carlsbad, CA: Hay House.

Cabrera, I. N., & Lee, M. H. M. (2000, April). Reducing noise pollution in the hospital setting by establishing a department of sound: A survey of recent research on the effects of noise and music in health care. *Preventive Medicine*, *30*(4), 339–345.

Campbell, D. (1995). *Music physician for times to come*. Wheaton, IL: Theosophical.

Campbell, D. (2001). *The Mozart effect*. New York: Quill.

Campbell, D. (2006). *The harmony of health.* Carlsbad, CA: Hay House.

Campbell, D. (2007). *Creating inner harmony: Using your voice and music to heal.* Carlsbad, CA: Hay House.

Cantello, M. (2004). *Communing with music: Practicing the art of conscious listening.* Camarillo, CA: DeVorss.

Crowe, B. J., & Scovel, M. (1996) Special feature—An overview of sound healing practices: Implications for the profession of music therapy. *Music Therapy Perspectives, 14*(1), 21–29.

Dotton, F. J., & Mandleco, B. (2007). Child and family communication. In N. Potts & B. Mandleco, *Pediatric nursing: Caring for children and their families* (2nd ed., pp. 359–379). Clifton Park, NY: Thomson Delmar Learning.

Emoto, M. (2006). *Water crystal healing: Music and images to restore your well-being.* New York: Atria Books.

Fein, J. (2007, May–June). The new supermarket of sound healing. *Spirituality and Health, 70,* 90–91.

Forbes, D., Peacock, S., & Morgan, D. (2005). Nonpharmacological management of agitated behaviours associated with dementia. *Geriatrics Aging, 8*(4), 26–30.

Freeman, L. (2004). *Mosby's complementary and alternative medicine: A research-based approach* (2nd ed.). St. Louis, MO: Mosby.

Gardner, J. (2006). *Vibrational healing through the chakras with light, color, sound, crystal, and aromatherapy.* Berkeley, CA: Crossing Press.

Gaynor, M. (2002). *The healing power of sound.* Boston: Shambhala.

Goldman, J. (2002) *Healing sounds: The power of harmonics.* Rochester, VT: Healing Arts Press.

Guzzetta, C. E. (2005). Music therapy: Hearing the melody of the soul. In B. M. Dossey, L. Keegan, & C. E. Guzzetta, *Holistic nursing: A handbook for practice* (4th ed., pp. 617–640). Sudbury, MA: Jones and Bartlett.

Hanser, S. B. (1999). *The new music therapist's handbook* (2nd ed.). Boston: Berklee Press.

Humphrey, M. A. (2000, June). Alzheimer's disease meets the "Mozart effect." *Nursing homes: Long term care management, 49*(6), 50–51.

Keegan, L. (2005). Environment. In B. M. Dossey, L. Keegan, & C. E. Guzzetta, *Holistic nursing: A handbook for practice* (4th ed., pp. 275–303). Sudbury, MA: Jones and Bartlett.

Kern, P., Wakeford, L., & Aldridge, D. (2007). Improving the performance of a young child with autism during self-care tasks using embedded song interventions: A case study. *Music Therapy Perspectives, 25*(1), 43–51.

Kligler, B., Newmark, S., Mehl-Madrona, L., Islam, J., & Gerik, S. (2004). Integrative approach to common pediatric conditions. In B. Kligler & R. Lee, *Integrative medicine: Principles for practice* (pp. 711–744). New York: McGraw-Hill.

Leddy, S. K. (2006). *Integrative health promotion: Conceptual bases for nursing practice* (2nd ed.). Sudbury, MA: Jones and Bartlett.

Leeds, J. (2001). *The power of sound*. Rochester, VT: Healing Arts Press.

Lichtman, N. (2006). Power chords: The healing power behind the music. *Current Health 2: A Weekly Reader Publication, 32*(5), 12.

Lingerman, H. A. (1995). *The healing energies of music*. Wheaton, IL: Theosophical.

Lippin, R. A., & Micozzi, M. S. (2006). Arts therapy. In M. S. Micozzi, *Fundamentals of complementary and integrative medicine* (3rd ed., pp. 332–350). St. Louis, MO: Saunders Elsevier.

Marchand, L. (2007). End-of-life care. In D. Rakel, *Integrative medicine* (2nd ed., pp. 873–888). Philadelphia: Saunders Elsevier.

Priesnitz, W. (2006, May–June). Music is medicine for body and soul. *Natural Life*, 10–11.

Romo, R., & Gifford, L. (2007). A cost-benefit analysis of music therapy in a home hospice. *Nursing Economic$, 25*(6), 353–358.

Schweitzer, M., Gilpin, L., & Frampton, S. (2004). Healing spaces: Elements of environmental design that make an impact on health. *Journal of Alternative and Complementary Medicine, 10*(Suppl. 1), S71–S83.

Seaward, B. L. (2005). *Achieving the mind-body-spirit connection: A stress management workbook*. Sudbury, MA: Jones and Bartlett.

Seaward, B. L. (2006). *Managing stress: Principles and strategies for health and well-being* (5th ed.). Sudbury, MA: Jones and Bartlett.

Storr, A. (1992). *Music and the mind*. New York: Free Press.

Vanweelden, K., & Cevasco, A. (2007). Repertoire recommendations by music therapists for geriatric clients during singing activities. *Music Therapy Perspectives, 25*(1), 4–12.

Wigram, T., Pedersen, I. N., & Bonde, L. O. (2004). *A comprehensive guide to music therapy: Theory, clinical practice, research, and training*. Philadelphia: Jessica Kingsley.

World Federation of Music Therapy. (1996). *Definition of music therapy*. Retrieved January 31, 2008, from http://www.musictherapyworld.de/

CHAPTER 10

Integrative Nutrition

Food is our common ground, a universal experience.
—JAMES BEARD

LEARNING OBJECTIVES

1. Describe the role of food and health in human history.
2. Identify the macronutrients and micronutrients and describe their role in nutrition and health.
3. Describe various diet types and their focus.
4. Describe the types and functions of nutraceuticals.
5. Identify the various toxins in our food chain.
6. Describe the role of herbs and herbalism in health care.
7. Explain the herbal production process.
8. Describe the levels of herbalists.
9. Identify the actions of herbs.
10. Describe the key concerns of herbalism today.

INTRODUCTION

How often have you heard, "You are what you eat"? Scientists now know that DNA and all other molecules that make up the cells are created from nutrients provided in the diet (Salguero, 2007). The old adage is now regarded as definitive, science-based knowledge.

Since the beginning of time, food has played an essential role in the survival of humankind. For many cultures, food is the center of social and family gatherings. Scientific research shows the therapeutic and preventive benefits of eating a variety of nutritious foods. Not only is *what* you eat important, but so are how and when you eat and how the food is grown or raised. In the modern world, the media are filled with the latest warnings about the dangers of one food or the virtues of another. Yet few people know how their food is processed or what has gone into the farming and raising of crops, and they barely take time to stop and savor the nutrients they eat.

Which foods should you eat? How should you prepare them? Which supplements are good for you? Learning about food and answering these questions can be daunting. As the understanding of nutrition evolves and the choices become more complex, nutrition therapy is more important than ever in assuring a healthy life. Integrative nutrition supports healthy eating habits by combining traditional concepts of nutrition with modern concepts of health (such as nutraceuticals) and the awareness of how food is grown or raised.

FOOD AND HEALTH

Food and nutrition are fundamental to all life. In addition to being a source of nutrition, food plays several other roles:

- *Spiritual*: Diets for religious purposes
- *Geographic:* Diets dependent on where people live and what is available
- *Economic:* Diets dependent on available financial resources
- *Physiological:* Diets for medical purposes
- *Social:* Diets for special occasions

As Micozzi (2006) states, "From birthday cake to bitter herbs of the Passover seder to Thanksgiving turkey to communion wafers, food helps form our social bonds, express our spirituality, and define who we are" (p. 256).

People often maintain specific food habits because they are practical or culturally symbolic. Cultural beliefs that influence nutrition and diet intake include:

- What is regarded as food and what is not
- How food is cultivated, harvested, prepared, and served
- How food is actually eaten
- Who prepares and serves it
- Which individuals eat together, where, and on what occasions
- The order of dishes served in a meal

Food is also a basic medium through which adult attitudes and sentiments are communicated, since eating can be associated with emotions like happiness, warmth, anger, or tension. Food can also be used as a pacifier and a relaxation technique, especially when people are under stress. In a movie theater, while watching a suspenseful movie, have you ever noticed the sound of people munching popcorn, eating candy, or sipping on their extra-large soft drinks? Have you ever been frustrated, angry, or bored, and just grabbed whatever was in your kitchen cupboard or workplace snack room and gobbled it up? Seaward (2006) asserts that "food and mood go together like peanut butter and jelly" (p. 498).

Food is basic to survival, meets security needs (through storage and hoarding), can be used as gifts or rewards, involves pride in preparation, and can help someone express self-actualization through its innovative use and new recipes. Food ideology is the comprehensive perspective of attitudes, beliefs, customs, and taboos affecting the diet. It is influenced by advertising and involves symbols associated with food such as prestige, power, status, lifestyles, and emotional fulfillment (Leddy, 2006). Because food habits and associations are learned early in life and tend to be long lasting and difficult to change, it is important to form sound nutritional practices when you are young.

Historical Perspectives

Human beings are omnivores and can eat almost anything found in nature, with the exception of grass or wood. For all but the last few moments of human history, our ancestors roamed the land as hunter-gatherers. Hunters brought home lean meat, and gatherers collected plants high in fiber and complex carbohydrates as well as vitamins and minerals. Life was challenging and physical, and getting enough calories was always a struggle. Food distribution was often based on social status. When agriculture was developed over 10,000 years ago, diets became relatively stabilized and seasonal crops became available. However, the quality of food did not change much, and the human diet consisted of natural foods until modern times (Micozzi, 2006).

Today, the typical American diet increasingly consists of more processed and contaminated foods than ever before. At the same time, Americans suffer from more degenerative lifestyle-related ailments (such as heart disease, some forms of cancer, diabetes, and stroke), causing many healthcare providers to suggest a link between what people eat and how they feel (Luck, 2005). Some believe that people are forced to overfeed themselves in order to get a little nourishment because foods are not as nutritionally complete as they were a hundred or more years ago. Many consider this "overconsumptive undernutrition" to be one of today's leading nutritional problems (Trivieri & Anderson, 2002).

Physiological Considerations

In the human body, cells are constantly being reproduced and molecules transformed and they are constantly in need of resources beyond the basic macronutrients (proteins, carbohydrates, and lipids) and their quality. A lack of appropriate micronutrients (such as folic acid, vitamin B12, niacin, ascorbic acid, tocopherols, iron, or zinc) has been shown to mimic radiation in damaging DNA by causing single- and double-strand breaks, oxidative lesions, or both (Salguero, 2007).

The lack of variety in foods, the overconsumption of foods with few nutrients, and too many empty calories in the form of refined sugar lead to a diet that lacks the necessary macronutrients and micronutrients to support a healthy body. For example, the consumption of appropriate amounts of fruit and vegetables is associated with a lower risk of degenerative diseases, including cancer, cardiovascular disuse, cataracts, and brain dysfunction (Salguero, 2007). Improvements in the foods served at schools have resulted in improved attendance, grades, and student interactions (Rindfleisch, 2007).

Another concept in food health that is gaining in importance is the glycemic index (GI). While not currently recognized by the American Diabetes Association (ADA) in the treatment of disease, it is nonetheless a useful nutritional concept. The GI chemically classifies carbohydrates as simple or complex, sugars or starches, and available or unavailable (Rindfleisch, 2007). This index measures how quickly a consumed carbohydrate affects postprandial serum glucose and insulin levels over a specific period of time, and it measures the relative glycemic response to dietary carbohydrates. In the glycemic index, glucose and white bread are the gold standard because they cause the fastest and most dramatic rise in glucose levels and so are assigned a value of 100, the highest possible index.

Several studies have associated a long-term, high-GI diet with an increased risk for developing type 2 diabetes mellitus, cardiovascular disease, and certain cancers (including gastric, colorectal, pancreatic, and endometrial cancers) (Rindfleisch, 2007).

DIETARY THEORY

Diet is the food people eat. *Nutrition* refers to the ingestion of foods and their relationship to health (Luck, 2005). Proper nutrition results primarily from food choices. Proper digestion, absorption, metabolism, and elimination require high-quality foods that contain optimum nutrients. The way food is prepared can affect the nutritional value of its nutrients, which must be broken down to be utilized effectively by the body. Nutrients provide the body with energy so it can build, repair, and renew tissues as needed (Eliopoulos, 2004).

Equally important as a food's preparation are its presentation, its smell and taste, and the emotional climate in which meals are eaten (including the surroundings, conversation, and other environmental sights and sounds). If food is eaten in an anxiety-ridden environment or state of mind, or if a meal is rushed, the result is different than if the food is delicious and eaten with friends in a relaxing, beautiful setting (Eliopoulos, 2004).

The Food Guide Pyramid

The Food Guide Pyramid is a widely recognized graphic providing guidelines about how much of each food group to ingest each day. Developed by the Food and Nutritional Board of the National Academies of Science (Eliopoulous, 2004), the graphic provides an easy way to make food choices from the six food groups: grains, vegetables, fruits, oils, milk, and meats and beans.

In addition to the foods listed on the Food Guide Pyramid, several essential dietary nutrients are absolutely necessary for human life; they fall into two categories called macronutrients (carbohydrates, proteins, fats, water, and fiber) and micronutrients (vitamins and minerals) (Eliopoulos, 2004; Leddy 2006).

Macronutrients

Carbohydrates

Carbohydrates provide the blood with glucose and allow the body to use protein for regeneration and repair (Eliopoulos, 2004; Micozzi, 2006). Carbohydrates provide energy and are comprised of two classes—complex and simple carbohydrates (Luck, 2005; Seaward, 2006).

Complex carbohydrates (fruits, vegetables, and grain products) contain starches and fiber. They are metabolized more slowly than simple sugars.

Simple carbohydrates include white table sugar (sucrose), the sugar in fruit (fructose), and the sugar in milk (lactose). Simple carbohydrates have fewer nutrients than complex carbohydrates and should be avoided, even though the body cannot distinguish between the two classes (Eliopoulos, 2004; Micozzi, 2006). In 1922, the average American consumed about 5 pounds of sugar per person per year. By 1990, that figure had skyrocketed to 135 pounds. In general, food that is canned, frozen, cured, and processed is likely to be high in sugar (Trivieri & Anderson, 2002).

Protein

Protein, the body's secondary energy source, must be present for the body to grow, repair damaged or injured tissue, create new tissue, and regulate water balance. It is a foundational element for the major organs, blood and blood clotting, muscles, skin, hair, nails, hormones, enzymes, and antibodies. It also helps maintain a proper balance of blood acidity and alkalinity (Eliopoulos, 2004; Micozzi, 2006; Seaward, 2006).

Amino acids are the building blocks of proteins. The essential ones are L-lycine, L-isoleucine, L-leucine, L-valine, L-methionine, L-threonine, L-phenylalanine, and L-tryptophan (Leddy 2006). Foods that consist of essential amino acids are considered complete proteins; examples include meats, dairy, fish, fowl, and eggs. Incomplete proteins are found in grains, beans, nuts, seeds, and leafy green vegetables. The body cannot store proteins for future use, so we must ingest them every day (Micozzi, 2006).

Fats

As a third energy source for the body, fats (lipids) are the most concentrated form of energy and account for more than 10% of the body weight of most adults (Luck, 2005). Fats supply greater energy (9 calories per gram) than carbohydrates or proteins (each with 4 calories per gram). They also supply the essential fatty acids, including linoleic and linolenic acid (found in seafood and unrefined vegetable oils), oleic and arachidonic acids (found in most organic fats and oils and peanuts) (Leddy 2006). One molecule of fat contains three molecules of fatty acids and one molecule of glycerol. This structure is known chemically as a triglyceride, and triglycerides comprise 90% of all dietary fat. The other two categories of fats are phospholipids and sterols (like cholesterol) (Leddy, 2006). The American Heart Association recommends that people consume fewer than 10% of their daily calories from saturated fats and fewer than 10% from polyunsaturated fats. Reducing the amount of animal foods in the diet is one way to achieve this level.

Fats perform two basic functions: they supply energy for prolonged, moderately intense activity and they provide cell membranes with the component necessary to regulate the membrane transport system (Seaward, 2006). Fats also help maintain healthy skin, regulate cholesterol metabolism, carry fat-soluble vitamins, act as a cushion and stabilizer for internal organs, and provide a protective layer that helps regulate body temperature and maintain heat (Eliopoulos, 2004). In particular, babies and children need fats for brain development.

Essential fatty acids (fats that the body is unable to make on its own) must be obtained through diet. Necessary for cell membrane integrity and chemical transport, they are also involved in the development of the central nervous system, energy production, oxygen transport, and inflammation regulation (Rakel & Rindfleisch, 2007). Essential fatty acids are classified as saturated (e.g., in beef and dairy fat), monosaturated (e.g., omega-9 fats such as those in olive, peanut, avocado, and canola oils), and polyunsaturated (essential fats of the omega-6 and omega-3 family) (Luck, 2005).

The more saturated the fat, the more stable it is at room temperature. Heating oils or fats may change them from their natural, more unstable form to a more stable (trans) form. During the 1950s, scientists discovered that partially hydrogenating (saturating) the fats or oils created a trans-fatty acid that allowed the fat to remain stable in a food for a long time—a benefit for foods that needed to be preserved. Partially hydrogenated vegetable oils eventually became the main oil used in cooking, and margarines replaced butter.

Hydrogenation, however, has an effect on human health. Partially hydrogenated oils (as well as animal products such as meat and dairy products) are a major source of omega-6 fatty acids, which are subunits of arachidonic acid (AA), a precursor to inflammatory processes in the body. The body has to use more energy to metabolize these fatty acids as an energy source because they are more stable. As a result of this metabolism, free radicals are released. Free radicals facilitate the mobilization of AA across the cell membrane, they raise levels of harmful low-density-lipoprotein (LDL) cholesterol, and they lower levels of the beneficial high-density lipoprotein (HDL). The more omega-6 fatty acids there are in the body, the less the body is able to utilize the beneficial influences of omega-3 fatty acids. A typical Western diet can have a ratio of omega-6 to omega-3 fatty acids as high as 25:1. Today, the recommended ratio is 4:1. It can take a person from 6 weeks to 6 months to change this ratio and experience clinical effects (Rakel & Rindfleisch, 2007).

Good sources of omega-3 fatty acids are cold-water fish (salmon, mackerel, sardines, herring, and albacore tuna) and fish oils with eicosapentaenoic acid (EPA) and docosahexaenoic acid (DHA). Flaxseed is also a rich source of omega-3 fatty acids, as are walnuts, dark green leafy vegetables, soybeans, algae, and hemp seeds. When buying fish, wild fish from northern waters are preferable to farm-raised fish because wild fish eat a lot of algae (a rich source of omega-3 fatty acids). Farm-raised fish are often fed cornmeal, which is low in omega-3 fatty acids (Rakel & Rindfleisch, 2007).

Water

Water, while not actually a macronutrient, is fundamental to life and critical for every bodily function and chemical reaction. The human body can survive up to 5 weeks without food but only a few days without water (Micozzi, 2006). Water comprises two-thirds of the body, maintains the body's temperature, transports nutrients to cells and toxins from them, lubricates joints, and transports oxygen through the blood and lymph tissues.

The quality of water varies by location. Filtration, distillation, and reverse osmosis are various ways to purify water and remove major contaminants (Eliopoulos, 2004). Experts suggest a minimum of eight glasses of water per day for optimal health (Seaward, 2006).

Fiber

Fiber, like water, is not truly a macronutrient but it is crucial to healthy diets. Fiber is found mainly in fruits, vegetables, and grains. It is not digested and is not an energy source for the body but it is essential for normal digestion; controlling blood glucose, blood pressure, and cholesterol levels; and for protecting against heart disease and cancer.

- *Insoluble fiber* decreases the transit time of food in the intestines and increases stool softness and weight. It is found in wheat bran, whole grains, fruits, vegetables, and nuts.
- *Soluble fiber* lowers the absorption of cholesterol, regulates blood sugar, and absorbs and removes toxic materials and carcinogens from the body (Luck, 2005). Oat bran, flax seeds, pectin (from apples), and psyllium seeds are examples of soluble fiber (Leddy, 2006).

The average intake of fiber in the United States, at 10–20 grams, is less than half the recommended daily intake of 30–50 grams per day (Eliopoulos, 2004; Leddy, 2006). Fiber intake should be increased gradually to avoid flatulence and bloating.

Micronutrients

Micronutrients (vitamins and minerals) are elements that occur naturally in food and allow the body to function properly. Needed in trace (small) amounts, vitamins and minerals work synergistically and should be obtained from whole foods as much as possible since foods contain hundreds of other compounds that allow the body to utilize the micronutrients better than when taken separately as supplements (Eliopoulos, 2004).

Essential vitamins are either fat soluble or water soluble.

- Fat-soluble vitamins (A, D, E, and K) are stored in the body for days or weeks.
- Water-soluble vitamins (C or ascorbic acid, B1 or thiamine, B2 or riboflavin, B3 or niacin, B5 panthothenic acid, B6 or pyridoxine, B12, folic acid, and biotin) dissolve quickly in the bloodstream and are removed by urine or sweat (Leddy 2006; Micozzi, 2006).

Essential minerals include (Leddy 2006; Luck, 2005):

- Macrominerals (calcium, magnesium, phosphorus, sodium, and potassium)
- Microminerals (iron, iodine, zinc, copper, manganese, chromium, silicon, fluoride, selenium, and molybdenum)

Other nutrients that support metabolism include vitamin C–complex factors choline and inositol as well as coenzyme Q10 and lipoic acid (Leddy, 2006).

Holistic Approach to Diet and Nutrition

A holistic approach to diet and nutrition consists of self-care, healthful foods, moderate intake, and balance. Nutritional intake should be varied and balanced with wholesome, quality, organic foods of varying tastes, textures, colors, and temperatures. Food should be eaten in a relaxed manner and with enjoyable company and surroundings to meet psychological, social, and cultural needs. The spiritual aspects of the meal can be met through rituals and family traditions. Eating at a consistent time is also important, because it allows the body time to rest between meals. Six small meals per day, beginning with breakfast, are recommended. Eating too much at a time or too late in the day can cause difficulty in digestion, poor sleep, and general uncomfortable sensations (Eliopoulos, 2004).

DIET TYPES

A number of therapeutic diets have been developed to prevent or treat various diseases or promote weight loss. Generally, the evidence shows that, regardless of the types of macronutrients ingested, diets that reduce caloric intake result in weight loss. Participation in a therapeutic dietary regimen should be overseen by a healthcare professional. The following sections describe some types of diets (Leddy, 2006).

High-Fiber, High-Carbohydrate, Low-Fat Diets

This category includes the macrobiotic diet, the Pritikin diet, the Ornish diet, and the Gerson diet.

- The *macrobiotic diet* consists of 50–60% whole grains, 20–25% vegetables, 5–10% beans and sea vegetables, and 5% vegetable soups. Nuts, seeds, fruits, and fish are eaten occasionally, and dietary needs are adjusted according to age, gender, climate, season, activity level, and other individual factors (Leddy, 2006). Developed in the 1950s by George Osawa, a Japanese educator and philosopher, the macrobiotic diet derives its name from the Greek words *macros* ("big" or "long") and *bios* ("life"). Macrobiotics advocates believe that all food has yin (calming) or yang (strengthening) properties and that people can rebalance their feelings and restore their physical well-being by eating the proper foods (Micozzi, 2006).

- The *Pritikin diet* is a low-fat, low-cholesterol, low-sodium, and high–complex carbohydrate diet combined with regular aerobic exercise. Protein is limited to 3.5 ounces of lean meat a day.
- The *Ornish diet*, developed to reverse the development of atherosclerosis and coronary heart disease, is similar to the Pritikin diet. The Ornish diet emphasizes gentle exercise and allows egg whites, nonfat yogurt, skim milk, and an occasional glass of wine. It excludes almost all other animal products and smoking.
- The *Gerson diet* is a vegetarian diet that includes raw vegetables or fruit juices and coffee enemas. It begins with a period of juice fasting and enemas, followed by a low-sodium, high-potassium diet (Leddy, 2006; Micozzi, 2006).

Atkins Diet

Developed in the 1970s, this diet is a high-protein, low-carbohydrate regimen with four stages: the induction diet, the ongoing weight loss diet, premaintenance, and maintenance. It emphasizes nutrient-dense, unprocessed foods; the avoidance of refined or processed carbohydrates; and the use of multivitamin and essential fatty acid supplements. Short-term weight loss has been demonstrated, but long-term health effects are still concerning for some (Leddy, 2006; Micozzi, 2006).

Moderate-Fat, Balanced-Nutrient, Reduction Diets

This category includes diets that contain 20–30% fats, 15–20% proteins, and 55–60% carbohydrates. Examples include Weight Watchers, Jenny Craig, and NutriSystem. The underlying premise of these diets is that caloric reduction results in weight loss. A wide range of food choices are available, and physical activity is promoted.

Raw Food Diet

Believing that raw foods are better for the human digestive system, provide better nutrition than cooked foods, and extend the life span, Swiss physician Max Bircher-Benner developed the raw food diet during the late 1800s. The diet includes 70% uncooked vegetables and fruits and 30% meat, dairy products, nuts, grains, and seeds (Micozzi, 2006).

Vegetarian and Vegan Diets

A vegetarian diet excludes meat, poultry, and fish but allows eggs and dairy products. This diet has been shown to lower the risk of heart disease, high blood pressure, diabetes, osteoporosis, gallbladder disease, colon cancer, and other conditions.

A vegan diet excludes all animal-based foods, including dairy products, eggs, and honey. The vegan diet has been useful in treating asthma, arthritis, hypertension, and angina. Vegans may need to use supplements to avoid the risk of vitamin B12 deficiency (Micozzi, 2006).

Elimination Diet

An elimination diet is an investigational, short-term or possibly lifelong eating plan. It usually omits one or more foods suspected or known to cause an adverse food reaction or allergic response. It can also serve as both a diagnostic and treatment strategy. Ayurvedic healing, for example, has promoted the practice of eliminating certain foods and emphasizing others for many centuries (see chapter 7 for more information about Ayurvedic medicine).

Elimination diets attempt to address adverse food reactions, which are divided into two groups: food allergies and food intolerances.

- *Food allergies* involve an immune-mediated reaction, usually to a glycoprotein found in the food.
- *Food intolerances* are any adverse physiologic responses to a food product and can be due to the presence of a toxic substance (e.g., food poisoning) or to pharmacologic properties (e.g., a headache from tyramine in cheese and wine). Some food intolerances are classified as disorders (such as lactose intolerance, celiac disease, gout, cholelithiasis, and gastroesophageal reflux disease), but others are more idiosyncratic in nature. The existence of a relationship between food intolerances and various diseases continues to be controversial.

Elimination diets have been most thoroughly evaluated when used to treat attention deficit-hyperactive disorder (ADHD), atopic dermatitis, irritable bowel disease, migraine headache, otitis media, and rheumatoid arthritis. When done properly and safely, the elimination diet is a simple way to determine whether foods affect an individual's health (Rindfleisch, 2007).

The typical elimination diet involves four phases:

1. During the *planning phase*, a thorough client history and dietary log are evaluated, and specific foods are identified for elimination.

2. The *avoidance phase* can involve low-, moderate-, or high-intensity elimination diets. Low-intensity elimination diets eliminate only a few foods or food groups; moderate-intensity diets eliminate multiple foods or food groups; and high-intensity elimination diets allow only the foods on a specific list.
3. During the *challenge phase*, small quantities of specific foods are reintroduced to the diet every 3–4 days. The reintroduced food is eaten for only 1 day and then it is eliminated again as other foods on the list are reintroduced.
4. The final phase involves *creating a long-term diet plan.*

The usual approach is to continue the elimination diet for at least 3–6 months, after which another challenge with the eliminated foods can be attempted (Rindfleisch, 2007).

Anti-inflammatory Diet

Chronic diseases affect more than 90 million Americans and are believed to account for 70% of all deaths and more than 75% of the nation's medical care costs. Inflammation is at the root of these health conditions, which include cardiovascular disease, cancer, stroke, and Alzheimer's disease. While the body has complex biochemical processes that have evolved as part of the body's defense mechanism and cause inflammation, at times these processes occur in excess and cause disease rather than promote healing (Rakel & Rindfleisch, 2007). Traditional allopathic treatment often involves medications to reduce inflammation or suppress the symptoms caused by inflammation (such as narcotics for pain control or antipyretics for a fever). However, dietary modifications may actually address the underlying cause of the problem and may result in fewer side effects.

Current research into the mechanisms suspected of influencing inflammation demonstrates that some foods contribute to the production of highly reactive compounds that can lead to significant inflammation and tissue damage; these same compounds can also help prevent infection. However, in individuals who take a lot of antioxidant supplements, the research shows an increase in inflammation, indicating that a high use of individual antioxidant supplements may not be as helpful as a *diet* with a varied mix of antioxidant-rich foods that protect against free radicals (Rakel & Rindfleisch, 2007).

Other studies have demonstrated a link between diets with a high dietary glycemic load and elevated inflammation in women. Type 2 diabetes mellitus also seems to be preceded by elevated inflammation markers. Levels of insulin can be dramatically affected by the foods a person eats, particularly foods with highly processed grains. Finally, certain foods and dietary supplements contain compounds that inhibit inflammation by acting on specific chemical pathways in the body. Turmeric, for example, is one of those (Rakel & Rindfleisch, 2007).

NUTRACEUTICALS

While scientists still recommend that people try to get as many nutrients as possible through a variety of nutrient-rich foods, this is not always possible for many reasons: a reduced-calorie diet, a dislike of certain foods, nutrient loss through cooking, a lack of knowledge or motivation, a lack of time to plan and prepare a balanced meal, and nutrient depletion because of stress, lifestyle, and certain medications (Trivieri & Anderson, 2002). Average Americans consume 18% of their calories from refined sugar, which is devoid of any vitamins or minerals. Another 18% of their diet consists of refined products that are particularly deficient in vitamin B (Luck, 2005).

Nutraceuticals are extracts of foods—usually in capsule, tablet, or powdered form in a prescribed dose—that are claimed to have a medicinal or physiological benefit or to provide protection against a chronic disease. Examples include antioxidants, phytonutrients, and supplements.

Antioxidants

Antioxidants are compounds that naturally protect the body from free radical damage and help depress the effects of metabolic by-products or environmental factors and toxins that cause degenerative changes related to aging. When the body uses oxygen to produce energy, the oxygen sometimes reacts with body compounds to produce unstable molecules with unpaired electrons (free radicals). Unpaired electrons are highly reactive and need to pair with other electrons to return to a stable state. Antioxidants neutralize free radicals by donating one of their electrons (Leddy, 2006).

Free radicals can result from improper nutrition, fatty foods, smoking, drinking, taking drugs, carcinogens, iron, smog, radiation, herbicides, and pesticides. They play a critical role in protecting or delaying the onset of cancers, heart disease, arthritis, stroke, immune problems, and premature aging. Although free radicals can be helpful in the body, at higher levels they can damage cells and tissues. Left unchecked, they damage cell structure, impair cell function, and damage DNA, leaving the body susceptible to viruses and bacteria. Free radical formation and the resulting damage are referred to as oxidative stress (Leddy, 2006).

Antioxidants are the body's protector nutrients. Vitamins A, B, C, E, and selenium assist the enzymes in fighting free radical damage (Eliopoulos, 2004).

Phytonutrients

Phytonutrients (or phytochemicals) are compounds that exist naturally in all plants and give foods that come from those plants their color, flavor, and aroma. Phytonutrients are biologically active and nonnutritive; they are not vitamins or minerals but they assist the immune system, act as antioxidants, balance hormone levels, and can protect against cancer (Leddy, 2006).

Phytochemicals are stored in plants as a result of complex interactions between the sun, soil, air, and water, and they exist as a result of the plant's own growth. Each plant can contain hundreds, maybe thousands, of different phytochemicals in various combinations. Examples of foods with these components include fruits, vegetables, grains, seeds, soy, licorice, and green tea. Phytoestrogens, soy, tomatoes, grapes, blueberries, cherries, whole grains, legumes, garlic, onions, cherries, tea, parsley, broccoli, and cauliflower all have these phytochemicals (Eliopoulos, 2004; Leddy, 2006).

Supplements

Supplements include vitamins, minerals, and other food factors that support good health and prevent or treat illness.

Years ago, when crop-growing soil was rich in nutrients, people widely believed that supplements were not necessary if they ate well-balanced meals. Nowadays, however, the soil is less nutrient rich, many individuals do not eat a balanced diet, and foods contain many other toxins and additives (Seaward, 2006). As a result, although the supplement industry is still in its infancy, it is growing exponentially because many people now believe they can make up for a poor diet by taking a multivitamin pill. Nutritional supplements have become a major business in the United States, where an estimated 80% of adults take them, many on a daily basis (Leddy, 2006; Trivieri & Anderson, 2002). Like other nutrients, supplements can be helpful or harmful. They are not a substitute for a healthy, sensible diet (Eliopoulos, 2004).

Forms of Supplements

Supplements can be purchased over the counter, over the Internet, by mail, and at many retail outlets. They come in many forms: tablets, capsules, soft gels, powders, and liquids. The United States Pharmacopeia (USP) oversees drug products and sets the standards for dietary supplements. All supplements require labels. The daily value (DV) listed on a label refers to the percentage of the recommended daily amount of a nutrient that one serving of the supplement provides. Individuals should receive 100% of the recommended nutrients each day; if they receive less, they need to determine whether they can meet the need through a dietary change. If they cannot, then supplementation may be necessary (Eliopoulos, 2004).

Not all supplements are created equal. They can be synthesized or crystallized, either of which involves heating, which can result in the loss of much of the supplement's beneficial qualities. They can also be freeze-dried or whole foods, and these are the best forms for absorption.

When taken in concentrated form, vitamins, minerals, and protein supplements can actually block the absorption of other essential nutrients. Individuals should consult a registered dietitian before taking supplements (Seaward, 2006).

Bacteria: Friend or Foe?

The body contains several trillion beneficial bacteria (totaling almost 2 pounds per person and comprising over 400 species) that are all necessary for health. Many of these "friendly" bacteria, also called probiotics, live in the intestines, where they are essential to the effective assimilation of nutrients. The most common are *Lactobacillus acidophilus* and *Bifidobacteria*. These friendly bacteria inhibit or kill pathogenic intestinal microbes such as *Salmonella*, *Shigella*, *Klebsiella*, *Pseudomonas*, *Vibrio*, and *Candida*. Prior to 1945, most Americans did not eat many processed foods and they got the necessary probiotics from their diet. Now supplementation of these bacteria may be necessary for people with an inadequate intake of fruits and vegetables (Orenstein, 2002; Trivieri & Anderson, 2002). The benefits attributed to healthy flora include lower cholesterol levels, partial relief from lactose intolerance, production of B-complex vitamins, control of bad breath and body odor, and possibly the relief of gastrointestinal symptoms such as diarrhea, constipation, and gas (Orenstein, 2002).

MODERN NUTRITION ISSUES

Today's consumers are increasingly aware of the importance of sound nutrition and its relationship to health, yet many believe that eating nutritiously means making sacrifices. The media contributes to this belief by overloading people with information about fast foods and specific foods, emphasizing preparation time rather than nutritional value. In addition, malnutrition, the social pressures to achieve a distorted body image, and obesity remain significant problems for youth and adolescents, as well as for adults, across all socioeconomic groups in the world today (Leddy, 2006).

Salguero (2007) states that "from 5% to almost half of the general population experiences suboptimal nutrient intake" (p. 26). While our hunter-gatherer and even our agricultural ancestors enjoyed natural foods, the diets of 20th-century human beings have been very different. Even 100 years ago, much of our food was unprocessed and unrefined; it was grown on clean, living (often virgin) soil with fresh air and pure water. No preservatives, pesticides, chemicals, or additives were used (Trivieri & Anderson, 2002).

Modern technology has tried to "improve" foods by using artificial chemicals, including pesticides, fungicides, ripening agents, and fumigants, all designed to make food grow more quickly so it can be shipped and stored more efficiently. Genetic engineering has changed the biological structure of plants in ways not fully understood. Some plants are irradiated (flooded with what is touted as harmless radiation) to lengthen shelf life. Animals are dosed with antibiotics and hormones to prevent disease and fatten them. Artificial sweeteners, "fake fats," and processed foods continue to raise questions about their safety. Many Americans sit down to a daily breakfast of pesticide-laden coffee and pastries made of refined flour, sugar, and margarine. They run to a fast food restaurant or grab a pre-made meal for lunch, and they cook frozen sauces and soups or chemically and hormonally treated meat for dinner (Trivieri & Anderson, 2002). The effects of all these processes on the human body are not fully known (Micozzi, 2006).

Toxins in the Food Chain

One of the greatest long-term problems faced by nutrition-conscious individuals is the pervasive use of contaminants in food. The Food and Drug Administration (FDA) and other government agencies have allowed the food industry to grow and process foods using hundreds of chemicals of questionable safety, including pesticides, herbicides, growth hormones, additives, stabilizers, and antibiotics. Many well-known experts in the field now believe that a lifetime of ingesting these can lead to cancers, neurotoxicity, birth defects, decreased immune function, food allergies, and chemical sensitivities (Trivieri & Anderson, 2002). They now recommend eating foods that are as low on the food chain as possible. For example, animals are high on the food chain and are often given growth hormones and antibiotics. In addition, the foods they consume are often sprayed with pesticides. Plants, which are lower on the food chain, are relatively less contaminated (Trivieri & Anderson, 2002).

Pesticides

Over 400 pesticides are currently licensed for use on foods. Every year, over 2.5 billion pounds are dumped on crops, forests, lawns, and fields, yet many of the pesticides and chemicals used in and on foods have never been tested for human safety. If a couple going out for dinner has a salad, a meat or fish main course, and dessert, the chances are high that they have consumed several types of pesticides. If they have a glass of wine or several glasses of water with their meal, they may ingest several more pesticides.

At present, the Office of Pesticide Programs at the Environmental Protection Agency does not count multiple exposures to the same pesticide when they calculate permitted levels. If they did, the totals could, at times, exceed 500% of the allowed daily intake. These "chemical cocktails" have demonstrated life-threatening and lethal effects in animal studies but, for obvious reasons, have not been tested in humans (Trivieri & Anderson, 2002).

Growth Hormones

The most common growth hormone is recombinant bovine growth hormone (BGH), which the FDA originally approved as a genetically engineered, synthetic version of the hormone naturally produced by cows. Recombinant BGH was designed to increase milk production by as much as 25%, which is economically unnecessary since American dairy farmers already produce a surplus of milk. The hormone is injected twice a month into approximately 30% of all milk-producing cows.

Some research has suggested links between BGH and prostate and breast cancers. The FDA does not require labeling of BGH-laced products (including yogurt, cheese, and other dairy products), and milk producers are not required to label their products as free of BGH even when they are (Trivieri & Anderson, 2002).

Additives

There are approximately 2,000 food-permitted additives (including artificial colors and flavors, stabilizing agents, texturizers, sweeteners, antimicrobials, and antioxidants) in the U.S. food supply. Red dye number 3 may interfere with brain neurotransmitters, and blue dyes number 1 and 2 are believed to be carcinogenic. Reducing the intake of nitrites, sugar, and other additives has shown to reduce adolescent antisocial behavior and raise test scores in schools (Trivieri & Anderson, 2002).

Irradiation

Irradiation kills insects, bacteria, molds, and fungi; prevents the sprouting of foods; and extends their shelf life. Irradiation also leads to the formation of toxic substances such as benzene and formaldehyde and has been shown to produce a higher incidence of tumors in mice than those fed nonradiated food.

While foods irradiated as a whole are required to be labeled with the distinct radiation symbol, irradiated ingredients within foods do not require such labeling (Trivieri & Anderson, 2002).

Genetically Altered Foods

Genetically engineered organisms (GEOs), or "Frankenfoods," are foods that have been genetically engineered in a process that alters their genetic code and often involves combining them with genes of dissimilar and unrelated species (Seaward, 2006; Trivieri & Anderson, 2002). In 2000, food scientists spliced a unique gene from a flounder into the DNA of tomatoes and the genes of Brazil nuts into the DNA of corn. The scientists went further by combining Roundup (a synthetic pesticide) with the DNA of corn, resulting in the mysterious death of thousands of migrating monarch butterflies and the recall of corn taco shells from Taco John restaurants and of corn flakes from the Kellogg Company (Seaward, 2006).

Foods are genetically altered to produce never-before-seen genetic combinations that can often be grown, transported, and stored for longer periods of time without losing the appearance of freshness. Only a small number of GEOs are created to improve nutritional value, yet over 65% of foods found in grocery stores have been genetically modified. Almost no safety testing has been done on these foods, and they don't have to be labeled as such (Trivieri & Anderson, 2002). One danger of GEOs occurs in people who are sensitive to a specific food and may not know they have ingested it. Because of the possibility of severe allergic reactions to such foods, choose whole foods with "certified organic" on their labels (Seaward, 2006).

Food Allergies

Approximately 108 million people have allergies, and 30 million of them have food-related allergies (Orenstein, 2002). Food allergies are considered the second most common type of ingested allergy. The great majority are to cow's milk, eggs, soybeans, chocolate, citrus, wheat, shellfish, food additives and preservatives, yeast, and corn (Micozzi, 2006).

The development of a food allergy is usually related to incomplete protein digestion. If the food is not properly broken down, the component parts are absorbed and perceived by the body's immune system as foreign substances. Repeated exposure to these food antigens sensitizes the immune system, resulting in a food sensitivity and food allergy.

How people experience a food allergy (e.g., headache or abdominal cramps) is largely determined by their genetic makeup (Orenstein, 2002).

Some theorize a possible psychological component and assert that, on some deep level, allergy sufferers may view the world as a hostile place due, for example, to a history of abuse (Micozzi, 2006).

SPIRITUAL NUTRITION

Nutrition is actually quite closely related to spirituality. Many people give thanks before beginning a meal. Eating can be a social or religious occasion that connects people to each other and often to their higher source (if they so believe). Several Eastern cultures believe that energy centers (chakras) run from the base of the spine to the top of the head, and Ayurvedic medicine suggests that people should eat specific foods and vegetables that correspond to these energy centers. Taoist philosophy advocates finding balance in food.

Gabriel Cousens, MD, founder and director of the Tree of Life Foundation, suggested eating in ways that support healthy living and being more harmonious with plants and the planet. His suggestions include (Seaward, 2006):

- Eating a variety of foods of all colors
- Avoiding big meals prior to meditation
- Undereating as a rule
- Drinking plenty of water to cleanse the body
- Getting plenty of sunlight and fresh air
- Achieving a good acid/alkaline balance in the diet (in terms of foods)
- Being fully present while eating, noting the taste, texture, temperature, and origin of the food (that is, being mindful of a spiritual experience)

HERBS AND HERBALISM

Modern medical miracles have provided antibiotics, magnetic resonance imaging (MRI) machines, laser surgery, organ transplants, and many other life-saving devices. However, these amazing advances have often made people lose sight of the history of healing. Humans have not always looked to technology to heal. During much of human existence, people relied on a connectedness to nature and its healing powers. Nature was part of everyday life, and people were intimately familiar with it. Plants, for example, have been used by humans for food, medicine, clothing, and tools, as well as in religious ceremonies, since before recorded history. Most traditional belief systems consider plants a gift of nature and access to them a basic human right. Even the World Health Organization (WHO) refers to herbs as "people's medicines."

For centuries, people believed that each herbal plant contained a sign left by God, intended to give humanity clues to its healing effects. This ancient philosophy, called the Doctrine of Signatures, said that God marked everything with a sign or signature designating its purpose. The Doctrine of Signatures indicates that plants have parts that resemble and are relevant to human body parts, animals, or objects. An example is the goldenseal, whose yellow-green root indicates its use for jaundice or lobelia and whose flowers are shaped like a stomach, reflecting its antiemetic properties (Freeman, 2004).

Throughout the last century, people lost much of their connectedness to nature as knowledge and fascination with the natural world took a back seat to advancements centered more on tools and equipment. This worldview is changing. With a renewed interest in less invasive, more holistic approaches to health care, people are rediscovering what is sometimes in their own backyards.

Definitions

The term *herb* originated with the Latin word *herba*, which refers to green crops and grasses. English use of the term can be traced to the 13th century, when it denoted a plant whose stem does not become woody but remains more or less soft and succulent, or one that dies to the ground or dies entirely after flowering (Leddy, 2006; Micozzi & Meserole, 2006).

Micozzi and Meserole (2006) define *herbalism* as "the study and practice of using plant material for food, medicine, and health promotion. This includes not only treatment of disease but also enhancement of quality of life, physically and spiritually" (p. 164). The use of herbs has been called the "art of simpling." Herbs were known as "simples" since a single herb could be used to treat many different health problems (Freeman, 2004; Tierra, 1998).

The term *herbalist* is now used to refer to early writers about plants as well as to someone who uses alternative medical therapy. Micozzi and Meserole (2006) define an *herbalist* or *herbal practitioner* as "someone who has undertaken specific study and supervised practical training to achieve competence in treating patients" (p. 164). Tierra (1998) adds that "the path of the herbalist is a cultivated attitude toward nature and all of creation" (p. xxiii). Herbalists view nature as a positive force, a provider, and a teacher.

The History of Herbalism

Flowers and herbs have formed the basis of medicine since the dawn of human history. For example, salicylic acid was derived from willow bark (Holt & Kouzi, 2002). Approximately 75% of all conventional medicines are derived from living plants (Airey & Houdret, 2006; Leddy, 2006). The word *drug* is derived from the old Dutch word *droog* meaning "to dry" because pharmacists, physicians, and ancient healers often dried the plants they used in medicines (Trivieri & Anderson, 2002).

In the United States, more than half of all healthcare consumers are estimated to have used herbs, herbal preparations, or natural product supplements alone or in combination with conventional medicines. Approximately 80% of the world's people incorporate phytomedicine, the use of plants or plant parts for therapeutic purposes, as their primary form of health care, yet modern medicine has veered away from the use of herbs in treating health disorders. Reasons for this include economic issues (since herbs cannot be patented), and the fact that the therapeutic value of many of these products is unproven. Some products may interfere with prescription medications and some may be harmful to clients with particular conditions. Many consumers who use these products never mention their use to their healthcare providers (Eliopoulos, 2004; Skidmore-Roth, 2001; Trivieri & Anderson, 2002).

Herbal medicine is one of the most ancient forms of treatment, evolving with humanity and involving almost every major culture and even some animal species (Holt & Kouzi, 2002; Micozzi & Meserole, 2006; Shealy, 1996). For example, 60,000-year-old ritual burials of Neanderthal humans contain seeds and pollen of medicinal herbs that are still used today (Freeman, 2004; Holt & Kouzi, 2002; Micozzi & Meserole, 2006). There is historical information about herbal medicine dating back to 3000 BC and the ancient Egyptians, and more recently to the first century BC in ancient Greek and Chinese culture (Busby, 1996; Shealy, 1996). Asclepius, the legendary first physician of ancient Greece (ca.1500 BC) achieved fame through his mastery of surgical skills and a knowledge of the curative power of plants (Holt & Kouzi, 2002). Paracelsus, an alchemist in the 1500s, believed in the Doctrine of Signatures and became the founder of modern pharmaceutical medicine. He is best remembered for prescribing laudanum (tincture of opium) (Freeman, 2004). Chinese herb guides from 2700 BC list 365 medicinal plants and herbs. A Chinese drug encyclopedia, *Pen ts'ao kang mu*, lists over 2,000 natural products used for healing and was compiled by Li Shih-Chen and published in AD 1596.

The ancient Romans are believed to have first brought herbs to northern Europe and herbalism was nurtured there by many other cultures, including the Arabs (Busby, 1996; Shealy, 1996). A collection of hymns from before 1000 BC includes more than 1,000 healing herbs, and even the Old Testament mentions the use of mandrake, vetch, caraway, wheat, barley, and rye (Holt & Kouzi, 2002).

In the Middle Ages, herbal lore was created around superstition and the belief that people had one of four bodily humors (cheerful, sluggish, hot tempered, or gloomy). Herbs were believed to have their own characteristics and were often prescribed to address incorrect balances in the humors (Eliopoulos,

2004; Freeman, 2004). Much of the information about herbs during the Middle Ages was preserved by monks of the various monasteries via hand-copied manuscripts (Holt & Kouzi, 2002). With the advent of the printing press, all of this knowledge and information could be printed, studied, and exchanged and herbalism flourished. In the early 1600s, Nicholas Culpepper, an English pharmacist, published *The English Physician*, an herbal book recommending that people grow their own herbs (Freeman, 2004).

In 19th-century North America, a form of herbalism known as physiomedicalism (referring to the study of healing through the use of organic substances) became the basis for modern herbalism as we know it in the United States today. Physiomedicalism includes elements of traditional Native American plant knowledge and rural settlers' folklore remedies (Shealy, 1996). The early physicians of North America were not trained in formal medical schools for almost 200 years after the arrival of the colonists so Native American medicines were important. More than 200 Native American herbs were included in the first edition of the *U.S. Pharmacopoeia* in 1820 and in the *National Formulary* in 1888, and thousands more were used unofficially (Holt & Kouzi, 2002).

Even when doctors became commonplace, they were often sought only after the problems were considered too serious for self-care or home remedies to treat. During the 18th and 19th centuries, people became concerned about the credentials of medical providers and the organized medical community insisted on regulations to protect the public from "quacks"' such as medicine shows and patent medicines. In the early 1800s, the Eclectic Movement became popular in the United States and tried to bridge the gap between traditional medical concepts and traditional herbal medicine. In the mid 1800s, the medical system we know as *biomedicine* began to dominate conventional medicine in the United States. The American Medical Association was formed in 1847 and sponsored legislation supporting state licensing laws for practitioners.

The future of competing forms of medicine was sealed with the release of a report by Abraham Flexner, an educator and founder of the Institute for Advanced Study at Princeton, New Jersey. This report was instrumental in upgrading medical school education, focusing greater attention on biomedicine research, and obtaining philanthropic support for medical education. Flexner's report indirectly led to the demise of more financially constrained schools of alternative medicine and it effectively stifled all competing schools of thought regarding the origins of illness and appropriate therapies (Freeman, 2004). By the end of the 19th century, the general public became discouraged with natural products. The use of medicinal and folk medicine declined as the emphasis on scientific medicine escalated (Holt & Kouzi, 2002).

Herbalism Today

Today, there are an estimated one million drug products in the United States. More than 300,000 over-the-counter (OTC) products are available, manufactured by 12,000 firms and containing about 800 active ingredients (Holt & Kouzi, 2002). Yet in 2000 Americans spent approximately $4.3 billion on herbs (Skidmore-Roth, 2001).

Reasons to Use Herbs

Americans are interested in the use of herbs for a variety of reasons. The term *self-care* refers to anything people do for themselves and others to promote or improve health; this concept is deeply rooted in American culture. The cherished value of freedom and independence is one reason that healthcare professionals are criticized for their control of healthcare products. Americans still prefer self-care practices because the concepts are relatively simple and seem more harmonious with life. However, self-care practices can pose a threat if professional help is actually needed (Holt & Kouzi, 2002).

Another reason for the interest in herbs is that pharmaceuticals are increasingly overprescribed, expensive, and dangerous. Herbal remedies are perceived as safer (especially if they are labeled "natural") and less toxic. People are increasingly interested in holistic approaches to health and preventative treatments, and they are willing to self-prescribe, investigate, and use herbs as adjuncts to other treatments, especially if they have been diagnosed with cancer, AIDS, arthritis, or diabetes (Leddy, 2006; Skidmore-Roth, 2001). Herbs are regulated as foods rather than as drugs, and many people think that because they occur naturally they are devoid of risks (Holt & Kouzi, 2002).

Benefits and Principles of Herbalism

Herbs, when used properly, cause fewer and milder side effects than traditional drugs, and they pose less risk overall. They are also lower in cost than prescription drugs and are more easily available since they can be purchased without a prescription at a variety of retail outlets as well as over the Internet. Access is virtually unrestricted and unlimited (Eliopoulos, 2004; Skidmore-Roth, 2001; Tierra, 1998).

There is no single, worldwide system of herbalism, but all herbal traditions share common themes (Micozzi & Meserole, 2006). They seek to optimize health and wellness, emphasize the whole person and the community, individualize care, enhance the quality of life, and promote simple self-treatment and preventive self-care (Leddy, 2006). Most traditions include specific systems of food, spice, and herb taboos and recommended inclusions and adherence to these to protect both practitioners and users from unwanted consequences. Attention is paid to finding and treating the root cause of a problem, not just the symptoms. There is a strong belief in the principle of duality, which asserts that natural law is greater than the will of the individual or community and that healing requires the healer, client, and community to be in alignment with natural forces (Micozzi & Meserole, 2006). Tierra (1998) asserts that when people use herbal therapy, "the body will become stronger and the individual will take the time to learn something about the factors that led to the disease in the first place, thus giving the opportunity to prevent reoccurrence" (p. xvi).

One of the key principles of herbalism is that of synergism, a belief that the strength of the sum of the parts is greater than the strength of the individual parts (Eliopoulos, 2004; Shealy, 1996). The herbalist may administer one or more herbs to bring the body back into balance, seeking to correct its underlying condition. This is in contrast with traditional drugs that are used mainly to treat symptoms without resolving the underlying health condition (Buhner, 2002; Eliopoulos, 2004; Skidmore-Roth, 2001; Tierra, 1998).

The premise that nature is inherently circular and repetitive leads to the common practice of offering a prayer in return for healing and a belief in the reality of the immeasurable and abstract. An openness to an exchange of knowledge, the regulation of the herbalist's practice through accountability, and humility on the part of the practitioner are essential (Micozzi & Meserole, 2006). Preventive care is promoted and guided, and simple treatments are utilized (Micozzi & Meserole, 2006). Of all the integrative health practices, "herbal medicine is probably the most popular, and the most ubiquitous" (Skidmore-Roth, 2001, p. x).

How Herbs Work

Herbs work in the same way as traditional pharmaceuticals: by means of their chemical constituents. Because herbs use an indirect route to the bloodstream and specific organs, their effects are usually slower in onset and less dramatic than the effects of purified drugs administered more directly. As a result, physicians and clients may become impatient with botanicals; however, their skillful selection and fewer side effects make herbs very effective in addressing chronic health issues (Trivieri & Anderson, 2002).

Most people are familiar with herbs used in cooking, such as basil, thyme, parsley, sage, mint, and chives. In fact, early botanic gardens started in Renaissance Italy and were called physic gardens because they were used to educate medical students of the day about medicinal plants. Physic gardens appeared in England in the 16th century and include the Oxford Physic Garden and the Chelsea Physic Garden.

Herbs, by definition, do not produce woody, persistent stems and they generally die back at the end of each growing season (Leddy, 2006), but in herbal medicine, herbs include a broader group of plants that are used to make medicine, spices, or aromatic oils for soaps and fragrances (Trivieri & Anderson, 2002). They occur naturally in many forms, including shrubs, flowering plants, trees, moss, lichen, fern, algae, seaweed, and fungus. The entire plant may be used as an herb or only specific parts can be utilized, like the flowers (marigolds and roses), fruits (lemons and rose hips), leaves, twigs, bark, roots, rhizomes, seeds, or exudates (such as tapped syrup). A combination of parts can also be used.

Nonplants are also used in many herbal traditions, and these include animal parts (bones, organs, and tissues), insects, animal or insect secretions, worm castings, shells, rocks, minerals, and gemstones (Leddy, 2006). Trivieri and Anderson (2002) note that "there are an estimated 250,000 to 500,000 plants on the earth today but only about 5,000 have been extensively studied for their medicinal applications" (p. 253). At this time, 121 prescription drugs come from only 90 species of plants, and 74% were discovered by listening to native folklore assertions. A jackpot of healing still waits to be discovered (Trivieri & Anderson, 2002).

Herb Production Process

While some herbs are used in their crude state, others go through various forms and degrees of refinement. Manufacturing processes vary widely, but the general steps used in herb production include the following (Skidmore-Roth, 2001).

- *Collecting/harvesting:* The natural harvesting of herbs is called wild crafting, but herbs can be harvested by hand or by machine. The time of harvest impacts the strength of the herb's properties, and the harvest method needs to ensure that the proper part of the plant is collected. Individuals who gather herbs on their own need to correctly identify the plant and be aware of possible chemical or pesticide use in areas where they pick.
- *Garbling:* The usable portion of the plant is separated from the nonusable portions or other materials, such as dirt and insect parts.
- *Drying:* Herbs are stored after harvesting to prevent the breakdown of their active components and contamination by microorganisms. Mild heat is used.
- *Grinding:* The herb is broken down mechanically into smaller pieces, ranging from coarse to fine depending on the intended use.

- *Extraction:* A solvent is used to separate the desired chemical components from the plant parts. In the United States, alcohol, water, a lipophilic solvent, or liquid carbon dioxide is often used. Extraction yields solutions such as tinctures, fluid extracts, or solid extracts.
- *Concentration:* Solutions produced by extraction may undergo evaporation to concentrate them and to remove the solvent, thus producing a pure extract.
- *Drying of extracts:* Freeze-drying or atomizing can dry extracts into a solid form. Once dried, these products are less susceptible to contamination by microorganisms.
- *Addition of excipients:* Herbal preparations are compounded into capsules or tablets using an inert ingredient such as starch.

Herb Preparation

Some herbs are used therapeutically or medicinally in a variety of forms such as whole plants, teas (infusions), decoctions (roots or barks simmered in water), capsules and tablets, tinctures (concentrated extracts of a herb in a solution of water and alcohol), elixirs, salves, balms, ointments, liniments, or infused oils. Herbs can also be added to bathwater for a therapeutic soak or to oils used for massage (Airey & Houdret, 2006).

- *Whole plants* are plants or plant parts that are dried and either cut or powdered. Some are used fresh, but they are highly perishable and so are not usually marketed this way.
- *Teas (infusions)* are either loose or in teabag form, dried, whole, or chopped. They are used to prepare the more delicate parts of the plants. Flowers, leaves, and powdered herbs (such as chamomile or peppermint) are infused while fruits, seeds, barks, and roots (such as rose hips, cinnamon bark, and licorice root) require decocting.
- *Decoctions* are simmered over low heat for about one hour and are stronger and more potent than teas. Distilled water is preferred, and glass or enamel containers best maintain the integrity of the medicine (Eliopoulos, 2004; Leddy, 2006; Tierra, 1998).
- *Capsules and tablets* are convenient forms of ingesting herbs without having to taste them. They may contain crushed, dried, or more concentrated powdered extracts (Eliopoulos, 2004).
- *Extracts and tinctures* provide a high concentration of the drug in low weight and space, making them easier to disintegrate and ingest. Fresh and dried herbs can be tinctured in alcohol, and some are put in vinegar. Others are active and well preserved as syrups, or glycerites (in veg-

etable glycerin). Extracts and tinctures are quickly assimilated by the body. Tinctures contain more alcohol than extracts. If the extract or tincture has known active ingredients, the strength is expressed in terms of the amount of active ingredient. Otherwise, it is expressed in terms of the concentration. Tinctures are usually a 1:5 concentration (one part herb, in grams, to five parts solvent). This expression does not provide an accurate measure of the potency because manufacturing techniques and the purity of raw materials vary.

- *Elixirs* are similar to tinctures except that they are sweet and use honey. They are often made with brandy and used as tonics (Leddy, 2006; Tierra, 1998; Trivieri & Anderson, 2002).
- *Salves, balms, poultices, and ointments* are made with dried herbs and vegetable oil or petroleum jelly (Trivieri & Anderson, 2002). Salves and ointments are semisolid preparations designed for application to the skin. They are not meant to blend into the skin but to form a protective outer layer that holds the medicine in place and prolongs the time the herb remains moist. They can also be called fomentations.
- *Liniments* are tinctures for external use only and they use isopropyl alcohol or sometimes vodka. They are prepared in the same way as tinctures, and the alcohol is quickly absorbed into the skin so the medicine is absorbed by the tissues.
- *Essential oils* are concentrated drops that are usually diluted in fatty oils or water before they are topically applied (Eliopoulos, 2004; Leddy, 2006; Tierra, 1998).

Herb Uses

Herbalists treat a wide variety of conditions in people of all ages. Herbal medicine is considered effective for many conditions including cardiovascular problems, migraines, and skin conditions. Treatment length varies according to individual needs; chronic problems can take several months to treat, while acute problems may respond within days to weeks (Busby, 1996).

The client's subjective experience is central to the diagnostic process, and a detailed case history is an important element of treatment. The case history provides the herbalist with a personal and social context for the individual's disease or illness.

Herbal treatments emphasize the individual's vital force, or life energy, and seek to mobilize the body's self-healing or homeostatic properties. The herbalist chooses plants that have either general actions (such as relaxants, tonics, and immune system enhancers) or specific actions (such as vasodilatory, hypertensive, anti-inflammatory, expectorant, and diuretic effects). Different portions of a prescription or parts of a single plant combine to produce a synergistic effect. For example, the aspirin-like salicylates of meadowsweet have anti-inflammatory actions that are buffered by other constituents that soothe and protect the mucosa of the digestive tract (Busby, 1996).

Because not all herbs are safe in all situations, there are some contraindications for their use. According to Busby (1996):

- Licorice should not be used for individuals with hypertension.
- Ginseng should not be taken by individuals with anxiety, tension, restlessness, or acute inflammation.
- Epilepsy cannot be effectively treated with herbs.
- Herbal treatment should be used only as a supportive treatment for those with mental illnesses or distress.
- Ephedra should be avoided by individuals using monoamine oxidase inhibitors (MAOIs)
- Some herbs containing cardioactive glycosides, such as lily of the valley, should not be prescribed in conjunction with digitalis as they potentiate each other.

Levels of Herbalists

There is currently no legally required standard training, official recognition, or licensing for herbalists in the United States or Canada, and training varies widely. Interested individuals can take weekend workshops or correspondence courses, or they can attend seminars or schools of herbalism. The American Herbalists Guild, established in 1989 and currently the only professional group of herbalists in the United States, bestows the title of Herbalists AHG on herbalists who have passed a peer-review process. Some naturopathic physicians who have graduated from 4-year accredited schools of naturopathic medicine use herbs and nutritional therapies as part of their practice (Leddy, 2006; Trivieri & Anderson, 2002).

Many types of practitioners have been trained in the use of herbs. According to Micozzi and Meserole (2006), each culture or medical system has different types. Most systems identify professional herbalists, lay herbalists, plant gatherer-growers, and medicine makers.

A professional herbalist undertakes formalized training or a long apprenticeship in plant and medical studies or in plant and spiritual or healing studies. This training includes extensive familiarity—or a relationship with—certain plants, including their identification, habitat, harvesting criteria, preparation, storage, therapeutic indications, contraindications, and dosing.

Herbalists may follow a family tradition or be selected at a young age to use plants as a healing aid. In the United States and Europe, this group includes officially trained medical herbalists, clinical herbalists, registered nurses, licensed naturopathic doctors specializing in botanical medicine, licensed acupuncturists, licensed Ayurvedic doctors, Native American herbalists and shamans, and Latin American curanderos (Leddy, 2006; Micozzi & Meserole, 2006).

Lay herbalists have a broad knowledge of plants used for health problems but do not have extensive training in medical or spiritual diagnosis and management. They can, however, evaluate medicinal plant quality, strength, uses, and doses (Leddy, 2006; Micozzi & Meserole, 2006).

Plant gatherers, plant growers, and medicine makers are like clinical pharmacists. Micozzi and Meserole (2006) explain, "In Chinese medicine, there is one specialist who produces and collects plants, one who processes and stores plants, and a clinical herbalist/doctor who prescribes the medicines" (p. 167). In systems where preparing and handling medicines are considered spiritual privileges, the medicines are handled only by the herbalist or healer (Micozzi & Meserole, 2006).

Although the unauthorized practice of medicine is illegal, professional nurses and physicians can use and prescribe herbs and botanical remedies, when authorized. As long as they have received the formal training and experience of a respected organization that provides exposure to the systems of herbology, licensed professional nurses can use herbs as a part of a plan to promote a client's well-being and quality of life (Leddy, 2006).

Systems of Herbology

Several healthcare systems use herbology.

- Traditional Chinese Medicine (TCM) focuses on restoring harmony in the body and gives medicines in balanced formulas rather than singly. In TCM, herbs are classified according to their energies, temperature (hot, warm, neutral, cool, or cold), and tastes. Each taste (such as bitter or sweet) has a particular medicinal action and can indicate the organ to which it has a natural affinity.
- Ayurvedic medicine is governed by three doshas (bioenergetic forces that determine an individual's physical constitution). The purpose of herbology is to balance the doshas, and herbal formulas are based on regulating the doshas.
- Western medicine views medicines as "magic bullets" and typically prescribes herbs individually according to their pharmacological (chemical) actions.

- Native American medicine supports respect for all living things and believes that an herb's therapeutic properties cannot be reduced to the sum of its qualities. Native American medicine emphasizes the physical and spiritually purifying and cleansing properties of herbs (Leddy, 2006; Shealy, 1996).

Actions of Herbs

Herbs can act in numerous ways. They can be (Eliopoulos, 2004; Leddy, 2006; Tierra, 1998; Trivieri & Anderson, 2002):

- *Adaptogenic:* They increase resilience and resistance to stress and enable the body to adapt to a problem. Adaptogens support the adrenal glands.
- *Alterative:* They gradually restore functioning of the blood (also known as blood purifiers).
- *Analgesic:* They relieve pain without causing loss of consciousness.
- *Antacid:* They neutralize excess acids in the stomach and intestines.
- *Anthelminitic:* They destroy or expel intestinal worms.
- *Anti-inflammatory:* They directly soothe or reduce tissue inflammation.
- *Antimicrobial (or antibiotic):* They destroy or resists pathogenic microorganisms and strengthens the body's resistance to infection.
- *Antispasmodic:* They ease cramps in smooth and skeletal muscles.
- *Antipyretic:* They reduce or prevent fevers.
- *Astringent:* They reduce irritation; create a barrier against infection; and have a binding action on mucous membranes, skin, and other tissues.
- *Bitter:* They stimulate appetite and digestive juices, aid in liver detoxification, and increase bile flow.
- *Carminative:* They stimulate the digestive system to work easily and properly and they soothe the gut wall and inflammation.
- *Demulcent:* They reduce irritation in the entire bowel, prevent diarrhea, and reduce gastric muscle spasms.
- *Diuretic:* They increase production and elimination of urine and support body cleansing.
- *Emetic:* They induce vomiting and cause the stomach to empty.
- *Emmenagogue:* They stimulate menstrual flow and support female reproductive function.
- *Emollient:* They soothe, soften, and protect the skin.
- *Expectorant:* They stimulate removal of mucus from the lungs, soothe bronchial spasms, and loosen secretions.
- *Hepatic:* They tone and strengthen the liver and can increase the flow of bile.

- *Hypertensive:* They lower blood pressure.
- *Laxative:* They promote bowel movements and either provide bulk, stimulate bile production, or trigger peristalsis.
- *Nervine:* They strengthen and restore the nervous system and reduce anxiety and tension.
- *Rubefacient:* They increase blood flow to the surface of the skin and produce redness where applied.
- *Sedative:* They quiet the nervous system.
- *Stimulating:* They quicken the metabolic and physiologic activity of the body.
- *Tonic:* They nurture and enliven the body, often as a preventative measure.
- *Vulnerary:* They encourage the healing of wounds by promoting cell growth and repair.

KEY CONCERNS

The key concerns regarding herbs and herbalism include the following:

- Limitations of current research
- Lack of regulation
- Lack of standardization among herbs and herb preparation
- Potential toxicity related to collection, harvesting, preparation, and administration

Limitations of the Research

Because of the exploding interest in this field and the rapidly increasing use of herbs by the general public, more and more efforts are being paid to their scientific study (Micozzi & Meserole, 2006; Skidmore-Roth, 2001). The amount of information available to healthcare providers about herbs and their effects is increasing but scanty because primary research is limited in the United States; much of the research exists outside the country and in languages other than English. The available information is anecdotal and largely unscientific, and it has not been subject to the same rigorous controls and replicative studies that prescription and over-the-counter drugs undergo. Inconsistencies in research designs and protocols among the various countries complicate the matter further.

Conducting research in a holistic context is essential and requires creative funding that is not likely to provide high-profit returns to a single source. Research on crude or extracted traditional plant remedies, however, is relatively inexpensive when compared to traditional drug development costs (Micozzi & Meserole, 2006).

Lack of Regulation

Skidmore-Roth (2001) notes that "lack of regulation is probably the single biggest factor affecting the reliability of commercial herbal products in the United States" (p. xiv). In the United States, clinical trials are used to demonstrate the safety, efficacy, and reliability of drugs. Expensive and time consuming, clinical trials can take anywhere from 8 to 18 years and cost hundreds of millions of dollars. As a result, manufacturers want to patent their products to recover their investment and make a profit. Naturally occurring herbs cannot be patented, so no economic incentive exists and only limited research is underway on whole plants or crude extracts (Freeman, 2004; Skidmore-Roth, 2001).

In the United States, the Food and Drug Act of 1906 addresses the quality issue of medicinal drugs. The Federal Food, Drug, and Cosmetic Act of 1938 addresses safety, and a 1962 amendment to the 1938 act requires proof of therapeutic efficacy. European and American phytomedical manufacturers petitioned the FDA to allow well-researched European herbs the status of "old drugs" so they would not have to undergo the prohibitively expensive new drug application process; to date, the FDA has not responded (Freeman, 2004).

Medicinal herbs are regulated as dietary supplements under the Dietary Supplement Health and Education Act (DSHEA) of 1994, which was amended in 1998. Medicinal herbs are considered safe unless proven unsafe by the Food and Drug Administration (FDA). Manufacturers are permitted to provide information about their herbs but are not allowed to endorse any particular product. The information may not be misleading, and it must be physically separated from the product. No medical claims are allowed on dietary supplement labels; the labels can state only the structure and function of the product. Labels must clearly contain directions for use, warnings, side effects, contraindications, safety data, and describe the properties of the product (Freeman, 2004; Holt & Kouzi, 2002; Skidmore-Roth, 2001). They must state that the product is a dietary supplement, contain a disclaimer that the FDA has not evaluated any health claims, and state, "This product is not intended to diagnose, treat, cure, or prevent any disease" (Skidmore-Roth, 2001).

Given the lack of regulation, the content and quality of active chemical constituents can vary widely from manufacturer to manufacturer (Holt & Kouzi, 2002). This is partly due to the fact that the way an herb is grown, harvested, processed, and stored affects its strength and quality. Some manufacturers voluntarily adhere to so-called good manufacturing practices (GMPs), but herbal products can be produced without meeting these compliance standards, and they can be marketed without prior approval of their efficacy and safety by the FDA (Leddy, 2006; Micozzi & Meserole, 2006; Skidmore-Roth, 2001).

The U.S. government has not supported the quality control or patenting of herbs because herbs have not been "discovered" and drug companies are therefore not motivated to invest much in testing or promoting them. There is also a limited supply of well-educated botanists and traditional healers and only a handful of ethnobotanists who can catalog the medicinal properties of plants (Leddy, 2006). Herbal medicine in the United States has therefore yet to be subjected to the same level of scientific scrutiny as traditional medical treatments and, as a result, has not gained wide acceptance by mainstream medicine. This might be one of the reasons that clients do not disclose their use to their healthcare practitioners (Skidmore-Roth, 2001).

In Europe, herbs are more readily accepted than in the United States. The *British Herbal Pharmacopoeia*, although not officially recognized by Parliament, is still the accepted publication in the field (Trivieri & Anderson, 2002). Germany is probably the world leader in developing herbal safety and efficacy (Freeman, 2004), and the German Commission E monographs are considered to be the definitive source of information on herbs. Commission E is a German governmental body like our FDA and is comprised of healthcare professionals including physicians, pharmacists, pharmacologists, and toxicologists, as well as representatives of the pharmaceutical industry and laypersons. The German Federal Health Agency established the commission in 1978 and charged it with investigating the safety and efficacy of herbal remedies. In 1998, the German Commission E's recommendations became available in English. As of 2001, 400 herbs had published monographs on them. The Commission E monographs are considered the most authoritative herbal evaluations currently available. German law allows manufacturers to market herbs with drug claims if the herb has proven safe and effective, and prescriptions for herbs in Germany are reimbursable by insurance (Freeman, 2004; Holt & Kouzi, 2002; Skidmore-Roth, 2001; Trivieri & Anderson, 2002).

The European Economic Community (EEC) developed a set of guidelines that outline standards for the quality, quantity, and production of herbal remedies and set forth labeling requirements for member countries to meet. These guidelines state that a substance's historical use is a valid way to document safety and efficacy in the absence of any contradictory scientific evidence. In Europe, herbal remedies fall into three categories (Leddy, 2006):

- *Prescription drugs*, which include injectable forms of phytomedicines (from plant sources) and those used to treat life-threatening diseases (This group is the most rigorously controlled.)
- *Over-the-counter (OTC) phytomedicines*
- *Herbal remedies*, including products that have not undergone rigorous clinical testing but have not demonstrated any serious incidents

In 1989, Europe formed the European Scientific Cooperative on Phytotherapy (ESCOP) to achieve consistent regulation of all drugs, including herbs. It has been developing monographs similar to Germany's, based on sound clinical and scientific evidence. Eventually, these monographs are slated to be integrated into the European Pharmacopeia (Skidmore-Roth, 2001; Trivieri & Anderson, 2002).

In China, herbal medicine is the backbone of the medicinal system. In 1984, the People's Republic of China implemented the Drug Administration Law, which characterized traditional herbal preparations as "old drugs," exempt from testing for efficacy or side effects. New herbal products are overseen by the Chinese Ministry of Public Health (Leddy, 2006).

Developing countries have minimal regulation and oversight regarding the use of their herbal remedies, even though they are a staple of medical treatment.

Many believe U.S. herbal regulations should be as liberal as those in Europe.

Lack of Standardization

When, where, and how an herb is grown can greatly affect the strength of its chemical components. Habitat, ambient temperature, rainfall, hours of daylight at the latitude where the plant is grown, altitude, wind conditions, and soil characteristics can all influence an herb's quality and potency. In addition, whether an herb is grown naturally in its native habitat or cultivated affects its potency (Micozzi and Meserole, 2006; Skidmore-Roth, 2001).

Complicating the standardization concern is the fact that healers often use crude drugs or unprocessed herbs (Leddy, 2006). Most herbs do not yet have standardized doses, and manufacturers do not always produce preparations with consistent strengths. Crude herbs can vary in chemical composition from batch to batch or from plant to plant, and even herbalists themselves disagree about dosages. Current research is insufficient to allow standardization (Skidmore-Roth, 2001).

Understanding the names of herbs can also be complicated since many names can be associated with a given plant, and in some cases a given name can refer to several species of plants. There is lack of agreement even in the scientific community about the formal names of plants (Holt & Kouzi, 2002).

Potential Toxicity

Herbs must be used with care. Many are toxic if used incorrectly; for example, one herb that is safe to use topically can be highly toxic if taken internally. Some herbs contain potent liver toxins, systemic toxins, carcinogens, mutagens, or teratogens. Special consideration needs to be given when treating pediatric, geriatric, or pregnant clients. The effects of herbs on children, for example, are mainly unknown and a few are outright dangerous. Commercial preparation may introduce toxic substances during the manufacturing process and, because of the lack of standardization, pose a real threat (Skidmore-Roth, 2001).

Americans have been conditioned to rely on synthetic, commercial drugs to provide quick relief. Herbal products can interact with either prescription or nonprescription drugs, and consumers often don't tell their healthcare providers about herbal therapies they are taking. "Natural" does not mean safe (Leddy, 2006). Although clients often self-diagnose and self-administer herbal products, the safest course of action is to use herbal preparations only under the supervision of a trained herbalist and to disclose all herbal medications to the healthcare provider.

All these concerns hold many challenges for the future of biodiversity and herbalism.

KEY CONCEPTS

1. For as long as humans have been alive, food has played a spiritual, geographic, economic, physiological, and social role. Food habits and associations are learned early in life and tend to be long lasting and difficult to change.
2. Flowers and herbs have formed the basis of medicine since the dawn of human history. Herbal medicine is one of the most ancient forms of treatment, evolving with humanity and involving almost every major culture and even some animal species.
3. Key concerns regarding herbs and herbalism include the limitations of current research; the lack of regulation; the lack of standardization of herbs and herb preparations; and the potential toxicity related to collection, harvesting, preparation, and administration.

QUESTIONS FOR REFLECTION

1. How does food affect people's health?
2. How do the toxins in the food chain potentially affect health?
3. What are the key concerns regarding herbs, herbalism, and nutraceuticals?

REFERENCES

Airey, R., & Houdret, J. (2006). *Natural healing therapies.* London: Anness.

Buhner, S. H. (2002). *The lost language of plants: The ecological importance of plant medicines to life on earth.* White River Junction, VT: Chelsea Green.

Busby, H. (1996). Herbal medicine. In D. F. Rankin-Box (Ed.), *The nurses' handbook of complementary therapies* (pp. 91–97). Edinburgh: Churchill Livingstone.

Eliopoulos, C. (2004). *Invitation to holistic health: A guide to living a balanced life.* Sudbury, MA: Jones and Bartlett.

Freeman, L. (2004). *Mosby's complementary and alternative medicine: A research-based approach* (2nd ed.). St. Louis, MO: Mosby.

Holt, G. A., & Kouzi, S. (2002). Herbs through the ages. In M. A. Bright, *Holistic health and healing* (pp. 135–160). Philadelphia: F. A. Davis.

Leddy, S. K. (2006). *Integrative health promotion: Conceptual bases for nursing practice* (2nd ed.). Sudbury, MA: Jones and Bartlett.

Luck, S. (2005). Nutrition. In B. M. Dossey, L. Keegan, & C. E. Guzzetta, *Holistic nursing: A handbook for practice* (4th ed., pp. 451–475). Sudbury, MA: Jones and Bartlett.

Micozzi, M. S. (2006). Nutrition. In M. S. Micozzi, *Fundamentals of complementary and integrative medicine* (3rd ed., pp. 256–268). St. Louis, MO: Saunders Elsevier.

Micozzi, M. S., & Meserole, L. (2006). Herbal medicine. In M. S. Micozzi (Ed.), *Fundamentals of complementary and integrative medicine* (3rd ed., pp.164–180). St. Louis, MO: Saunders Elsevier.

Orenstein, N. S. (2002). Nutrition. In M. A. Bright, *Holistic health and healing* (pp. 121–133). Philadelphia: F. A. Davis.

Rakel, D., & Rindfleisch, J. A. (2007). The anti-inflammatory diet. In D. Rakel, *Integrative medicine* (2nd ed., pp. 961–971). Philadelphia: Saunders Elsevier.

Rindfleisch, J. A. (2007). Adverse food reactions and the elimination diet. In D. Rakel, *Integrative medicine* (2nd ed., pp. 941–950). Philadelphia: Saunders Elsevier.

Salguero, M. L. (2007). Environment and gene expression. In D. Rakel, *Integrative medicine* (2nd ed., pp. 23–30). Philadelphia: Saunders Elsevier.

Seaward, B. L. (2006). *Managing stress: Principles and strategies for health and well-being* (5th ed.). Sudbury, MA: Jones and Bartlett.

Shealy, C. N. (Ed.). (1996). *The complete family guide to alternative medicine: An illustrated encyclopedia of natural healing.* Shaftesbury, Dorset, UK: Element Books.

Skidmore-Roth, L. (2001). *Mosby's handbook of herbs and natural supplements.* St. Louis, MO: Mosby.

Tierra, M. (1998). *The way of herbs.* New York: Pocket Books.

Trivieri, L., Jr., & Anderson, J. W. (Eds.). (2002). *Alternative medicine: The definitive guide* (2nd ed.). Berkeley, CA: Celestial Arts.

CHAPTER 11

Therapeutic Massage and Bodywork Healing Therapies

Oh, that the water softens the rocks with time,
may thy hands craft my body soft like the weathered rock.
—ANONYMOUS

LEARNING OBJECTIVES

1. Describe cultural variations in bodywork.
2. List the principles or techniques of contemporary and traditional bodywork.
3. Describe the benefits of therapeutic massage.
4. Explain the therapeutic massage modalities of Swedish massage, sports massage, neuromuscular massage, and Aston patterning.
5. Describe the Eastern, meridian-based, and point therapies of acupressure, shiatsu, Jin Shin Jyutsu, and reflexology.
6. Explain the emotional bodywork therapies of Rolfing and Hellerwork.
7. Describe the manipulative therapies of chiropractic and osteopathy.
8. Identify the cautions and contraindications for massage and bodywork.

INTRODUCTION

Human touch is one of the most primal needs. Research has demonstrated that touch can enhance health and heal the body and mind (Freeman, 2004). As health care evolves and integrates the worlds of alternative and allopathic practitioners, therapeutic massage and bodywork healing methods are being integrated with health care in hospitals, nursing homes, hospice centers, and other healthcare facilities.

Trivieri and Anderson (2002) define the term *bodywork* as "therapies such as massage, deep tissue manipulation, movement awareness, and bioenergetic therapies, which are employed to improve the structure and functioning of the body" (p. 119). They add that the benefits of bodywork include pain reduction, musculoskeletal tension relief, improved blood and lymphatic circulation, and the promotion of deep relaxation. Shealy (1996) defines massage as soft tissue manipulation, including holding, causing movement, and/or applying pressure to the body.

Massage has a complex and extensive history, with over 75 different types of massage and bodywork therapies. First practiced over 5,000 years ago in China and Mesopotamia, massage is a therapy that applies manual techniques and may apply additional alternative and complementary therapies with the intent to positively affect an individual's health. One of the oldest forms of health practice, massage is derived from the Arabic, Greek, Hindi, and French words associated with touch, pressing, or shampooing. Both the Bible and the Koran refer to anointing the skin with oil. Various techniques were used in Japanese and Middle Eastern cultures as part of their health and hygiene routines, and by the Greeks and Romans when preparing their soldiers and gladiators for battle (Rankin-Box, 1996). During the Middle Ages, religious dogma and superstition regarded massage as sinful because it was related to physical and emotional pleasure. Massage was introduced to the United States from Europe in 1879, and nurses and physiotherapists used massage on injured soldiers during both world wars (Rankin-Box, 1996).

Although the techniques for massage and bodywork vary among practitioners, the objectives are similar: to relax, soothe, stimulate, and relieve physical, mental, emotional, and/or spiritual discomfort (Dossey, Keegan, & Guzzetta, 2005). Touching and stroking are important to the health of infants, children, and adults. Regular massage improves overall health, eases tension in muscles, promotes circulation of the blood, and stimulates lymphatic drainage to encourage the elimination of waste from the body.

Most bodywork practitioners employ a combination of bodywork methods (Moore & Schmais, 2000; Shealy, 1996). Swedish massage, reflexology, shiatsu, sports massage, and Rolfing are some examples of massage and bodywork modalities used to promote general relaxation, relieve muscle tension, and improve circulation and range of motion.

Despite differences in techniques, all massage therapists must understand the following three concepts (Werner, 2005):

- How the human body works when it is healthy
- How the body works in the context of disease or dysfunction
- How a particular bodywork modality may influence those processes

Werner (2005) provides a comprehensive text entitled *A Massage Therapist's Guide to Pathology* to help bodywork practitioners make informed choices when selecting modalities for clients who may not be in perfect health.

CULTURAL VARIATIONS IN BODYWORK

Both ancient and modern cultures have developed some form of touch therapy that involves rubbing, pressing, massaging, and holding. Although attitudes toward touch vary from one culture to another, the widespread use of bodywork practices indicates that these are natural manifestations of the desire to heal and care for one another (Keegan & Shames, 2005).

Nevertheless, cultural differences have influenced the development of touch. For example, whereas the Eastern worldview is founded on the concept of energy, the Western worldview is based on the reductionism of matter. This cultural difference has created a variety of different approaches to the use of touch, and the blending of Eastern and Western techniques has resulted in an explosion of new bodywork healing modalities. This may be due, in part, to a healthy response to the fast-paced technologic revolution and the desire to provide individuals with a sense of balance and caring (Keegan & Shames, 2005).

BODYWORK APPROACH TO AWARENESS AND PHYSICAL HEALTH

Both contemporary and traditional bodywork therapies are based on one or more of the following principles or techniques (Clay & Pounds, 2008; Trivieri & Anderson, 2002):

- The individual is a whole organism (everything is connected).
- Shortened muscle tissue can do no work.
- The soft tissues of the body respond to touch.
- Pressure or deep friction can be used to alter muscular and soft tissue structures.
- Movement can be used to affect physiological structure and functioning.
- Education and awareness can be used to change or enhance physiological function.
- Breathing and emotional expression can be used to eliminate tension and change physiological functioning.

THERAPEUTIC MASSAGE

Therapeutic massage is undergoing a renaissance, and massage therapy is one of the fastest-growing healthcare professions in the United States (Clay & Pounds, 2008). An overwhelming accumulation of scientific evidence supports the claim that massage therapy can be beneficial in healing injuries, treating certain chronic and acute conditions, dealing with the stress of daily life, and maintaining good health. As individuals look for alternative or complementary therapies to supplement their medical treatments, many choose therapeutic massage.

The therapeutic use of massage has been around for centuries. It is one of the oldest known forms of healing (Vaughan, 2002). Massage was first practiced in a structured way in China and Mesopotamia more than 5,000 years ago (Shealy, 1996). Hippocrates, generally recognized as the father of Western medicine, considered massage of prime importance in any health regimen. Most modern methods of massage are derived mainly from Swedish massage, originally developed in the late 18th century.

Today therapeutic massage includes Swedish massage, sports massage, Esalen massage, neuromuscular therapy, and Aston patterning, as well as deep tissue, trigger point, and myofascial massage.

Definition of Therapeutic Massage

Therapeutic massage is the systematic and scientific manipulation of the soft tissues and muscles of the body for the purpose of improving, maintaining, and assisting the body in healing. It can also be defined as organized, intentional touch (Eliopoulos, 2004; Salvo, 1999). Massage therapy is a profession in which the practitioner applies manual techniques and may apply adjunctive therapies with the intention of positively affecting the health and well-being of the client.

Benefits of Therapeutic Massage

Systemic Benefits

By the response it creates within the body, massage has the ability to affect the physiologic functioning of a number of systems. The scientific application of massage therapy can best be understood by examining its beneficial aspects on the following body systems (Eliopoulos, 2004; Freeman, 2004; Salvo, 1999; Vaughn, 2002):

- *Circulatory:* Massage is known to increase venous blood flow back to the heart, thus improving circulation.
- *Digestive:* Massage promotes the activation of the parasympathetic nervous system, which stimulates digestion, helps promote evacuation of the colon, and promotes peristaltic activity in the large intestine.
- *Endocrine:* Massage decreases pain by releasing endorphins, enkephalins, and other pain-reducing neurochemicals.

- *Excretory:* Massage promotes autonomic nervous system functioning; an increase in the production of gastric juices, saliva, and urine; and general homeostasis.
- *Integumentary:* Massage improves the skin's condition, texture, and tone by stimulating the sebaceous glands, causing an increase in sebum production.
- *Muscular:* Massage relieves muscular tightness, stiffness, and spasms; it promotes muscular relaxation and enhances blood circulation, thus increasing the amount of oxygen and nutrients available to the muscles.
- *Nervous:* Because massage activates the sensory receptors, the nervous system can be stimulated or soothed, depending on the massage stroke used and the amount of pressure applied. Massage also stimulates the parasympathetic nervous system, resulting in relaxation.
- *Respiratory:* Massage slows down the rate of respiration by reducing the stimulation of the sympathetic nervous system. By decreasing tightness in respiratory muscles and fascia, massage may be used to increase vital capacity and pulmonary function.
- *Skeletal (connective):* Massage is indicated for musculoskeletal discomfort. It can increase joint mobility and flexibility by reducing hyperplasia (thickening) of connective tissue and freeing fascial restrictions.

Physical, Mental, and Emotional Benefits

Many people use massage therapy simply for relaxation, restoration, and pain relief. To best understand how massage works, it is important to understand the physical, mental, and emotional benefits of therapeutic massage (Holey & Cook, 1998; Salvo, 1999; Seaward, 2006).

Massage has physical benefits because it:

- Relieves stress and aids relaxation
- Helps relieve muscle tension and stiffness
- Fosters faster healing of strained muscles and sprained ligaments, reduces pain and swelling, and reduces the formation of excessive scar tissue
- Reduces muscle spasms
- Increases joint flexibility and range of motion
- Enhances athletic performance
- Promotes deeper and easier breathing
- Improves the circulation of blood and the movement of lymph fluids
- Reduces blood pressure
- Helps relieve tension-related headaches and the effects of eyestrain
- Enhances the health and nourishment of skin

- Improves posture
- Strengthens the immune system

The mental benefits of massage include:

- Fostering peace of mind
- Promoting a relaxed state of mental alertness
- Helping to relieve mental stress
- Improving the ability to monitor stress signals and respond appropriately
- Enhancing the capacity for calm thinking and creativity

The emotional benefits include:

- Helping to satisfy the needs for caring
- Nurturing touch
- Fostering a feeling of well-being
- Reducing levels of anxiety
- Increasing awareness of the mind-body connection.

Help with Medical Conditions

Individuals with the following medical conditions may benefit from therapeutic massage (Shealy, 1996; Trivieri & Anderson, 2002):

- Allergies
- Anxiety and depression
- Arthritis (both osteoarthritis and rheumatoid arthritis)
- Asthma and bronchitis
- Back and neck pain
- Carpal tunnel syndrome
- Circulatory problems
- Digestive disorders, including spastic colon, constipation, and diarrhea
- Headache, especially when due to muscle tension
- Insomnia
- Reduced range of motion

Swedish Massage

Pehr Henrik Ling, a Swedish physiologist and gymnastics instructor, developed the system of Swedish massage (Salvo, 1999). The most widely known and widely used system of massage in the United States, Swedish massage involves the manipulation of soft tissues for therapeutic purposes (Freeman, 2004). This system uses long strokes, kneading, and friction techniques on the more superficial layers of the muscles, combined with active and passive movements of the joints.

Each stroke and manipulation of Swedish massage is intended to have a specific therapeutic benefit. Five basic strokes or movements are used to administer a Swedish massage (Salvo, 1999; Seaward, 2006; Vaughn, 2002):

- *Effleurage:* A light, purposeful, gliding movement that focuses pressure horizontally in the direction of the client's muscle fibers
- *Petrissage:* A cycle of rhythmic lifting of the muscle tissues away from the bone or underlying structures with the hollow of the palm(s), followed by firmly kneading or squeezing the muscle with a gentle pull toward the therapist, and ending with a release of the tissue
- *Friction:* A brisk, often heat-producing compressive stroke that may be delivered either superficially to the skin or to deeper tissue layers of muscle
- *Tapotement:* An application of downward vertical pressure with an abrupt release
- *Vibration:* Shaking, trembling, or oscillating movements applied with full hands, fingertips, or a mechanical device for the purpose of inducing relaxation

The strokes and manipulations of Swedish massage have specific therapeutic benefits. One of the primary goals is to increase the speed of the venous return of unoxygenated blood and circulatory waste products and toxins from the extremities.

Other benefits of Swedish massage include:

- An increase in circulation without increasing heart load
- A shortened recovery time from muscular strain
- An increase in tendon and ligament suppleness secondary to stretching
- A reduction of emotional and physical stress
- A feeling of general relaxation
- An elimination of waste products from the tissues

Sports Massage

One of the most visible specialties in therapeutic massage today, sports massage is the specific application of purposefully timed massage techniques, hydrotherapy protocol, range of motion and flexibility procedures, and strength and endurance training principles for athletes in competitive and recreational settings. The techniques are similar to those used in Swedish massage and have been adapted to meet the athlete's special needs (Gottlieb,

1995). Whether used by professional athletes or weekend exercisers, sports massage is an effective way to help people stay healthy and injury free (Trivieri & Anderson, 2002). Sports massage should be tailored to the individual (Salvo, 1999).

Common injuries that benefit from sports massage include the following:

- *Strain:* A partial or complete muscle or tendinous tear
- *Sprain:* A partial or complete ligamentous tear caused by an overstretch injury
- *Bursitis:* Inflammation of the bursa

Sports massage can help heal strained muscles and allow healthy ones to reach and maintain peak action, with less risk of injury. The most commonly acknowledged purposes of sports massage include the following (Holey & Cook, 1998; Trivieri & Anderson, 2002):

- Improving athletic training
- Treating sports injuries and rehabilitation
- Enhancing athletic performance
- Reducing muscle soreness and recovery time
- Assisting recovery from fatigue
- Eliminating buildup of lactic acid
- Facilitating the healing of damaged tissues
- Restoring muscle tone and mobility after vigorous workouts
- Promoting local and general relaxation

The components of sports massage include an understanding of when and when not to petrissage a sore muscle; which specific techniques to use for treating tendonitis (and how to prevent its return); why delayed muscle soreness occurs; when to schedule a session for an athlete who works out 10–12 times per week; and where to look for adhesions, trigger points, or other ischemic pockets that are particular to a given sport.

Neuromuscular Massage Therapy

Neuromuscular massage therapy applies deep tissue massage to specific muscles using concentrated finger pressure. Used to increase blood flow, reduce pain, and release pressure on nerves caused by injuries to muscles and other soft tissue, neuromuscular massage helps release trigger points, those intense knots of tense muscle that can also refer pain to other parts of the body. For example, relieving a tense trigger point in a client's back can help to ease pain in his or her shoulder. Trigger point massage and myotherapy are varieties of neuromuscular massage (Gottlieb, 1995; Salvo, 1999).

Aston Patterning

Aston patterning uses posture reeducation and stresses physical fitness techniques (Gottlieb, 1995). Working with Ida Rolf, the developer of Rolfing, Judith Aston developed Aston patterning in its current form in 1977. Aston patterning was developed to teach people to maintain the improved alignment they received through Rolfing. Unlike Rolf's model and its focus on body symmetry and alignment, Aston noted that all movement is naturally asymmetrical and that a healthy body develops asymmetrically through adaptation to the kinds of work, recreation, sports, and other daily activities it performs (Trivieri & Anderson, 2002).

Aston patterning focuses on four areas:

- Movement reeducation
- Massage and soft tissue bodywork
- Fitness training
- Environmental design (for example, altering the height of an office chair to suit a particular body type)

Aston patterning is beneficial for improved movement and coordination and for managing painful conditions such as backaches, headaches, and tennis elbow.

EASTERN, MERIDIAN-BASED, AND POINT THERAPIES

This category includes the bodywork modalities of acupressure, shiatsu, Jin Shin Jyutsu, and reflexology.

Acupressure

Unlike acupuncture, which uses needles, acupressure applies finger and/or thumb pressure to specific sites along the body's energy meridians (the invisible channels of energy flow in the body) to relieve tension, reestablish the flow of energy along the meridian lines, and restore balance to the human energy system (Eliopoulos, 2004; Keegan & Shames, 2005). Acupressure is older than acupuncture and continues to be an effective self-care and preventive health-care treatment for tension-related ailments (Trivieri & Anderson, 2002).

Acupressure may be even more effective than acupuncture for relieving everyday aches, pain, and stress such as headaches, backaches, sinus pain, neck pain, eyestrain, and menstrual cramps. Acupressure can also reduce the pain of ulcers, help heal sports injuries, relieve insomnia, and alleviate constipation and other digestive problems (Gottlieb, 1995). Research has demonstrated that acupressure is a preventive measure against nausea and vomiting after surgery, two common side effects of general anesthesia (Trivieri & Anderson, 2002).

Shiatsu

Shiatsu is an ancient form of pressure-point massage that has been practiced for centuries in Japan. The name literally means "finger pressure" or "thumb pressure" (Micozzi, 2006). A contemplative form of massage, shiatsu is based on the theory of the circulation of energy (qi) and the principles of the Chinese discipline of acupuncture. Micozzi (2006) explains shiatsu as follows:

> The major underlying principle of shiatsu, derived from the tenets of Asian medicine, is actually a reflection of scientific thought. Simply stated, "Everything is energy." When considered in the context of molecular structure, all matter is a manifestation of energy. Shiatsu interacts directly with this energy, and therefore with life itself. (p. 439)

In shiatsu, the systematic use of the thumb, finger, and/or heel of the hand for deep pressure is exerted on specific points along acupuncture meridians, usually for 3–10 seconds. Unlike Swedish massage, shiatsu requires the client's participation in coordinating breathing with the manipulations (Gottlieb, 1995; Keegan & Shames, 2005; Salvo, 1999).

Jin Shin Jyutsu

Translated as the art of compassionate spirit, Jin Shin Jyutsu is a gentle acupressure-type of healing approach (Keegan & Shames, 2005). Developed in Japan by Jiro Murai, this Japanese form of self-help acupressure has the goal of harmonizing the body, mind, and spirit by touching 26 points known as safety energy locks and found along energy pathways in the body. This method involves gentle touching or cradling of the body rather than massage-like movements. Treatment can involve a series of touches, or it can be as simple as holding one finger. Jin Shin Jyutsu is beneficial for relieving pain and muscular discomfort, correcting imbalances, and preventing illness. The system is a synthesis of acupuncture, acupressure, Taoist breathing exercises, and Western psychotherapeutic theory (Gottlieb, 1995; Trivieri & Anderson, 2002).

Reflexology

Reflexology dates back to the ancient Egyptians, Greeks, possibly the Chinese, and native peoples of North and South America. Modern reflexology stems from the work of two Americans, Dr. William Fitzgerald and Eunice Ingham. Dr. Fitzgerald proposed the theory that "the body is divided into ten equal zones that extend the length of the body from head to toe, and that stimulating an area of the foot in one zone affects other parts of the body in the same zone" (Shealy, 1996, p. 52).

According to Trivieri and Anderson (2002), "Reflexology states that there are reflex areas in the hands and feet that correspond to every part of the body, including organs and glands, and that these parts can be affected by stimulating the appropriate reflex areas" (p. 129). A specialized massage for the hands and feet, reflexology is also known as zone therapy and is based on the Chinese idea that stimulating particular points on the surface of the body affects other areas of the body. Reflexology relates specific zones of the hands and feet to specific organs in the body and is based on the theory that 10 equal longitudinal zones run the length of the body from the top of the head to the tip of the toes (Keegan & Shames, 2005). Congestion or tension in any part of a zone affects the entire zone running laterally throughout the body.

Reflexologists believe that energy pathways exist throughout the body. The entire body, including organs, glands, and body parts, has reflex points located on the feet and, to a lesser extent, on the hands. More than 72,000 nerves in the body terminate in the feet (Keegan & Shames, 2005). By applying pressure to these points, reflexologists release blockages around the corresponding body part and rebalance the entire body (Eliopoulos, 2004; Salvo, 1999). Therapists use many methods to apply pressure to the reflex points, including rubbing and rotating movements, compression, and tissue rolling, but they usually begin with firm but gentle stroking movements over the feet (Shealy, 1996; Vaughn, 2002).

Reflexology aims to correct the three negative factors involved in the disease process: congestion, inflammation, and tension (Gillanders, 1995). Reported results of reflexology include pain relief and relief from the effects of stroke, hypertension, anxiety, sinusitis, sciatica, menstrual disorders, digestive problems, stress, fatigue, and general aches and pains (Shealy, 1996; Trivieri & Anderson, 2002).

ENERGY-BASED THERAPIES

The use of energy-based interventions is rapidly increasing, and new types of energy-based therapies are being used in bodywork. Energy-based therapies such as Therapeutic Touch, Reiki, and Healing Touch are discussed in chapter 3.

EMOTIONAL BODYWORK THERAPIES

Some of these modalities are derived from ancient traditions and others from established health fields such as chiropractic (Keegan & Shames, 2005). This category of bodywork includes techniques that combine psychotherapy and bodywork, such as Rolfing and Hellerwork, among other techniques.

Rolfing

Developed by Ida Rolf, this technique helps clients establish structural relationships deep within the body and manipulates muscles for balance and symmetry (Keegan & Shames, 2005). The cornerstone of Rolf's work is that the body's structure profoundly affects all physiological and psychological processes and that human function is improved when the segments of the body (head, torso, pelvis, legs, and feet) are properly aligned (Trivieri & Anderson, 2002).

Rolfing attempts to reeducate the body about proper posture. Poor posture is reflected in a number of health problems, such as backaches, headaches, and joint pain. Rolfing seeks to realign the body by working and massaging the myofascia (the connective tissue that surrounds the muscles and helps to hold the body together) through the application of sliding pressure to the affected area with the fingers, thumbs, and occasionally elbows. Once considered painful, Rolfing now includes new techniques that are quite painless (Gottlieb, 1995).

Rolfing reduces chronic stress, promotes changes in body structure, and enhances neurological functioning. Individuals suffering from pain and stiffness related to mechanical imbalances and poor posture often benefit from Rolfing (Trivieri & Anderson, 2002).

Hellerwork

Developed by Joseph Heller, Hellerwork combines deep touch, movement education, and verbal dialogue. Hellerwork can improve body alignment and flexibility and specifically addresses the mechanical, psychological, and energetic functioning of the body. The mechanical aspect of Hellerwork, patterned after Rolfing, is designed to properly align the body with the earth's gravitational field.

Hellerwork includes emotional content as part of the treatment (Trivieri & Anderson, 2002). For example, the first of 11 Hellerwork sessions is designed to unlock tension and unconscious breath-holding patterns in the chest to allow for fuller and more natural breathing. The client engages in a dialogue intended to emphasize the emotions and attitudes that may affect the physiological process of breathing.

Hellerwork adds both mental and movement reeducation to the physical work. In the 11-session series, instruction is provided on the process of breaking bad posture habits. Hellerwork utilizes movement and awareness to teach clients how to sit, stand, walk, lift, or run in ways that that are appropriate to the body's natural design. In addition, massage focuses on returning muscles and other tissue to their proper positions. The results can be dramatic (Gottlieb, 1995).

The benefits of Hellerwork include improved body alignment and flexibility, increased vitality, and greater emotional clarity. This form of therapy is beneficial for individuals suffering from stiff, painful muscles due to structural imbalances or conditions that may be the result of injury, emotional trauma, or sustained stress.

MANIPULATIVE THERAPIES

The goal of manipulative therapies is to restore health and well-being by looking at the relationship between the structure and the function of the body (Erickson, Rosner, & Rainone, 2004). Manipulative therapies include chiropractic and osteopathy.

Chiropractic Medicine

According to history, the Chinese used manipulation healing techniques as early as 2700 BC, the Greeks in 1500 BC, and Hippocrates in 460 BC.

Founded by David Palmer in 1895, chiropractic is the fourth largest health profession in the United States (Eliopoulos, 2004) and the second largest primary healthcare field in the world. The popularity of chiropractic is due to an increased interest in wellness and holistic health, the risks of many conventional procedures and drugs, and a very high client satisfaction rating (Trivieri & Anderson, 2002).

Chiropractic is the science that investigates the relationship between the human body's structure (primarily of the spine) and function (primarily of the nervous system) to restore and preserve health. Chiropractors do not use medications or surgery, but they do employ, in conjunction with manual spinal alignment techniques, a variety of complementary treatments such as exercise and lifestyle recommendations, nutritional counseling, and massage. They may also use laboratory tests and X-rays for diagnosis (Gazdar, 2004; Trivieri & Anderson, 2002).

Sierpina (2001) explains that "the central concept in chiropractic thought is that disturbances of the body's structural and functional interrelationships may induce or aggravate disturbances in other organ systems or body areas" (p. 226). Trivieri and Anderson (2002) add, "When there is nerve interference caused by misalignments in the spine, known as subluxations, tension and/or pain can occur and the body's defense can be diminished. By adjusting the spine to remove subluxations, normal nerve function can be restored" (p. 154). Subluxations can be caused by five types of factors: physical (which includes trauma), mental (such as stress), genetic predispositions, chemical (imbalance or toxicity), and thermal (includes extreme changes in temperature) (Trivieri & Anderson, 2002).

Chiropractic philosophy and practice emphasize four major points:

- The human body has an innate self-healing ability and seeks to maintain homeostasis, or balance.
- The nervous system is highly developed in humans and influences all other systems in the body, thereby playing a significant role in health and disease.
- Joint dysfunction and subluxation may interfere with the ability of the neuromusculoskeletal system to act efficiently and may lead to or be concomitant with disease.
- Treatment is based on the chiropractic physician's ability to diagnose and treat existing pathologies and dysfunctions through appropriate manual and physiological procedures.

The word *chiropractic*, which means "manually effective," describes a system of healing that believes humans are integrated beings with strong relationships between their spinal, musculoskeletal, neurological, vascular, nutritional, emotional, and environmental components. Pain and disease are considered the results of pressure on the nervous system caused by mechanical, chemical, or psychological factors. Through a series of special examination and manipulative techniques, chiropractic practitioners apply this knowledge to diagnose, treat, and rehabilitate structural dysfunctions affecting the nervous system without the use of medications or surgery (Gazdar, 2004; Shealy, 1996).

Chiropractic may benefit many conditions, such as arthritic conditions, asthma, back pain, headaches, stiffness, digestive difficulties, muscle strains and joint sprains, and sciatica. It may also help relieve muscular pain in the neck, shoulder, or upper arm (Eliopoulos, 2004; Gazdar, 2004; Shealy, 1996; Trivieri & Anderson, 2002).

Osteopathy

Osteopathy is the oldest complete system of health care to originate in the United States. It is a philosophy, an art, and a science, emphasizing soft tissue work, skeletal manipulation, and pulses (Keegan & Shames, 2005). A form of bodywork, osteopathy helps restore the structural balance of the musculoskeletal system by combining joint manipulation, physical therapy, and postural reeducation.

Trivieri and Anderson (2002) explain that "doctors of osteopathic medicine (D.O.s, also known as osteopaths) believe that the structure of the body is intimately related to its function and that both structure and function are subject to a wide range of disorders" (p. 413). Osteopathic physicians focus on preventive health care and the treatment of the whole person and their environments. Osteopathic physicians use their hands to diagnose injury and illness and to encourage the body's natural tendency toward good health (Leddy, 2006; Micozzi, 2006). Their training incorporates osteopathic manipulative treatment (OMT) as well as standard medical procedures; they are therefore are accorded unlimited licensure and full medical and surgical privileges, serve as primary providers and medical specialists, and are frequently considered mainstream practitioners (Alexander & Goldman, 2002; Bright, 2002).

The effectiveness of osteopathic treatment depends on the following factors:

- The level of organic disease
- The level of musculoskeletal involvement
- The client's nutritional status
- The effectiveness of the body's healing mechanisms

Osteopathy is effective in treating spinal and joint difficulties, arthritis, digestive disorders, menstrual problems, and chronic pain. Osteopathy has also benefited clients with allergies, cardiac diseases, breathing dysfunctions, chronic fatigue syndrome, hiatal hernia, high blood pressure, headaches, sciatica, and various other neuritis disorders (Trivieri & Anderson, 2002).

The various types of manipulative approaches utilized in osteopathy include the following (Leddy, 2006; Trivieri & Anderson, 2002):

- *Gentle mobilization:* This involves moving a joint slowly through its range of motion, gradually increasing the motion to free it from restrictions.
- *Articulation:* When motion is severely limited, a quick thrust of movement is sometimes used.
- *Functional and positional release methods:* The client is placed in a specific position to allow the body to relax and to release muscular spasms that may have been caused by strain or injury.

- *Muscle energy technique:* This involves gently tensing and releasing specific muscles to produce relaxation.
- *Cranial manipulation:* Gentle and subtle cranial techniques are used to treat conditions such as headaches, strokes, spinal cord injury, and temporomandibular joint dysfunction (TMJ). Cranial osteopathy can also benefit young children who suffer from hyperactivity, mood disorder, dizziness, or dyslexia.

The principles and philosophy of osteopathy emphasize the following major points about health and illness:

- Structure and function are interdependent. Behavior involves complex interactions in which psychosocial influences can affect both anatomy (structure) and physiology (function). All these relationships are fundamentally designed to work in harmony.
- The body has the ability to heal itself, and the role of the osteopathic physician is to enhance the healing process as much as possible. Diseases, impairments, and disabilities arise from disruptions of the normal interaction of anatomy, physiology, and behavior.
- Appropriate treatment is based on the practitioner's ability to understand, diagnose, and treat by whatever methods are available, including manually applied procedures. When hands-on procedures are used to identify somatic dysfunction, the practitioner determines whether the observed pattern of somatic dysfunction can be related to any visceral, neuromusculoskeletal, or behavioral dysfunction.

CAUTIONS AND CONTRAINDICATIONS TO BODYWORK

Bodywork is not appropriate for everyone. Individuals with the following conditions should check with their physicians before undergoing massage (Micozzi, 2006; Sierpina, 2001):

- *Vascular conditions:* Clients with vascular conditions have a tendency to bruise, form clots or thrombi, or rupture blood vessels, and they may be adversely affected by massage therapy. Contraindicated vascular conditions include varicosities, embolus, phlebitis, thrombosis, aneurysm, atherosclerosis, hypertension, and Raynaud's phenomenon.
- *Infectious diseases:* Infectious diseases such as cold, flu, measles, mumps, and scarlet fever are caused by an infectious agent such as a virus or a bacterium and are highly contagious. They could be transmitted to the massage therapist or to other clients.

- *Certain forms of cancer:* Many cancers spread lymphatically, and massage increases circulation of the lymph.
- *Some skin conditions:* Conditions such as rashes, poison ivy, poison oak, sumac, impetigo, athlete's foot, ringworm, scabies, blisters, abnormal lumps, warts, herpes simplex, herpes zoster, large or loose moles, and skin ulcerations should not be massaged. As well as being contagious, several of these conditions may be worsened and spread by massage therapy.
- *Some cardiac problems:* Massage increases circulation and may overburden a failing heart. It may also increase the risks of developing a thrombus or embolus.

In addition, bodywork may be contraindicated for the following conditions unless the client's physician gives approval (Salvo, 1999):

- *Fever:* A rise in body temperature (fever) is often a symptom of other conditions, such as infections caused by the presence of foreign bacteria or viruses. There is a risk of spreading such an infection as a result of increased circulation during bodywork.
- *Recent injury:* Because of the possibility of internal vascular bleeding, individuals should wait at least 72 hours after minor injuries before having a massage.
- *Recent surgery:* After surgery, a physician's medical clearance is necessary before massage therapy can begin.
- *Multiple sclerosis:* Alteration in sensation occurs in many clients with multiple sclerosis, and they may be sensitive to touch. The typical hour-long massage may be too long for these clients, causing them to feel overstimulated. Because of their nerve damage, external heat is not used when massaging these clients.
- *Diabetes:* Clients with diabetes are prone to atherosclerosis, hypertension, and edema. A medical referral is necessary because these clients typically lose sensation in extremities in advanced stages of diabetes, and any loss of sensory nerve function must be taken into consideration prior to receiving a massage. If the client is receiving insulin therapy by injection, massaging the area of recent injection sites should be avoided.
- *Fractures:* Healing fracture areas should not be massaged until the fracture is completely healed and medical clearance is obtained.
- *Pregnancy:* Bodywork is not recommended during the early stages (the first trimester) of pregnancy. During the last trimester, however, gentle stroking can help ease backache and promote relaxation, although more vigorous movements should be avoided. Preeclampsia, a complex

condition of pregnancy, is a contraindication for massage therapy unless approved by the client's attending physician.

- *Hepatitis:* Bodywork is usually contraindicated in the client with hepatitis because it increases circulation and may stress an already debilitated liver.

KEY CONCEPTS

1. Massage and bodywork therapies are based on the physical manipulation of body structures; some are based on the manipulation of the body's energy fields.
2. Massage and bodywork therapies use awareness and learning as the basis for improving body movement and functioning and integrating the mind and body for healing.
3. It is important for the healthcare professional to understand massage and bodywork, not only to use with clients but also to educate them about massage and bodywork therapeutic modalities.

QUESTIONS FOR REFLECTION

1. What are the benefits of therapeutic massage?
2. How many of the massage and bodywork healing therapies have you experienced?
3. What are the cautions and contraindications for massage and bodywork?

REFERENCES

Alexander, J., & Goldman, A. (2002). Osteopathy. In M. A. Bright, *Holistic health and healing* (pp. 227–237). Philadelphia: F. A. Davis.

Bright, M. A. (2002). *Holistic health and healing*. Philadelphia: F. A. Davis.

Clay, J. H., & Pounds, D. M. (2008). *Basic clinical massage therapy: Integrating anatomy and treatment.* Philadelphia: Lippincott Williams and Wilkins.

Dossey, B. M., Keegan, L., & Guzzetta, C. E. (2005). *Holistic nursing: A handbook for practice* (4th ed.). Sudbury, MA: Jones and Bartlett.

Eliopoulos, C. (2004). *Invitation to holistic health: A guide to living a balanced life.* Sudbury, MA: Jones and Bartlett.

Erickson, K., Rosner, A., & Rainone, F. (2004). Chiropractic and osteopathic care. In B. Kligler & R. Lee, *Integrative medicine: Principles for practice* (pp. 153–176). New York: McGraw-Hill.

Freeman, L. (2004). *Mosby's complementary and alternative medicine: A research-based approach* (2nd ed.). St. Louis, MO: Mosby.

Gazdar, M. (2004). *Taking your back to the future.* Walnut Creek, CA: John Muir Chiropractic Center.

Gillanders, A. (1995). *The joy of reflexology.* London: Gaia Books.

Gottlieb, B. (Ed.). (1995) *New choices in natural healing.* Emmaus, PA: Rodale Press.

Holey, E., & Cook, E. (1998). *Therapeutic massage.* Philadelphia: W. B. Saunders.

Keegan, L., & Shames, K. (2005). Touch: Connecting with the healing power. In B. M. Dossey, L. Keegan, & C. E. Guzzetta, *Holistic nursing: A handbook for practice* (4th ed., pp. 643–666). Sudbury, MA: Jones and Bartlett.

Leddy, S. K. (2006). *Integrative health promotion: Conceptual bases for nursing practice* (2nd ed.). Sudbury, MA: Jones and Bartlett.

Micozzi, M. S. (2006). *Fundamentals of complementary and integrative medicine* (3rd ed.). St. Louis, MO: Saunders Elsevier.

Moore, K., & Schmais, L. (2000). The ABCs of complementary and alternative therapies and cancer treatment. *Oncology Issues, 15*(6), 20–22.

Rankin-Box, D. F. (Ed.). (1996). *The nurses' handbook of complementary therapies.* Edinburgh: Churchill Livingstone.

Salvo, S. G. (1999). *Massage therapy: Principles and practice.* Philadelphia: W. B. Saunders.

Seaward, B. L. (2006). *Managing stress: Principles and strategies for health and well-being* (5th ed.). Sudbury, MA: Jones and Bartlett.

Shealy, C. N. (Ed.). (1996). *The complete family guide to alternative medicine: An illustrated encyclopedia of natural healing.* Shaftesbury, Dorset, UK: Element Books.

Sierpina, V. (2001). *Integrative health care: Complementary and alternative therapies for the whole person.* Philadelphia: F. A. Davis.

Trivieri, L., Jr., & Anderson, J. W. (Eds.). (2002). *Alternative medicine: The definitive guide* (2nd ed.). Berkeley, CA: Celestial Arts.

Vaughan, V. (2002). Therapeutic massage. In M. A. Bright, *Holistic health and healing* (pp. 161–169). Philadelphia: F. A. Davis.

Werner, R. (2005). *A massage therapist's guide to pathology.* Philadelphia: Lippincott Williams and Wilkins.

CHAPTER 12

Healing Effects of Physical Activity and Movement

A sound mind in a sound body.
—JUVENAL

LEARNING OBJECTIVES

1. Describe the types of physical activity and their associated risks.
2. Explain the physiological benefits of physical activity and movement.
3. Explain the psychological benefits of physical activity and movement.
4. Describe the mechanics of breathing.
5. Explain the philosophical basis of yoga.
6. Explain the philosophical basis of Tai Chi Chuan.
7. Describe important steps in initiating a physical activity program.

INTRODUCTION

The human body is an amazing, complex phenomenon with approximately 60 trillion cells (Eliopoulos, 2004). It's made to move; it's that simple. From the high school coach who said sports builds character to the way you feel on the dance floor boogying with your friends to tossing a Frisbee at a park, moving feels good. Even as you sit and read this book, your heart pumps blood across miles of arteries and veins, your eyes move across the page, your lungs expand and contract, and neurons in your brain fire. Every time you move a muscle, your cells mobilize energy and remove waste products. Thousands of processes occur in your body to support the essence of who you are.

Human survival has been based on a fight-or-flight response that involves hormones producing an increase in blood pressure to shunt blood from the body's core to its periphery and allow major muscles to help people escape their real (or imagined) enemies (Eliopoulos, 2004).

Freeman (2004) quotes Hippocrates, the father of modern medicine, who once stated:

> All parts of the body which have a function, if used in moderation and exercised in labours in which each is accustomed, become thereby healthy, well-developed and age more slowly, but if unused and left idle, they become liable to disease, defective in growth, and age quickly. (p. 483)

Although people once used muscles as part of their everyday lives in farming, cooking, and cleaning, less than 1% of all energy used in factories, workshops, and farms today comes from human muscles. While increasing numbers of people exercise regularly, few exercise at the intensity or frequency needed to obtain maximal health benefits (Rose & Keegan, 2005). Low levels of physical activity continue to be a major public health challenge in almost every population group, despite the fact that incorporating physical activity into all areas of daily living is critical.

In the 1960s, President John F. Kennedy launched the President's Council on Physical Fitness and officially began the fitness craze. In the first organized effort to encourage children to get up and move, children of all ages were tested to see how well they could climb a rope, perform sit-ups and push-ups, and run specific distances. Today's children struggle with an ever-increasing sedentary lifestyle and unprecedented obesity (Eliopoulos, 2004). The lack of physical activity starts early in life. By age 10, more than one-third of children have already adopted a sedentary lifestyle (Leddy, 2006).

For those interested in improving the aging process, improved physical fitness is a priority. In fact, the U.S. Congress even broadened its definition of the Older Americans Act (in 1975) to include services that enable older persons to attain and maintain physical and mental well-being through programs of regular physical activity (Eliopoulos, 2004).

Once thought to be necessary only for athletes in training, exercise is now known to be good for everyone. Fitness is not limited to any particular age, ethnic, or cultural group, and physical limitations do not mean that someone cannot engage in health-promoting movement activity. In fact, it is a myth that someone who is aging or who has a health condition must experience physical decline, physical dysfunction, or dependency. These conditions result from stagnation and inactivity, not from age (Eliopoulos, 2004).

Some variations in exercise participation accompany ethnic, gender, educational, and occupational characteristics. For example, according to Leddy (2006), African-American and other ethnic minorities are less active than white Americans. White-collar workers and higher-educated people are more active than those with less education. Men are more active than women, and younger individuals are more active than older adults. People with a negative health status (e.g., smokers and overweight individuals) are more likely to be sedentary, and even their knowledge of their risk status does not motivate them to remain active.

It is amazing how much better people feel when they exercise regularly and "move creatively to the rhythm of life" (Rose & Keegan, 2005, p. 477). The ancient Greek ideal of sound mind in a strong, sound body is once again important to the development of total health. Eliopoulos (2004) notes that "muscles are made to work and just as the human spirit thrives when given a task or job to do, so does the body when put into motion" (p. 75). A healthy physical body is a temple for the mind-spirit, and the way people care for their physical bodies affects all aspects of their lives—self-esteem, self-care practices, longevity, and the ability to care for or serve others (Rose & Keegan, 2005).

THE PHYSIOLOGY OF EXERCISE

Rose and Keegan (2005) define exercise as "any form of movement in a continuum from active physical exertion to subtle motions that are only slightly perceptible" (p. 480).

Muscles perform their work through the contractions of microscopic fibers. Muscles that contract are composed of two different types of rod-like protein filaments, or myofilaments, called actin and myosin. The energy required for contracting is obtained by hydrolysis of the adenosine triphosphate (ATP) nucleotide. Since the availability of ATP is limited and its effects are transient, ATP must constantly be synthesized in working skeletal muscles for the muscles to work properly. ATP is synthesized primarily from carbohydrates and fats (Freeman, 2004).

Muscles are composed largely of protein. Exercise affects protein synthesis to such a degree that even in the absence of growth hormone, insulin, or adequate food intake, exercise stills result in muscle strengthening or hypertrophy (Freeman, 2004).

Types of Physical Activity

A subset of physical activity, physical exercise is planned, structured, repetitive, and associated with specific outcomes such as the improvement or maintenance of physical fitness, flexibility, and balance. Being fit is associated with being able to carry out daily tasks with vigor and alertness, without undue fatigue, with enough energy to deal with emergencies as they arise, and to enjoy leisure pursuits (Leddy, 2006).

There are six components of a well-rounded fitness program and two categories of physical activity (Leddy, 2006; Seaward, 2006). The first three types of fitness (cardiovascular endurance, muscular strength and endurance, and flexibility) are considered to be the most important aspects, while the last three (agility, power, and balance) supplement them.

- *Cardiovascular endurance* is the ability of the heart, lungs, and blood vessels to transport oxygenated blood to the working muscles for energy metabolism.
- *Muscular strength* is the power of muscle groups or the ability to exert maximal force against resistance. *Muscular endurance* is the ability to sustain repeated contractions over a prolonged period of time.
- *Flexibility* is the ability to use a muscle group throughout its entire range of motion without undue stress and to maintain some degree of elasticity of major muscle groups.
- *Agility* is the maneuverability and coordination of fine and gross motor movements.
- *Power* is force times distance over time.
- *Balance* is the ability to maintain equilibrium in motion.

The many types of physical activity (including swimming, golfing, yoga, walking, biking, etc.) fall into two main categories: anaerobic and aerobic.

Anaerobic Activity

Seaward (2006) defines anaerobic activity as "a physical motion intense in power and strength, yet short in duration" (p. 523). Anaerobic activity develops speed, strength, and power and can be done for only a limited amount of time (Sacks, 1993). This type of activity is, theoretically, the type used in the fight part of the fight-or-flight response. The term *anaerobic* means "without oxygen," and anaerobic activity stimulates the hypertrophy of muscle fibers (Seaward, 2006).

There are two types of anaerobic energy systems.

- The adenosine triphosphate phosphocreatine system (ATP-PC) lasts 1–10 seconds.
- The anaerobic glycolysis (lactic acid) system continues after the ATP-PC system for approximately 5–6 minutes, then activity is suspended because of either extreme fatigue or the beginning of the aerobic energy system.

Lactic acid builds up and causes muscle fatigue. Depending on the individual's physical condition, blood redistribution can take anywhere from 4 to 6 minutes. Since the initial oxygen supply does not last for long, the body needs an immediate and easily metabolized energy source (carbohydrates). Anaerobic activity thus involves only short bursts of activity; sprinting and weightlifting are examples.

Aerobic Activity

Aerobic exercise, often known as cardiovascular exercise, includes such repetitive movement and activities as running, swimming, walking, cycling, and cross-country skiing (Freeman, 2004). Aerobic exercise is one of the most important and efficient methods of attaining muscular and cardiovascular fitness. Defined as "sustained muscle activity within the target heart range that challenges the cardiovascular system to meet the muscles' needs for oxygen" (Rose & Keegan, 2005, p. 479), the term was first coined in the 1970s by physician Kenneth Cooper. At that time, aerobic exercise was described as a biological reaction that uses oxygen for metabolism. Jackie Sorenson, the originator of aerobic dance, used the term to describe her exercise routines using dance. It became an extremely popular alternative to running, and the term *aerobics* became a household term in the United States (Seaward, 2006).

Aerobic activity is theoretically the type used in the flight part of the fight-or-flight response. While anaerobic activity primarily uses carbohydrates for fuel, aerobic activity uses fats. Aerobic activity challenges the cardiovascular and pulmonary systems, lowers the risk of heart disease, reduces body fat, and decreases physical arousal due to stress (Seaward, 2006).

Aerobic exercise is intense enough to lead to a significant increase in muscle oxygen uptake. The heart rate is a simple measure of whether exercise is aerobic (Leddy, 2006). The recommendation for aerobic exercise is a heart rate between 65% and 85% of maximal intensity, with the average at about 75% for healthy individuals. This target heart rate is calculated by subtracting an individual's age from 220, then multiplying that number by 0.65 and 0.85. The resulting numbers provide a heart rate range within which the individual receives the most cardiovascular benefits. For example, a 50-year-old woman would subtract 50 from 220 and multiply that number (170) by 0.65 and 0.85. The results, 111 and 145, constitute her heart rate range for maximal cardiovascular benefits. If she goes above that range, her aerobic energy system is phased out and the anaerobic energy system begins; however, it does not last long because muscle fatigue begins.

Recommended Levels of Exercise

A universal formula for exercise programs for all individuals involves four factors:

- Intensity
- Frequency
- Duration
- Mode of exercise

Intensity

Intensity is the stress placed on a specific physiological system involved in an activity (Seaward, 2006). It is measured in terms of heartbeats per minute or the volume of oxygen consumed in liters per minute.

- *Moderate-intensity activity* is equivalent to a brisk walk and noticeably accelerates the heart rate.
- *Vigorous-intensity activity* is equivalent to jogging and causes rapid breathing and a substantial increase in heart rate.
- Both moderate- and vigorous-intensity activity recommendations are in addition to routine activities of daily living, which are considered *light-intensity* (e.g., self-care, cooking, casual walking, or shopping) or lasting less than 10 minutes in duration (e.g., walking around the home or office, walking from the parking lot) (Haskell et al., 2007).

Aerobic activities are rhythmic and continuous, and they involve moderate intensity for prolonged periods of time. The recommended levels of exercise needed to develop and maintain cardiovascular fitness include engaging in moderate-intensity aerobic exercise 3–5 days per week at an intensity of 55–90% of the maximum heart rate for 30–60 minutes (or a minimum of three 20-minute vigorous-intensity episodes during the week).

Even intermittent episodes of activity can be beneficial. Those who perform light-intensity exercise should do them more often, or for longer periods of time, or both. Any level of activity above the sedentary is beneficial for weight loss. However, to reduce the long-term risk of cardiovascular disease, aerobic exercise is necessary (Leddy, 2006).

Frequency

Frequency is the number of exercise sessions per week, and the minimum recommendation is three. A day of rest between aerobic exercise sessions is advisable for beginners so their bodies can recover with less risk of strain on muscles, ligaments, and tendons.

Duration and Mode

Duration is the length of time the individual is involved with the activity. The minimum duration for health benefits is 20–30 minutes, and the heart rate should remain elevated during that time.

The mode of exercise is the type of activity chosen (such as walking, running, skiing, swimming, weightlifting, or dancing).

Workout Formula

Workouts also have a specified formula to ensure safety. The components include a warm-up period, a stimulus period, and a cool-down period (Seaward, 2006).

The warm-up prepares the body for exercise and lasts approximately 5–10 minutes. This time allows the body's heart rate to increase slowly, muscles to become saturated with oxygenated blood, and ligaments to warm. If this component is bypassed, small muscle tears can occur because the muscles are not pliable. The more fit and flexible an individual is, the more quickly the individual warms up. Many injuries take place during warm-up phases, especially as a result of overstretching before blood has had a chance to be adequately distributed throughout the muscles and body.

The stimulus period is the essence of the workout and the most intense time for the body's systems. It should last for a minimum of 20 minutes for aerobic or anaerobic workouts (Seaward, 2006).

The cool-down period is the ending of the workout and provides one of the most important times for the body to return to its normal resting state. This period allows blood to be pumped back to the heart and should consist of approximately 5–10 minutes of decreasing intensity of activity, as well as stretching. If a workout is stopped during the stimulus period, blood pools in the extremities, and the body has to work harder to circulate it and eliminate metabolic by-products. Most exercise fatalities occur during this time if the cool-down has been inadequate (Seaward, 2006).

Also part of the workout formula, stretching and resistance training for the major muscle groups should be done 2–3 days a week. Stretching should be done after a slight warm-up and during cool-downs. Resistance training is considered one set of 8–10 exercises with 8–12 repetitions per exercise. Resistance training, or muscle-strengthening activities, include progressive weight training programs, weight-bearing calisthenics, stair climbing, and similar resistance exercises that use the major muscle groups (Haskell et al., 2007; Rose & Keegan, 2005).

PHYSIOLOGICAL EFFECTS OF EXERCISE ON HEALTH

Benefits

Oxygen is the essence of the life force; every cell in the body needs it to function properly. With physical activity and movement, the body's cells draw in oxygen, receive the nourishment they need, and eliminate waste. Blood vessels dilate as the demand for oxygen increases, allowing more blood to surround tissues and bathe cells. The increased demand for blood flow carries oxygenated, nutrition-filled blood and lymphatic fluids to every cell in the body.

Lymph fluid differs from blood in that it is not *pumped* like blood but rather *undulates*, moving in wavelike motion in response to muscle contractions. Lymph pathways form a lace-like network throughout the body and function to remove excess fluid from body tissues, absorb and transport fatty acids to the circulatory system, and produce immune cells. Physical activity stimulates bone marrow to produce more oxygen-carrying cells. Cells become stronger, and both the heart and lungs become more efficient. As time goes on, this increased efficiency means that, at rest, these organs do not have to work as hard to function properly (Eliopoulos, 2004).

Regular physical activity improves muscle tone and strength. Body image, appearance, posture, and the ability to engage in self-care activities all improve. Exercise helps regulate hormone and blood glucose levels, and it improves insulin regulation and utilization. With exercise, cortisol (one of the important stress hormones, produced by the adrenal glands) is much better modulated, thereby reducing the detrimental effects of stress (Eliopoulos, 2004).

The short-term effects of exercise (both neural and hormonal) last about 36 hours, but the long-term benefits require continuous training to obtain and maintain. As Seaward (2006) states, "Exercise, like money in the bank, can be considered an investment in health . . . unlike money, it accrues very little, if any, tangible interest" (p. 524). If training is stopped or interrupted for longer than 2 weeks, approximately 10% of cardiovascular gains can be lost. When inactivity continues for a month's time, up to 40% can be lost. However, if cardiovascular training is maintained, impressive physiological changes occur after 6 weeks. These include high-quality sleep and improved immunity, as well as decreased resting heart rate, resting blood pressure, muscle tension, cholesterol and triglyceride levels, and glucose levels.

Additional benefits from habitual cardiovascular exercise include decreased body fat, improved body composition and heart rate efficiency, decreased risk of osteoporosis, increased tolerance to heat and cold, reduced chronic pain (including headaches, joint stiffness, and premenstrual cramping), and decreased rate of aging (especially cognitively) (Eliopoulos, 2004; Freeman, 2004; Leddy; 2006; Rose & Keegan, 2005; Seaward, 2006). Regular exercise improves immune system functioning, although excessive exercise can actually decrease it (Sacks, 1993).

In aging adults, physical exercise can improve bone mass, mobility, flexibility, strength, balance, and muscular endurance, and it can reduce the risk of falls due to loss of lower-extremity strength (Freeman, 2004). Lower back pain can be reduced with activity and appropriate rehabilitation. In asthmatic clients, deep diaphragmatic training reduces both the amount of medication needed and the intensity of the asthmatic symptoms. Diabetes control also improves with regular aerobic exercise as well as yoga and therapeutic movement (Haskell et al., 2007; Leddy, 2006; Rose & Keegan, 2005). Chronic pain associated with lower back and spine problems often improves through the use of Pilates, a form of exercised developed several decades ago by Joe Pilates as a way to strengthen core body muscles. Originally used by dancers and athletes to prevent and rehabilitate injuries, Pilates is now commonly taught at fitness centers throughout the country (Seaward, 2006).

Risks

Exercise has its risks. Physically active adults tend to have a higher injury rate during their sport and leisure-time activities, while physically inactive adults report more injuries during nonsport and nonleisure time. Although the risk of sudden cardiac arrest or myocardial infarction is very low in generally healthy adults during moderate-intensity activities, exercise poses potential risks for individuals with the following conditions (Haskell et al., 2007; Leddy, 2006):

- A previous myocardial infarction
- Exertion chest pain or pressure
- Severe shortness of breath
- Pulmonary disease
- Bone, joint, or other musculoskeletal disease
- Hypertension
- A history of cigarette smoking
- High blood cholesterol
- Prescription medication use
- Drug or alcohol abuse
- Chronic illnesses

Certain activities have intrinsic injury risks, such as shin splints for those who run; they can be decreased or prevented by using proper equipment and correct technique. Extrinsic risks, such as being hit by a car while riding a bicycle or sustaining an overuse injury caused by doing too much, too fast, too frequently, can often be managed by choosing a different sport, revising the workout schedule, or maintaining moderation in distance, intensity, and speed (Leddy, 2006).

Given the complexities of both the positive and negative factors for physical exercise, an effective program for activity must be reviewed, designed, and personalized based on the individual's preferences and needs before beginning.

The American College of Sports Medicine recommends a physician-supervised stress test for individuals over 50 years of age who wish to undertake a vigorous training program (Freeman, 2004).

PSYCHOLOGICAL EFFECTS OF EXERCISE ON HEALTH

Among the psychological effects of exercise on the stress response is an important concept called parasympathetic rebound. When the body anticipates movement, the central nervous system releases epinephrine and norepinephrine. Throughout the activity, catecholamine levels remain elevated. When the activity ceases, the parasympathetic nervous system inhibits the secretion of epinephrine and norepinephrine, bringing about a calming response (Freeman, 2004; Seaward, 2006). Physically fit individuals have been found to return to their resting heart rates and serum catecholamine levels sooner than sedentary individuals; the values actually continue to decrease below pre-activity states in conditioned individuals (Seaward, 2006).

Those who exercise also tend to experience less depression than those who do not. While exercise alone cannot eliminate depression or help someone in an acute phase of depression, it has been very helpful for those with milder cases or for those with acute feelings of sadness, discouragement, and self-deprecation (Freeman, 2004; Leddy, 2006; Sacks, 1993).

According to Seaward (2006), when the fitness movement exploded in the 1970s, valium was the most prescribed drug in the country. Clinical medicine was caught off guard by the enthusiasm for exercising and the concurrent drop in tranquilizer use. People began talking about the Zen-like quality of the "runner's high" and using their exercise time to sort out personal problems and reflect on their lives and relationships. Many people stopped taking their prescription tranquilizers, and running in particular was reported to have an addictive quality.

In the early 1980s, a new human neuropeptide was discovered and shown to have qualities much like morphine. Beta-endorphin was shown to be the body's own natural opiate, reducing sensations of pain and promoting feelings of exhilaration and euphoria. Endorphins have an addictive quality. Inactive people show signs of depression. When they become more active, they exhibit improved mood, due in part to the euphoria resulting from the production of endorphins. Certain cardiovascular activities, such as swimming and walking, have demonstrated this effect.

Physical activity and movement can actually produce a tranquilizing effect on the body that can last for 4 hours or so. According to Sacks (1993), people who struggle with the physical symptoms of anxiety (such as gastrointestinal problems, sweating, palpitations, pacing, etc.) are especially likely to benefit from exercise.

Physical activity has also been shown to promote fantasies and daydreams and to support imagination, all of which are wonderful psychological benefits and play a vital role in health. Some people daydream while they exercise. Others experience a rhythm, flow, or sense of "being on" that can bring an intense feeling of elation. Sacks (1993) says, "This playful suspension of the real world, together with the expression of the physical exuberance of childhood, is at the psychological core of exercise" (p. 327).

Exercises like cycling, running, or swimming can offer a meditative form of awareness because of their inherent rhythmic, repetitive motion. This rhythmic activity is said to shift the brain's dominant hemisphere from the left to the right brain, possibly resulting in heightened mental receptivity and alertness, increased perception and information processing, greater imagination and creativity, improved problem solving, and improved self-esteem. Additional benefits include improved self-reliance and self-efficacy, increased perception of acceptance by others, decreased feelings of depression and anxiety, and a reduction in the overall sense of stress and tension (Seaward, 2006).

MECHANICS OF BREATHING

Breathing is an essential component to exercise and movement. The word *spirit* in many cultures is described as "the first breath" (Seaward, 2006). Each breath is an opportunity to "inspire the life force," "bring in spirit," and allow the body as well as the soul to be nourished and energized. Breath signifies vital energy; by controlling it, people can control their bodies and gain control over their minds (Copp, 2007).

Under normal circumstances, the average person breathes 14–16 times per minute. When people are anxious or aroused, their breathing is faster and shallower. During heavy exercise, people can breathe as many as 60 breaths per minute as the body tries to meet oxygen demand. When people are relaxed, their breathing slows and deepens.

The main muscles involved in breathing include the diaphragm (the large, dome-shaped partition separating the abdominal and chest cavities) and the intercostals (the muscles between the rib bones). Together, they work to draw oxygenated air into the lungs and release deoxygenated air from the body. With each inspiration, the diaphragm contracts and flattens downward, increasing the size of the chest cavity, creating negative pressure in the lungs, and beginning the breathing cycle. The air sacs (alveoli) of the lungs fill with air as the lungs expand into the enlarged chest cavity. Oxygenated air circulates throughout the body and returns to the lungs to be expelled (Eliopoulos, 2004).

Diaphragmatic breathing is one of the easiest methods of relaxation. A deep sigh, or big breath taken to regroup or relax, it involves the movement of the lower abdomen. Most people breathe using the upper chest and thoracic cavity, a practice that is believed to be the result of cultural preferences for a large chest and small waist (Seaward, 2006).

One way to experience the effectiveness of breathing properly is simply to start by breathing deeply, concentrating on the breath as you fill your lungs. Picture it moving throughout your body. If your mind wanders, just refocus on your breathing. Take several deep, conscious breaths this way. With each one, picture the breath as light-like energy that fills your entire body. With each exhalation, breathe out your stress.

Diaphragmatic breathing is a potent health-promoting exercise with many benefits beyond providing the body with life-sustaining oxygen (Eliopoulos, 2004). Focusing on your breath for a few minutes each day can improve how you respond to stress. It can slow the heart and breathing rate, lower blood pressure, reduce the body's need for oxygen, increase blood flow to the major muscles, and reduce muscle tension. It can also provide increased energy, improved coordination, and an increased ability to address daily activities more efficiently (Copp, 2007).

Many people never stop to think about the importance of proper breathing and its impact on exercise and movement, but conscious breathing is incorporated into many activities such as walking, yoga, meditation, dancing, swimming, or jogging.

MOVEMENT

A commonly held but limited image of exercise is that of a strenuous weightlifting or calisthenics session that leaves the individual breathless, sweating, and exhausted. The more current perspective emphasizes the importance of movement: activities that engage the muscles and take the form of gentler, deeper forms of exercise that can last a lifetime. How a person holds and carries his or her body and how groups communicate through body language are also characteristics of movement.

The various aspects of movement found in sport, dance, swimming, and theater are integral parts of rituals, celebrations, and healing rites that have always been part of human existence. Rose and Keegan (2005) note that "movement ranges from the rapid motions of active dance or acrobatics, to the subtle rhythm characterized by breathing and choral singing, to the slow, careful movements of Tai Chi" (p. 484). Yoga and Tai Chi Chuan are two ancient forms of movement that enhance overall health. Aimed at developing the energy that flows through the body, they are based on total concentration, strength, relaxation, and symbolic movement (Rose & Keegan, 2005). Eastern approaches to exercise and movement—distinctly different from their Western counterparts—have broadened the once narrow definition of exercise held in the West. Practices such as yoga and Tai Chi Chuan promote movement to support or restore health. Breathing exercises, stretching, poses, and spiritual practices are central to these approaches.

Yoga

Yoga is an ancient practice of linking mind, body, and spirit through a combination of postures, breathing, and conscious relaxation and meditation. Iyengar (2005) explains that yoga's goal "is nothing less than to attain the integrity of oneness—oneness with ourselves and as a consequence oneness with all that lies beyond ourselves. We become the harmonious microcosm in the universal macrocosm. Oneness, what I often call *integration*, is the foundation for wholeness, inner peace, and ultimate freedom" (p. xiv).

Derived from a Sanskrit word meaning "yoke," "constellation," "conjunction," or "union," yoga is the integration of physical, mental, and spiritual energies that enhance health and well-being (Copp, 2007; Leddy, 2006; Micozzi & Singh, 2006; Seaward, 2006). It is a way to live in harmony with nature, and good health is the result. Yoga has also been described as a balance between active and passive that teaches people how to work with their bodies and relax (Copp, 2007). By emphasizing postures (to strengthen the body), controlled breathing (to create a chemical and emotional balance in the body and mind), and meditation (as a form of prayer), yoga stimulates powerful healing abilities in its practitioners (Massey, 2007). One of its greatest gifts is an increased body awareness as practitioners link their movements with their breathing. As Iyengar (2005) says, "The yogic journey guides us from our periphery, the body, to the center of our being, the soul. The aim is to integrate the various layers so that the inner divinity shines out as through clear glass" (p. 3).

Origins of Yoga

Yoga is believed to have originated in India and is considered an ancient form of active meditation in the Hindu and Buddhist traditions (Benson, 1993). The Rig Veda (Hindu scriptures translated as "knowledge of praise") defines yoga as a means of deliverance from pain, suffering, and sorrow through the mastery of whatever disturbs an individual's peace and harmony on the path to a perfect union with God or the universal spirit (Leddy, 2006; Micozzi &

Singh, 2006). The Bhagavad Gita (Lord's Song), the most popular and treasured of all yoga scriptures, dates back approximately 2,500 years; Mahatma Gandhi called it "my mother." Hatha yoga (or forceful yoga), an important tradition of yoga that emerged in the 11th century under the influence of Tantrism, has its own scriptures (Micozzi & Singh, 2006).

Yoga has probably been practiced for more than 5,000 years and is believed to be a path by which its practitioners could transcend the human experience. Scholars have traced the roots of yoga as far back as the sixth century BC to the teachings of the Hindu philosopher Kapila. These teachings, along with those attributed to the Hindu deity Krishna, laid the foundation of yoga (Seaward, 2006). Over the millennia, yoga has evolved into a way to develop the self mentally, physically, and spiritually and, through discipline, to achieve spiritual enlightenment. Seaward (2006) notes that, "The premise of this mind-body-spirit union . . . is that humanity's most salient nature is of a divine quality. The abyss that separates the corporeal and incorporeal is the wall of conscious intellect, or ego censorship" (p. 384). The philosophy of yoga is traditionally passed down from teacher to student through physical instruction and oral discussion.

Swami Vivekananda introduced yoga in the United States when he made a presentation to the World Parliament of Religions in Chicago in 1893 and later toured the country for 2 years. By the end of the 19th century, two ashrams (yoga centers) were established in California. Yoga gained popularity in the 1960s when people began to take interest in Eastern cultures and holistic medicines. In the 1970s, Swami Rama, a yogi master from the Himalayan Institute, was invited to the Menninger Foundation in Topeka, Kansas. He demonstrated an almost unbelievable control over his autonomic functions (respiration, heart rate, and blood flow) and indicated to researchers that bodily functions once thought to be involuntary could be controlled (Seaward, 2006). Today, yoga is a $3 billion industry in the United States and approximately 16.5 million people practice it. One reason for its popularity is that many people live fast-paced lives, filled with pressure and stress. As the stress and pressure affect their mental and physical beings, and as they come to accept the connection between mind and body, more and more people seek holistic approaches to manage their stress (Copp, 2007).

Components of Yoga

Approximately 2,000 years ago, the sage Patanjali described the eight limbs of yoga in his text, the *Yoga Sutra*, and these limbs serve as a practical guide to self-development. They outline specific lifestyle, hygiene, and detoxification regimens, as well as physical and psychological practices that can lead to integrated personal development (Leddy, 2006). The limbs are not designed to serve as a step-by-step approach to yoga; instead, students can start at any limb. The eight limbs are (Copp, 2007; Leddy, 2006; Micozzi & Singh, 2006):

- *Yamas:* Moral restraint from violence, lying, stealing, casual sex, and hoarding
- *Niyamas:* Observance of purity, contentment, discipline, reflection, and devotion
- *Asana:* Practicing postures or yoga poses
- *Pranayama:* Controlled breathing
- *Pratyahara:* Withdrawing the mind from the senses in preparation for meditation
- *Dharana:* Concentrating on one object for a length of time
- *Dhyana:* Practicing a progressive deepening of concentration through meditation
- *Samadhi:* Self-actualization or enlightenment

Yoga consists of five principles that apply to daily life and enhance well-being (Massey, 2007):

- Proper relaxation (savasana)
- Proper exercise (asanas)
- Proper breathing (pranayama)
- Proper diet (vegetarian)
- Meditation (dhyana)

Categories of Yoga

There are several categories of yoga (Copp, 2007; Leddy, 2006; Massey, 2007; Micozzi & Singh, 2006; Shealy, 1996):

- *Ananda yoga* is a gentle, classical style of yoga. Not athletic or aerobic, it is designed to maintain relaxation.
- *Ashtanga yoga* is a dynamic, physically demanding, and fast-paced practice that uses breath to link the flow from one movement to another. It is also called power yoga and participants jump from one posture to another.
- *Anusara yoga* (*anusara* means "flowing with grace") is a spiritually oriented yoga using postures with a mind-body emphasis.
- *Bhakti yoga* (*bhakti* means "devotion") seeks the pathway to God through devotion and love. The practices take on the form of ritual, love-intoxicated chanting, singing, dancing, and meditation.
- *Bikram yoga* is practiced in a room heated to at least 100 degrees Fahrenheit. The goal is to cleanse the body and increase flexibility.

Consisting of 26 postures that are always done twice and in the same sequence, this is a challenging form of yoga that can also be called hot yoga.

- *Hatha yoga* (*hatha* means "force") uses physical purification and body strengthening as an arduous means of self-transformation and transcendence. This form of yoga is based on the development of Tantrism (techniques and rituals outlined in Hindu or Buddhist scriptures). Many of its practices attempt to stimulate the chakras and to clean and improve the condition of various physical organs.
- *Iyengar yoga* is a slower paced form of yoga that focuses on the precise alignment of the feet and body. Blocks, belts, bolsters, and other props are used to achieve this alignment.
- *Jnana yoga*, the yoga of the intellect, has the goal of attaining prajna, or transcendental wisdom through meditation and thought.
- *Karma yoga* is a yoga of service, emphasizing doing for others as a remembrance of God. The individual who practices this form of yoga acts in daily life to lessen lawlessness and restore virtue and harmony.
- *Kripalu yoga* uses traditional sitting postures (asanas) but emphasizes meditation and reflection by encouraging self-acceptance, objectively observing the mind's activity, and applying what is learned in class to daily living.
- *Kundalini yoga* incorporates chanting with powerful breath work and specific postures designed to awaken the energy ("serpent power") in the sacrum.
- *Mantra or nada yoga* focuses on the vibrations and radiations of life energy using sound.
- *Raja yoga* ("royal union"), formulated about 200 BC, is an orthodox system of Hindu philosophy. In this form of yoga, the mind is king, and the body must first be tamed through self-discipline and purification. Social and personal codes of conduct prepare the mind and body for the higher stages of meditation by reducing attachment and inducing tranquility.
- *Yin yoga* focuses heavily on stretching the joints and connective tissue. Poses are passive and often held for long periods.

Although the forms of yoga vary in terms of their rituals and religiousness, all are spiritual and may be regarded as India's common brand of spiritualism.

Yoga in the West

The same range of expressions reflected in the different types of yoga can be found in the spiritual traditions of Judaism, Islam, and Roman Catholicism (Micozzi & Singh, 2006).

According to Leddy (2006), the West has primarily adopted three aspects of entirely different yoga practices: the breathing techniques of prana yoga, meditation, and the asanas of hatha yoga.

- *Prana yoga:* This form of yoga emphasizes pranayama, or yogic breathing. The name of this ancient form of deep breathing literally means regulation or control of prana, the life force or universal energy (Micozzi & Singh, 2006). Through deep breathing techniques, the life force is brought into the body. The practice involves taking an initial breath and blowing it out through the mouth, then inhaling through the nose to the count of four, holding it without tension to a count of eight, and exhaling through the nose to a count of eight. This cycle is repeated seven times. The practice is done in preparation for meditation.
- *Meditation:* The final stage of yoga is Samadhi, or spiritual realization. This stage requires long, dedicated, disciplined practice and is said to be a stage in which the individual enters the fourth state of consciousness, separate from and beyond the ordinary states of wakefulness, sleep, and dreams (Leddy, 2006).
- *Asanas:* While yoga postures may involve very little movement, the mind is involved in every asana. This awareness and discipline help circulate qi.

Benefits and Risks

Yoga needs to be performed correctly. If done incorrectly, for too long, or too strenuously, it can cause physical damage, particularly to the back. For example, individuals with sciatica should not perform forward bends or intense stretching. Menstruating women, those who are pregnant, or anyone with glaucoma or ear congestion should avoid inverted poses and breath retention (Leddy, 2006).

Despite the fact that yoga has been practiced for nearly 100 years in the United States, there is little clinical research to substantiate claims that it improves overall health (Seaward, 2006). Without any doubt, yoga builds strength, stamina, and flexibility. It enhances body awareness and improves concentration. It may reduce high blood pressure, insulin resistance, and chronic pain, and it may improve coronary function (Copp, 2007; Micozzi & Singh, 2006; Seaward, 2006). As a form of exercise and stress reduction, yoga has been found to be beneficial in reducing the symptoms of asthma and in reducing the risk of many diseases such as diabetes mellitus, heart disease, cancer, and even Alzheimer's disease. It has also been effective in reducing medication use and improving nerve function (Massey, 2007; Shealy, 1996).

More high-quality, randomized, controlled studies are needed to support the use of yoga as an important medical therapy. Massey (2007) notes that, "Given the nature of chronic disease, yoga may play a role in treatment and, more important, prevention" (p. 1006).

Tai Chi Chuan

Understanding Tai Chi Chuan means first understanding the cultural context in which it originated. Westerners have often viewed health as the absence of disease and illness. The Chinese view health as an unrestricted current of subtle energy throughout the body. When qi (chi) is restricted, illness results. As Seaward (2006) explains:

> There is a life force or subtle energy that surrounds and permeates all of us, which the Chinese call *chi*. To harmonize with the universe, to move in unison with this energy, to move as freely as running water is to be at peace or one with the universe. This harmony of energy promotes tranquility and inner peace. (pp. 454–455)

Some forms of exercise actually occur in the energy body rather than the physical body. Tai Chi Chuan is such an exercise (Leddy, 2006). This traditional Chinese exercise involves "a series of individual dancelike movements linked together in a continuous, smooth-flowing sequence" (Rose & Keegan, 2005, p. 484). These fluid, graceful, dance-like postures are performed in movements known as forms, whose softness, continuity, and relaxation allow qi to move freely along meridians. Translated as "the ultimate" or "supreme ultimate," the name *Tai Chi Chuan* means improving and progressing toward the unlimited. It seeks to integrate the connections between mind, body, and spirit in a quest for the highest form of harmony in life by combining meditation and exercise (Leddy, 2006).

Origins of Tai Chi Chuan

Believed to originate from observations of the movements of animals, plants, and even water, Tai Chi Chuan focuses on balancing the flexibility, strength, and speed found in nature (Massey, 2007). Dating back thousands of years, Tai Chi Chuan promotes the peaceful flow of energy throughout the body, helping practitioners to maintain a state of good health (Seaward, 2006).

Tai Chi Chuan is a form of martial arts, the basis of which is to support a path to physical, mental, and spiritual health. Although the histories of most martial arts are vague because they have been passed down orally from master to student (Massey, 2007), in Asia martial arts and medicine have been inseparable for thousands of years. The origins of Tai Chi Chuan are thousands of years old and believed to be a blend of Chinese philosophy and physical survival. Legend has it that a man once observed a fight between a crane and a serpent. The crane repeatedly tried to strike the serpent to defeat him but was unsuccessful. The snake, in a series of calculated maneuvers, simply shifted its body weight at the right time and remained free of harm. Ultimately, the crane tired of this, gave up, and left.

What makes Tai Chi Chuan different from other forms of martial arts is its basis in philosophy (Seaward, 2006). According to Massey (2007), martial arts are commonly divided into two main categories with extensive overlap.

- *External* martial arts include karate and tae kwon do. The movements and exercises primarily affect the muscles, are relatively ballistic, and use linear snapping motions to create speed and strength.
- *Internal* martial arts, such as Tai Chi Chuan, kung fu, and bagwa, emphasize circular movements at a slower pace. Internal martial arts support strength, speed, and balance, and they reduce stress, support the health of the joints and internal organs, and focus on enhancing the production and flow of bioenergy (qi).

In both the internal and external forms, a specific pattern of breathing is believed to be vital for health and it is the foundation for most martial arts. When the flow of energy is good, the body is healthy.

What Is Tai Chi Chuan?

In Taoist philosophy the Tai Chi, or the source and end of the universe manifested as unity, is composed of two interacting and complementary forces called yin and yang (heaven and earth). Meditation seeks to increase yang (masculine) and reduce yin (feminine), while exercise seeks to reduce yang and increase yin. Tai Chi Chuan is a method of moving meditation. Although outwardly at rest, the individual is inwardly peaceful and quiet, using breathing and mental concentration to facilitate the flow of energy throughout the body (Leddy, 2006). As a metaphor for life, Tai Chi Chuan represents moving with the flow, not against it.

Tai Chi Chuan can be practiced anyplace, at any time, and without any equipment. There are five main schools of Tai Chi Chuan, each named after the style's founding family: Chen, Yang, Sun, Wu (Jian Qian), and Wu (He Qin). The Yang style is the most popular style practiced today (Leddy, 2006).

Tai Chi Chuan involves the manipulation of force by yielding to become part of it and by controlling the self (Seaward, 2006). Tai Chi Chuan expresses force through a "beautiful, coordinated series of postures that through regular practice, develop and coordinate the body, under the control of qi, to a level of perfection not otherwise attainable" (Eliopoulos, 2004, p. 82). The body is properly aligned and the mind stilled through the slowness of movement.

Concepts and Principles of Tai Chi Chuan

Tai Chi Chuan is based on four basic philosophical concepts (Seaward, 2006):

- *Fasting the heart* explains the flow of life's energy, finding comfort in solitude and silence. Fasting means silence, the language of the soul.
- *Returning to nature* is a way of describing a regression to the joys of childhood, embracing innocence, joy, laughter, and play. As adults, we tend to lose this ability.
- *Wu-wei* is the philosophy of nothing-doing, nothing-knowing. It means to act without forcing and to move in accordance with nature's flow. For example, before you may take, you must give.
- *Winning by losing* advocates the success of failure. When failure is acknowledged, it becomes the first step to success. This is an expression of unconditional acceptance. True understanding comes by emptying the mind and lowering the walls of the ego; the human spirit is liberated and can unite with the universal life force.

Tai Chi Chuan also has several principles of practice (Leddy, 2006).

- Loose-fitting clothing and soft shoes or bare feet are essential.
- The movements are best learned from an instructor at first, and can then be performed alone or in a group.
- Relaxed, natural breathing is important.
- Shoulders are relaxed, knees are slightly bent, and movements are slow and fluid.
- The circulation of qi can be noted by the amount of tingling felt in the fingers and hands.
- The practice should take place for approximately 25–30 minutes daily (Leddy, 2006; Shealy, 1996).

Benefits of Tai Chi Chuan

An excellent activity for aging adults, Tai Chi Chuan has been shown to improve balance and strength in the elderly and may be instrumental in preventing falls. Other benefits include enhanced flexibility and immune function, improved cardiovascular and pulmonary function, improved lymph functioning, increased energy flow, reduced chronic pain, improved mental alertness and creativity, reduced stress and anxiety, and the cultivation of poise and a "tranquil spirit" (Leddy, 2006; Massey, 2007; Shealy, 1996).

INITIATING A FITNESS TRAINING PROGRAM

Physical exercise is a tremendous stress-reduction technique and has many health benefits. However, physical activity has to be done correctly, or it can pose a serious threat to health. For maximum benefits, physical activity must be done at the right intensity, frequency, and duration, and it should be the appropriate mode of exercise for the specific individual. Most people make the mistake of trying to do too much, too soon. New Year's resolutions, for example, can cause people to jump into a program with all kinds of excitement and goals and go overboard with their activity. For years, the catchphrase used in gyms was "no pain, no gain." This dangerous concept can result in injuries (including muscle and tendon damage) and burnout (Seaward, 2006).

Initiating an exercise program can be difficult. Approximately 41% of adults are sedentary, and of those already regularly engaged in activities, about 50% will discontinue activity at some time in the coming year (Leddy, 2006). Most individuals have busy lives, with long work days and families to manage, and the last thing they often want to do is add another task to their to-do lists. In addition, the current, typically commercial idea of a perfect body is unrealistic and often discourages people from being active because the vision is unattainable (Eliopoulos, 2004).

Motivation

Internal and external motivation can be difficult to attain, and because changes don't happen overnight, maintaining motivation can prove challenging. Motivation peaks about 3–7 days after the start of a fitness program and then rapidly declines (Seaward, 2006). Because of the loss of motivation, the rate of participation in an exercise program typically drops within the first 3–6 months, then plateaus and continues in a gradually decreasing pattern over the next 12–24 months. Individuals who are still active after 6 months are likely to remain active a year later (Leddy, 2006).

Motivation is influenced by a number of factors, including belief in the health benefits of exercise, understanding the risks of not participating in an exercise or activity, a history of past participation in exercise or sports, social support, convenience, the perception of being in good health, and the individual's degree of self-confidence in his or her ability to participate in a broad range of healthful behaviors (Leddy, 2006).

One way to help maintain motivation is to set goals and prescribe specific exercise programs tailored to the individual's lifestyle. Other motivational ideas include individual education about the benefits of activity, addressing costs and affordability, addressing safety, treating concurrent morbidities, facilitating empowerment, promoting socialization, providing physical and occupational therapy, and giving the individual a written prescription on a prescription pad (Leddy, 2006).

Overcoming Barriers to a Physical Activity Program

Factors that make it challenging for individuals to exercise include (Leddy, 2006):

- Environmental barriers (such as safety, availability and location of facilities, weather, financial considerations, work, and childcare issues)
- A lack of time and energy
- Limited access to training and information about physical activity
- A lack of readiness to exercise
- A lack of role models
- A lack of encouragement by healthcare providers
- A lack of self-regulatory skills (interventions that teach goal setting, planning, self-monitoring, self-rewards, and what to do in case of a relapse)
- Disruption of the exercise routine

Recommendations for successfully developing and maintaining an effective exercise program include the following (Haskell et al., 2007; Leddy, 2006; Sacks, 1993; Seaward, 2006; Shea, 2008):

- *Start cautiously and progress moderately.* One of the most important aspects of beginning an exercise routine is a physical examination by a qualified medical provider. The healthcare provider should prescribe targets for the program, including target heart rate; individual goals; a mode of exercise best suited for you; and the intensity, frequency, and duration of a workout. People who view physical exercise as a process, not as an outcome, are often better able to incorporate it into all aspects of their lives. Many former athletes get frustrated because they cannot easily do the things they did 5, 10, or 15 years ago. Don't be in a hurry, and don't compete with an image of yourself from the past. Listen to your body! One rule of thumb is that you should be able to carry on a conversation when exercising. If you are out of breath and cannot hold a conversation, you are probably pushing too hard.
- *Change your definition of exercise.* Any form of movement can be considered exercise. Exercise must be an integral part of personal lifestyle if it is to have optimum effects on health. Energy begets energy, and falling into a slothful way of life is easy, particularly when the seasons change. How often have you found it difficult to get moving after a nice dinner on

a dark winter evening? If you have been more sedentary than you would like to be, start thinking outside the box. If you normally work out at the gym each day for 45 minutes and think that is the only form of exercise worth any respect, think again! Cleaning the house, shopping, or raking leaves are all ways that you can increase your movement quotient. In addition, changing your routine to include other types of movement activities, such as yoga, Tai Chi Chuan, dance, swimming, or long walks with your dog, can help you achieve your goals. Make your exercise time a time of renewal—a time just for you. It can be a time to connect with others or a time to spend with yourself.

- *Set personal fitness goals for yourself.* Setting achievable goals is one of the surest ways to stay motivated with a fitness program. (Marking your progress on a calendar is the most common method.) Whether it is losing weight, losing inches, running a marathon, or having abs of steel, once the goals are set, tracking them is a positive way to help achieve them. Stand firm on your commitment because this commitment is for you. An important part of goal setting is to reward yourself when you achieve your goals.
- *Select an activity you enjoy.* This is probably one of the most important aspects of exercise. Be playful. Engaging in an activity you like to do is critical to continuing it. If you hate jogging, don't jog. Some people may go to the dance studio, while others may surf in the ocean to wash away their anxiety. One of the wonderful benefits of exercise is the related release of endorphins. These happy hormones provide a sense of joy and sometimes of pain relief during an activity. They are enhanced if you like the activity you are engaged in. Selecting alternative activities is a good way to prevent burnout. It also prevents injuries because many episodes of chronic pain result from too much physical activity or overuse syndrome. Complementary exercises, such as walking or biking, can provide an effective alternative when you need a rest from your primary activity. Picking an exercise that does not involve competition or ego boosting also keeps motivation high. Taking your dog with you can also make your exercise fun; it's hard to resist that big doggy smile when your pet sees you get the leash. Other ways to make exercise fun are to listen to music, news, or talk shows; exercise outdoors; have a positive attitude; and periodically reward yourself when you achieve your goals.
- *Select a time of day to exercise.* By making a commitment to selecting a specific time of day to exercise, you make yourself a priority. Exercise time is for you and you alone, and all your other responsibilities and

commitments fade away, at least temporarily. Many people select the morning because it precedes work or school, and the activity helps them meet the challenges of the day. However, mornings can be difficult for people who like to sleep in late. Others prefer an afternoon or evening option; this can be difficult if your work or school day has been long or tiring, but the activity helps release all that pent-up energy. For still others, the lunch hour is perfect and provides a much-needed boost for the remainder of the day. The minimum time needed to obtain benefits is 3 days a week for at least 30 minutes each time. If you are unable to make your commitment for a few days, just do what you can. You will feel much better about getting some exercise versus none.

- *Choose the right equipment and clothes.* When you are exercising, the type of clothing you wear, especially your shoes, can make a big difference in how you feel. Shoes that support your feet, ankles, knees, hips, and back are critical, so footwear is probably one area where less is definitely not more. Spending money on a high-quality pair of shoes can mean the difference between stability, safety, and pain-free exercising and the less optimal alternatives. In addition, clothing that wicks moisture away from your body or that can be peeled off in layers if you get too hot can make workouts much more comfortable.
- *Develop a support group.* Exercising with a group of individuals is a great way to get you through the tough times. On those days when the thought of exercising is just more than you can bear or when you're struggling to reach a goal, having a fitness buddy can make all the difference. Having a group or class format for exercising is another way to promote exercise. Groups or class formats are often more cost effective, provide visual modeling by the instructor on safe techniques, and have a set structure with respect to location, time, and day. However, for some the structure can be confining and expensive, provide only a limited variety of formats, and be discouraging in terms of social comparisons.
- *Prevent the occurrence of injuries.* Preventing injury is, of course, the best way to achieve your goals. If you suffer an injury, take care of it right away. Pain is not a gain, and pain should be treated with respect. An injury may be treated with something as simple as ice, or it may require medical attention. More physicians specialize in sports medicine than ever before, so it should be easy to find a qualified professional. Exercise physiologists and other qualified personnel are also available to assist you as you begin your program.

KEY CONCEPTS

1. Physical activity and movement are important elements in obtaining and maintaining good health and well-being.
2. The major types of physical activity include aerobic and anaerobic activity. Muscular strength and endurance, flexibility, agility, power, and balance are important aspects of fitness as well.
3. Yoga and Tai Chi Chuan are forms of physical activity that combine breathing, movement, and meditation.

QUESTIONS FOR REFLECTION

1. How do lifestyle behaviors like exercise and movement affect a person's general sense of well-being?
2. How does exercise contribute to physiological and psychological well-being?
3. What is the philosophical basis for yoga? For Tai Chi Chuan?

REFERENCES

Benson, H. (1993). The relaxation response. In D. Goleman & J. Gurin (Eds.), *Mind body medicine: How to use your mind for better health* (pp. 233–257). Yonkers, NY: Consumer Reports Books.

Copp, M. (2007, Winter). Breathing room: Give yourself the space to rejuvenate with yoga. *Massage Therapy Journal*, *46*(4), 66–78.

Eliopoulos, C. (2004). *Invitation to holistic health: A guide to living a balanced life.* Sudbury, MA: Jones and Bartlett.

Freeman, L. (Ed.). (2004). *Mosby's complementary and alternative medicine: A research-based approach* (2nd ed.). St. Louis, MO: Mosby.

Haskell, W. L., Lee, I., Pate, R. R., Powell, K. E., Blair, S. N., Franklin, B. A., et al. (2007, August). Physical activity and public health: Updated recommendations for adults from the American College of Sports Medicine and the American Heart Association. *Medicine Science and Sports Exercise*, *39*, 1423–1434.

Iyengar, B. K. S. (2005). *Light on life: The yoga journey to wholeness, inner peace, and ultimate freedom.* Emmaus, PA: Rodale Books.

Leddy, S. K. (2006). *Integrative health promotion: Conceptual bases for nursing practice* (2nd ed.). Sudbury, MA: Jones and Bartlett.

Massey, P. B. (2007). Prescribing movement therapies. In D. Rakel (Ed.), *Integrative medicine* (2nd ed., pp. 999–1007). Philadelphia: Saunders Elsevier.

Micozzi, M. S., & Singh, D. (2006). Yoga. In M. S. Micozzi, *Fundamentals of complementary and integrative medicine* (pp. 508–517). St. Louis, MO: Saunders Elsevier.

Rose, B. H. C., & Keegan, L. (2005). Exercise and movement. In B. M. Dossey, L. Keegan, & C. E. Guzzetta, *Holistic nursing: A handbook for practice* (4th ed., pp. 479–493). Sudbury, MA: Jones and Bartlett.

Sacks, M. H. (1993). Exercise for stress control. In D. Goleman & J. Gurin (Eds.), *Mind body medicine: How to use your mind for better health* (pp. 315–327). Yonkers, NY: Consumer Reports Books.

Seaward, B. L. (2006). *Managing stress: Principles and strategies for health and well-being* (5th ed.). Sudbury, MA: Jones and Bartlett.

Shea, S. B. (2008, December/January). Merry fitness. *Natural Health, 38*(1), 76–82.

Shealy, C. N. (Ed.). (1996). *The complete family guide to alternative medicine: An illustrated encyclopedia of natural healing.* Shaftesbury, Dorset, UK: Element Books.

Index

NOTE: *t* with page number indicates tables.

B

F

I

Q

R

T